Vitamins & Supplements

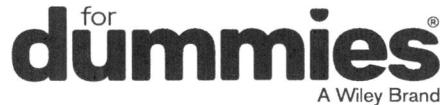

for
dummies®
A Wiley Brand

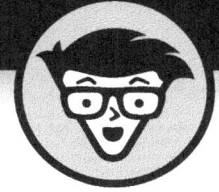

Vitamins & Supplements

By Shelley B. Weinstock, PhD, CNS, FACN

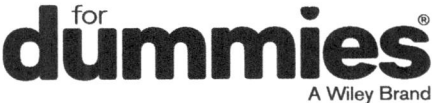

Vitamins & Supplements For Dummies®

Published by: **John Wiley & Sons, Inc.**, 111 River Street, Hoboken, NJ 07030-5774, www.wiley.com

Contents at a Glance

Table of Contents

Introduction

'm guessing that you bought this book because you are concerned about your health and want to do whatever you can to prevent disease and lead an active and healthy life. You may be very good at researching the internet for information on vitamins and supplements that would be good for you to take, but you're finding an overabundance of information of questionable accuracy and informativeness. You may be looking for a bottom line, truthful recommendation to help you decide which vitamins and supplements you may need.

My goal with *Vitamins & Supplements For Dummies is* to clarify the gigantic field of vitamins and supplements so that you a health-conscious consumer — can spend your money wisely and be as healthy as you can be. I was just a rebellious 14-year-old when I started my health-conscious journey. I became a vegetarian, cooked my own meals, and tried to use whole foods instead of processed products. It was a good start, but I ended up with some vitamin deficiencies because, at that age, I didn't know any better. The internet didn't exist, so research was far more difficult to do.

I studied nutritional biochemistry for my PhD, which enlightened me to the inner workings of our cells and organs and the thousands of metabolic pathways that keep our bodies functioning and healthy. Those studies were based on the burst of scientific research about vitamin and mineral metabolism, their function, and their link to diseases that has happened in the last 100 years or so. Now, it's almost impossible to keep up with the science and fiction around vitamins and supplement information that's available.

In this book, I hope to present current evidence-based information to help you determine whether you need vitamins and how to choose from the myriad products on the market. In the process, I talk about the importance of understanding food and nutrition and how supplements can enhance your health. Lastly, I help you distinguish between good and bad products and how they are regulated by the government for Good Manufacturing Practice (GMP), safety, purity, and labeling.

About This Book

The information in this book spans from basic biochemistry to considering the options available on the supplement shelf at the store (or online). I include information on as many supplements and types of products as I could fit in these pages. Given that there are an estimated 80,000 products on the market, though, it's not a 100 percent exhaustive reference.

Foolish Assumptions

As I wrote, I made some assumptions about you, the reader, and what you may be thinking:

>> You want to understand the pros and cons of supplements and why you should or shouldn't take them.

>> You're having trouble navigating the nutrition aisles at the supermarkets and other stores.

>> You're probably not a biochemist or at least not one who specializes in nutritional biochemistry.

>> You know of many self-proclaimed "experts," and it's hard to know who to believe.

>> The internet information is too overwhelming and confusing to make sense of and distinguish among the products.

I'm also thinking you may be assuming the following:

>> You may believe that all advertisements or claims about supplements are evidence based.

>> You may have a "why not just try supplements — they can't hurt" attitude.

>> All vitamin brands are equal in quality.

The above statements are not true and need more explanation. I'm hoping that this book provides the education you need to decide for yourself, given your health status, lifestyle, and goals.

Icons Used in This Book

The icons in this book alert you to information of special importance or that you may find interesting.

REMEMBER

This icon means that the information is important, so you should be aware of it.

TECHNICAL STUFF

This icon gives you technical information or terminology that may be helpful to understanding the topic being discussed.

TIP

This icon marks important information that may help you save time and energy.

WARNING

This icon warns against potential problems.

Beyond the Book

There are numerous resources out there to consult as you go beyond this book. I've listed what I believe are the most reliable websites in Chapter 17. Always do your research and try to check out any science behind a particular product. Don't necessarily believe the marketing hype! The dietary supplement business is a big machine worth about $44 billion in North America and $177 billion globally.

The online Cheat Sheet offers quick guides to essential vitamins and minerals, their functions, food sources, and signs to look for potential deficiencies. I list some common supplements and botanicals and their uses. I also present some topics for you to discuss with your doctor or healthcare provider to help you decide if you need supplements and how to take them safely. Visit www.dummies.com and search for **Vitamins & Minerals For Dummies** to access this valuable information.

Aside from this book and its online cheat sheet, the following experts can be helpful. Knowledgeable and often licensed professionals include the following:

>> **Nutritionists:** A nutritionist is a professional who can advise you on improving your overall health and managing your medical conditions, and they can provide personalized nutrition plans based on scientifically backed information.

They can help you achieve fitness and lifestyle goals and make informed dietary and supplement choices. The best certification program is the Certified Nutrition Specialist controlled by the American Nutrition Association. A CNS must have a master's degree or PhD as well as a certification. Nutritionists are trained to conduct medical nutrition therapy (MNT), which is covered by some insurance companies. Always check credentials before choosing a nutritionist.

>> **Dietitians:** Registered Dietitian (RD) or Registered Dietitian Nutritionist (RDN) is a nationally recognized degree that's regulated and licensed in every state. Dietitians are health professionals who specialize in food, nutrition, and dietetics, and they're trained to help you manage your health and prevent or treat illnesses through personalized nutrition plans. Like certified nutrition specialists, they offer MNT. Dietitians also often consult for hospital and nursing home food services.

>> **Functional medicine practitioners:** People with MD, DO, MS, PhD, CNS, and RD after their name and other qualified professional healthcare professionals can be trained in functional medicine, which is a holistic approach of treating the root causes of disease. They integrate their knowledge of biology, physiology, genetics, social and environmental determinants of health, and mental health to work with patients to come up with personalized plans. Their focus is to integrate conventional treatments with nutrition, lifestyle changes, and supplements

>> **Pharmacists:** Pharmacists are trained to dispense and consult about medications, but they are also educated in vitamins, minerals, and other supplements. You may not realize that your pharmacist is a great source for advice about choosing supplements, but they are knowledgeable about supplement uses, doses, and interactions with medications. Some may know a lot about herbal and botanicals depending on their training.

>> **Chiropractors:** A chiropractor's training includes basic principles of diet and nutrition, but it's not as in depth as a nutritionist or dietician. Their focus is typically on musculoskeletal health and the nervous system. Chiropractors often offer some nutrition counselling and supplement prescriptions, but their education doesn't generally go to the level required for complex medical nutrition therapy or disease-specific dietary interventions.

>> **Acupuncturists:** Acupuncturists, especially those trained in traditional Chinese medicine, may offer some nutrition and herbal and supplement recommendations along with their holistic approach to health. Acupuncturists trained in the Western tradition may also get some nutrition education in their programs. The level of knowledge is not as great as a nutritionist or dietitian.

>> **Naturopathic doctors:** These physicians are trained in a medical system that uses natural remedies to help prevent disease. They treat holistically, meaning they consider the mind, body, and spirit. As they focus on education and prevention, their advice may address diet, exercise, and stress management. They may use homeopathy, herbal medicine, and acupuncture as well as herbs, massage, exercise, and nutritional counseling as part of a treatment plan.

TIP

Some MDs, DOs, or chiropractors may have additional degrees in nutrition, so check for credentials.

REMEMBER

Even among experts, there may be different opinions and philosophies so be sure to do your own evaluation before spending your hard-earned money on supplements.

Where to Go from Here

You can start anywhere in this book if you're looking for specific information. Check out the index or table of contents to find a topic and jump right to it. You can also start at the beginning to get a good overall understanding of vitamins and supplements because there is a lot to know!

1

Getting Started with the Basics

Chapter **1**

The ABC's of Vitamins, Minerals, and Supplements

The interest in dietary supplements has grown since the 1970s and has especially picked up since 2020 due to the COVID-19 pandemic. Consequently, the dietary supplement market has become huge. Some estimates predict it will reach more than $200 billion by 2029.

The purpose of dietary supplements is to complement your diet by providing nutrients that may be lacking or insufficient in your normal food intake. They're intended to help promote overall health and long-term well-being. It's a broad category of products that contain one or more ingredients such as vitamins, minerals, herbals, botanicals, amino acids, fatty acids, algae, fungi, bacteria, synthetic products, metabolites, and more. They are sold as capsules, soft gels, gelcaps, tablets, powders, gummies, and liquids — any form that's ingestible. Essential vitamin and mineral supplements are often used along with your food intake to meet daily the Recommended Dietary Allowance (RDA). Other supplements may be consumed to round out your diet to fulfill additional basic nutritional requirements during different life stages, if you're taking certain medications, or if you're an athlete — basically, in any situation where a person needs to bring their cellular levels of nutrients to normal levels. However, some people take dietary supplements for a variety of other reasons, such as reducing risk of certain diseases, protecting bodily tissues, enhancing athletic performance, improving mood, and increasing energy.

The increase in intake of dietary supplements may be in part due to their availability in supermarkets, drugstores, convenience stores, and online. They're everywhere! There are an estimated 80,000 supplement products on the market and a lot of books, websites, publications, and other information to sift through to determine if you need or desire a supplement. In this chapter, I introduce some basics about supplements.

Defining the Terminology

Dietary supplements include vitamins, minerals, herbs, botanicals, amino acids, proteins, fats, and more. There are many terms used throughout this book that are defined in the text, and some are also in the glossary at the end of the book. In this section, I introduce vitamins, minerals, additional supplements, and the regulatory process.

Vitamins

Vitamins are organic compounds, meaning they contain carbon and are produced by plants or animals. The first part of the word *vitamin* — *vita-* — is derived from Latin and means *life*. The rest of the word — *-amin* — is from *amine* because researchers originally thought that all vitamins contain amino acids (nitrogen- and carbon-containing molecules that are building blocks of proteins).

Vitamins are essential (necessary) for normal growth and nutrition. You need them in small amounts to maintain various bodily functions such as immune health, energy production, and wound healing. Your body can't make these compounds, so you must get them from food or supplements.

Vitamins are divided into two categories:

>> **Fat-soluble vitamins:** This group includes vitamins A, D, E, K. These are stored in body fat and in the liver and can accumulate if you have too much.

>> **Water-soluble vitamins:** All the B vitamins and vitamin C are water soluble. Your body doesn't retain these. Instead, you excrete them in your urine. You need to continuously replenish these by consuming foods rich in them or with supplements.

Minerals

Minerals are naturally occurring, inorganic elements formed in the earth through geological processes. They are vital components in foods that your body needs to develop and function normally. Some minerals are essential (necessary for life) for building bones, facilitating nerve function, regulating water balance, and supporting the immune system.

There are 13 essential minerals summarized in the following list (and covered in more detail later in this book). Some of these are needed in relatively large amounts, and others are considered "trace minerals" that you need in very small amounts.

WARNING

It's critical to understand doses of any supplement that you take. Some are measured in milligram doses (mg), and others are in microgram doses (mcg).

These are the essential minerals:

» **Calcium:** Builds strong bones and teeth and helps in muscle contraction, blood clotting, nerve transmission, cell signaling, and regulation of metabolism

» **Chloride:** With sodium, maintains the normal fluid balance in the body

» **Copper:** Trace mineral that participates in energy production and facilitates iron uptake from the gut

» **Magnesium:** Essential in several biochemical reactions, including synthesis of deoxyribonucleic acid (DA) and some antioxidants

» **Iron:** Trace mineral necessary for hemoglobin formation, which carries oxygen in the blood

» **Iodine:** Trace mineral used to produce thyroid hormones and essential for metabolism and physical and mental development

» **Manganese:** Trace mineral that plays an important role in protein, carbohydrate, and cholesterol breakdown, and cell division, and blood clotting

» **Phosphorus:** Helps build and repair bones and teeth, facilitates nerve function, and aids in muscle contraction

» **Potassium:** Maintains fluid balance and aids in muscle contraction and nerve impulse conduction

» **Selenium:** Trace mineral that helps prevent oxidative damage to the cells and aids in thyroid hormone metabolism

>> **Sodium:** Important in contracting muscles, conducting nerve impulses, and controlling fluid balance in the body

>> **Sulfur:** Has antibacterial properties, helps fight acne-causing bacteria in the skin, and repairs DNA damage

>> **Zinc:** Trace mineral that aids in cell division, immunity, and wound healing

Supplements

Dietary supplements are products that are meant to add nutrients to the diet. Vitamins, minerals, herbs, other botanicals, amino acids, and proteins are included in this category. Supplements can fill any gaps in your intake of nutrients from other sources — mainly food. They are identified by a dietary supplement label and intended to be taken orally. They come in many forms, including tablets, capsules, gummies, powders, drinks, and bars. There are over 80,000 supplements on the market, so this book covers some but certainly not all of the available options.

WARNING

Supplements should never replace a balanced diet. You should take them with caution to avoid overdosing on certain nutrients. The Supplement Facts label lists active ingredients, dose, fillers, binders, and flavoring. The FDA does not determine whether supplements are effective before they're produced and marketed. Therefore, safety of taking supplements is in your hands.

TIP

Understanding what your nutrient needs are and what constitutes a healthy diet is important when you're considering supplements. Two good resources are the Dietary Guidelines for Americans (https://dietaryguidelines.gov) and MyPlate (https://myplate.gov) websites. A good source for information on supplements is the Office of Dietary Supplements (ODS) of the National Institutes of Health (NIH) (https://ods.od.nih.gov).

TIP

Before taking supplements, it is always important to consult with a healthcare professional so that you can be sure that the supplements support your health concerns, you're taking the correct nutrients, know the best dose for you, and have no interactions with any medications you're taking. Also, if you're undergoing a surgical procedure, you may need to alter your intake temporarily.

Manufacturers may also fortify foods that you eat, so it's good to be aware of those foods that are fortified so that you can add this to your understanding of your total intake. For example, iron and B vitamins are added to many breakfast cereals, which is a great source for these nutrients. Make sure to consider how much you're getting if you eat cereal because you may not need to supplement some of these nutrients.

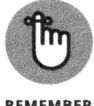

REMEMBER

The FDA has established Good Manufacturing Practices (GMP) that companies are required to follow to ensure identity, purity, strength, and composition of supplements. Some products are marked with the GMP symbol to confirm that the manufacturer complies with all FDA standards, procedures, and documentation regarding its identity, strength, purity, and more. These are manufacturing requirements, but the FDA doesn't test products on these qualities unless there are consumer complaints or issues with the product after production and marketing. The FDA also doesn't ensure the effectiveness of supplements, so you will need to rely on marketing information and your own research.

TIP

There are three major independent or third-party organizations that check the quality, purity, dose stated on the label of supplements. They are ConsumerLab. com, NSF International, and US Pharmacopeia. These are discussed later in the book in Chapter 13. For now, know that it is always best to look for products with one of these certifications to ensure that what you're buying is what is truly in the supplement. In addition, there are other independent certifications, including USDA Organic, Certified Vegan, International Fish Oil Standards (IFOS), Non-GMO Project Verified, and Informed Sport.

IMPORTANT GOVERNMENT REGULATORY AND INFORMATION AGENCIES

There are government sites that are involved in regulating and provide information on dietary supplements.

- **Federal Drug Agency (FDA)** issues rules and regulations and oversees dietary supplement labeling, marketing, and safety. Recall notices are also posted on the FDA's website.

- **Federal Trade Commission (FTC)** regulates health and safety claims made in advertising for dietary supplements.

- **U.S. Department of Agriculture (USDA)** provides information on food and nutrition topics.

- **U.S. Department of Health and Human Services (HHS)** provides personal health tools, news, and information on wellness

Looking at the Nature of Vitamins and Supplements

Throughout this book, I cover how vitamins and supplements function to keep you healthy. To help you understand which supplements will be beneficial, you need to have some understanding of how and why they're important and how they function in your body.

Each vitamin, mineral, botanical, or other supplement is unique in how it works. Essential vitamins and minerals are important because they are vital for bodily functions and health and can't be made by your body; therefore, you must get them from foods. Supplements are supposed to add to (*supplement*) your dietary intake to help you get complete nutrition for good health or added benefits.

In this section, I introduce what is meant by "essential" vitamins and minerals.

Knowing why vitamins are essential

Essential vitamins and minerals must be obtained from food and supplements because your body doesn't produce them. This discovery was made early on when certain diseases, such as scurvy and goiter, were found to be related to deficiencies in Vitamin C and iodine, respectively. Simply supplementing the diet cured these diseases, which plagued people a century ago.

Each vitamin and mineral has one or many specific roles in bodily function. In this book, I talk about metabolism, which is a series of thousands of biochemical reactions that take place in your cells to process food you eat for energy and building and maintaining tissues and organs. Vitamins and minerals are vital components of these processes.

Vitamins and minerals are essential because they're critical to maintaining normal body function and health. Here are some ways they are essential:

>> Participating in metabolic processes that produce energy and are important for body functions. Vitamins act as cofactors (support) for enzymes in biochemical reactions.

>> Being precursors for enzymes or biochemicals involved in metabolism.

>> Supporting cell division, growth, and development.

>> Preventing deficiency diseases such as scurvy, rickets, goiter, and anemia.

>> Regulating hormonal balance.

>> Maintaining and strengthening immune function.

>> Supporting bone and tissue health.

>> Participating in antioxidant and anti-inflammatory processes.

>> Supporting neurological and cognitive development and function.

>> Healing wounds.

>> Supporting skin, hair, and nail health.

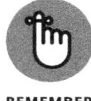

REMEMBER

You may experience vitamin and mineral deficiencies in your life at different life stages or if you have health issues. There are certain life stages when you need more nutrients, such as if you're pregnant or lactating and as you age. Vitamin and mineral deficiencies can also happen if you eat a poor diet low in nutrients for too long of a time. Medications may reduce your body of some nutrients and can also interact with some supplements. Talk with your doctor to find out which vitamins and supplements are best for your situation.

OVERFED AND UNDERNOURISHED

Perhaps you have seen the 2004 movie called *Supersize Me* directed by and starring Morgan Spurlock, an American independent filmmaker. He ate only McDonald's restaurant food, three meals a day for 30 days, resulting in about 5,000 calories per day and a lot of sugar and fat. In that time, he gained weight and developed fatty liver. He was monitored by a physician, a nutritionist, and other health professionals who were surprised by the quick negative effects of this diet.

Although this was just one example (and the film and the director received some criticism for how the experiment was conducted, the issue that Spurlock brought to the public view was and still is very real. The negative effects demonstrate how you can eat a lot, but if the calories and nutrients come from the wrong foods, your body can still be lacking nutrients and be undernourished. The Standard American Diet (SAD) is a dietary pattern of many people in the United States that is based on ultraprocessed foods, added sugar, fat, and sodium. It lacks the correct amount of fruits, vegetables, whole grains, and lean protein. There are long-term health effects of this diet, including diabetes, heart disease, and obesity. Some Americans become deficient in nutrients including vitamins D, E, and C, fiber, calcium, and potassium.

Vitamin and mineral deficiency can lead to poor health and needs to be addressed by diet and supplements. To avoid deficiencies, follow healthy–eating guidelines such as these:

>> Dietary Guidelines for Americans is a large document that's updated every five years. It provides advice on what to eat and drink to meet nutrient needs, prevent disease, and promote health.

>> The MyPlate website describes a healthy way of eating called the "Healthy US–Style (HUSS) dietary pattern, which is a more balanced alternative than the SAD. It includes nutrient-dense foods like fruits, vegetables, lean protein, grains, and low-fat dairy with limited sugar and fat.

>> The Mediterranean, DASH, MIND, and vegetarian diets are also excellent ways of eating that promote health and reduce risk of obesity and chronic disease.

Seeing why supplements are extra

Depending on what you eat, how much you eat, your stage of life, and perhaps what health issues you have, you may need more nutrients than you can get from your diet. Supplements are "extra" because you use them in addition to the nutrients that you already get in your foods. Extra can bring you up to normal RDA levels.

Extra can also mean going above and beyond these essential nutrients. Extra vitamins might be vitamin C if you are trying to reduce the severity of a cold. It could mean echinacea or another herbal or botanical for immunity or other purposes. Extra could mean more protein if you are trying to build muscles or are athletic.

Here are some examples of how supplements may be used:

>> Correcting deficiencies, such as low vitamin D, B12, or iron.

>> Preventing health conditions, such as anemia (low iron) or osteoporosis (taking calcium)

>> Supporting health goals — for example, taking glucosamine for joint health

>> Enhancing performance, such as when athletes take supplements for energy and improving muscle strength.

REMEMBER

Supplements can help in a variety of health situations, but you should always talk to your healthcare provider before taking supplements.

Here are some other situations where you may need supplements:

» Different life stages

- *Infants:* Infants may need vitamin D, iron, maybe B12 and choline. This will depend on the maternal diet if the baby is breastfed.

- *Toddlers and older children:* If toddlers are not getting enough from their food intake plus breast milk or formula, they may need vitamins A, D, iron, and zinc. Older children may also need these supplements for growth and development if they don't get enough from foods.

- *Pregnant and lactating women:* Prenatal vitamin containing folate, other nutrients critical for fetal growth and development and maternal health

- *Adults older than 50:* A multivitamin, calcium, vitamin D, and B12 because absorption of some vitamins decreases with age, more D and calcium are needed for bone support, and sometimes older people eat less and do not get everything they need from food

- *Athletes or people in physically demanding jobs:* Extra protein and energy (carbohydrates) to improve muscle strength and energy, respectively

» Certain lifestyles:

- *Vegetarian:* B12 and omega-3

- *Vegan:* Calcium, B12, omega-3, and vitamin D

- *Busy people who eat on the go:* A multivitamin to fill in gaps in a diet that may lack nutrient-rich foods

» People with health-related deficiencies or health-related goals

- *Limited sun exposure:* Vitamin D

- *Anemia or during menstruation:* Iron or B vitamins depending on the type of anemia.

- *Poor iron absorption or for a fruit-poor diet:* Vitamin C

- *Heart and brain support:* Omega-3 fatty acids

- *Poor gut health and gastrointestinal issues:* Probiotics

- *Anti-inflammation:* antioxidants such as vitamins A, E, C, and green tea extract

- Glucosamine and chondroitin sulfate: Joint health

» Addressing prevention and certain diseases states

- *Bone health/osteoporosis:* Calcium and vitamin D

- *Heart health:* Omega-3 fatty acids (fish oil or plant based), CoQ10 if taking statins

- *Spina bifida in infants:* Maternal folate supplements

- *Vision:* Vitamin A, C, E, beta-carotene, zinc, omega-3 fatty acids, lutein zeaxanthin, bilberry extract

- *Cognitive and mental health:* B vitamins important in nerve function and metabolism, magnesium, ashwagandha

- *Enhanced immunity:* Vitamins A, C, D; zinc; elderberry; echinacea

Recognizing the limitations of supplements

There are some limitations to supplements:

» **Toxicity:** It's possible to overconsume vitamins, particularly the fat-soluble vitamins, which are A, D, E, and K. When you take too much, they can accumulate in the body and can cause damage. Each vitamin has an upper limit (UL), beyond which toxicity can occur.

Be sure to follow the Recommended Dietary Allowance (RDA) for any supplement, which is defined as "the levels of intake of essential nutrients that, on the basis of scientific knowledge, are judged by the Food and Nutrition Board to be adequate to meet the known nutrient needs of practically all healthy persons."

TIP

The Food and Nutrition Board is part of the National Academies, a nonprofit, nongovernmental organization committed to evidence-based information and leadership.

» **Bioavailability:** Vitamins are generally more available to your body when you get them from foods. Supplements that are chemically synthesized may not be as available for use as food-based vitamins.

» **Quality control:** There are FDA guidelines that manufacturers are required to follow for supplement labeling, marketing, and safety, but the products are not approved by the FDA before marketing. The FDA does not require that supplements are effective, but the FTC regulates health and safety claims. Look for the seals from third-party certifiers to decide which products to buy. (Read more in Chapter 13.)

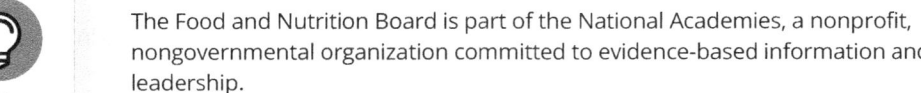

TIP

Supplements' presentation, labeling, and advertising must not claim or imply that they can prevent, treat, or cure human disease.

DISTINGUISHING BETWEEN NUTRIENTS FROM FOODS AND SUPPLEMENTS

Because your body cannot make the essential vitamins and minerals, you must get them by ingesting from foods or supplements. If you get enough from your food, then you do not need supplements. If you have a limited diet for any reason, though, you must supplement with the necessary vitamins to make sure that you're getting the RDA for all these essential micronutrients.

Protein, carbohydrates, and fats (the macronutrients) also have recommended amounts:

- **Proteins:** The recommended amount is 0.8 gram per kilogram of body weight or 0.36 gram per pound of body weight. You can also roughly calculate the amount at between 10 percent and 35 percent of your daily calorie intake.

- **Carbohydrates:** This category of macronutrient should make up 40 percent to 60 percent of your daily calorie intake.

- **Fats:** The recommended amount of dietary fat is 20 percent to 35 percent of your daily calorie intake.

Understanding the Science and Business of Supplements

The global vitamin and dietary supplement market is growing. Between 2012 and 2022, there were more than 69,000 scientific articles on dietary supplements published, and there were many more marketing publications produced by manufacturing and sales companies.

The growth of the market means that supplements are widely available from all kinds of retailers. You can find them at online retailers such as Amazon. Direct-to-consumer brands often have personalized nutrition models and sell subscriptions based on your need. The traditional way to buy vitamins is strong as well; retailers such as Costco, CVS, and Walgreens have their own labels but also sell products from major brands such as Centrum, Nature Made, and GNC. Supplements are being manufactured by pharmaceutical and food companies such as Nestle, Pfizer, and Abbott. There is an abundance of supplement companies, such as NOW, Garden of Life, New Chapter, Gaia, MegaFoods, Metagenics, Pure Encapsulation, Life Extension, and many more. Herbalife and Amway are also still big players.

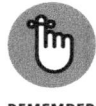

Buying from a reputable company is always important, but even then, you need to do your research, read labels, understand health claims, and match your needs with the product. Some brands may contain unwanted dyes or fillers.

Supplements are also being sold illegally worldwide, which increases the risk for adulteration and possibly dangerous side effects. Certain types of supplements are more prone to online sales and marketing and may contain ingredients that are not included in the labeling or may exceed upper limits of safety. Some online products have been shown to contain things like lead or arsenic or to be adulterated with dangerous compounds. Be especially careful with supplements in the following categories: sexual enhancement, weight loss, and body building. I always recommend buying from well-known and reliable sources.

Here are some of the growing areas of nutrition and supplements and future areas of interest:

>> **Personalized nutrition:** This is understanding a person's genetics, health, and lifestyle and deciding which supplements are appropriate based on this evaluation.

>> **Nutrition and genetic testing:** Micronutrient testing, genetic testing, microbiome analysis, and food allergy testing help to personalize nutrition and supplement recommendations.

>> **Gut health:** Probiotics and prebiotics sales are growing due to supportive evidence of their role in digestive health and mental health.

>> **Herbal and botanical supplements:** These are used in a variety of preventative and health issues. A program called CARBoN (Consortium for Advancing Research on Botanical and Other Natural Products) through the ODS promotes research on the safety and effectiveness of botanicals and how they work to benefit health. They can act as antioxidants and aid with immunity, digestive health, sleep, and more.

>> **Products with sustainably sourced ingredients and responsible packaging:** These include food-based supplements and products with fewer additives and fillers. They may be organic, gluten free, or kosher.

>> **Weight loss:** Specialized vitamins are being developed as more people start GLP-1s medications and undergo surgery for weight loss.

Chapter **2**

Taking a Closer Look at Nutritional Biochemistry

When I earned my PhD in nutritional biochemistry and nutrition from the (no longer in existence) department of food science and nutrition at MIT, it was the late 1970s and early '80s. It may be hard to believe, but what I learned then as it relates to health and wellness hasn't changed that much!

What has changed dramatically is that more people all over the world are suffering from obesity and chronic diseases. Another thing that's changed is the food supply, which is different in terms of the number of products on the market, the increase in processed foods, larger portion sizes, and the amount of takeout and restaurant food people eat. All of this has led to many people being overfed and undernourished and experiencing vitamin deficiencies and metabolic disorders.

Nutritional biochemistry is the scientific study of how nutrients and food components interact with your biological processes. It focuses on nutrient absorption, biochemical processes, metabolism, and the impact on health and disease. It's the study of how nutrients such as proteins, fats, carbohydrates, vitamins, and minerals are digested, absorbed into the blood, and used in the body to create energy, build tissues, and function in the numerous bodily functions. Nutritional biochemistry is based in science. By understanding it and your metabolism, you can personalize and optimize your nutrition to support your health and longevity.

These days, I focus on metabolic health, with the goal of helping people keep their metabolism working efficiently. Metabolism in your cells and organs refers to thousands of processes that turn food into energy that can be used or stored. It also refers to the creation of building blocks or intermediates of metabolism that are used to create things like muscles and bones.

In this chapter, you find out how complex human metabolism is and how the essential vitamins and minerals are an integral part of biochemistry of our cells. These can come from food or supplements. For example, vitamins and minerals are essential for enzymes to work or for hormones to be synthesized. I hope to give you a better understanding of why nutrients from foods and supplements are important to everyday working of your body and general health and wellness. Throughout this book, you discover more about nutritional biochemistry and how to optimize your health through food and use of supplements.

Examining Biochemistry in Our Cells

Biochemistry is the area of science that refers to the plethora of interactions and transformations of molecules that happen inside the cells of an organism — many of them simultaneously. It's the understanding of life processes that support your body at the cellular level. *Metabolism* is the sum of all the biochemical reactions in your cells — which might be millions.

Understanding biochemical reactions and enzymes

A biochemical reaction is when two or more molecules (called reactants) act together to create a new set of molecules (called the products). The reactions of metabolism are organized into metabolic pathways, in which one chemical — such as a fat, carb, or protein — is converted to its breakdown products through multiple steps.

Each step is catalyzed by an enzyme to speed up the reaction. An enzyme is a protein that has a very specific action of bringing together molecules in a way that makes them react with each other to form something new. Enzymatic reactions often have complex mechanisms that require helpers in the form of cofactors or coenzymes. These are often vitamins or minerals and are necessary for the reaction to occur.

There are many types of metabolic reactions. They can be categorized as anabolic or catabolic. (See Figure 2-1.)

>> **Anabolic reactions** are those that build a larger molecule from smaller ones and require energy. An example is that you make cholesterol in your body and hormones from it! Cholesterol is the precursor to steroid hormones, testosterone, estradiol (estrogen), progesterone, cortisol, and aldosterone. Other examples of these anabolic reactions are the biosynthesis of DNA/RNA, protein, carbohydrates, or lipids.

>> **Catabolic reactions** are those that break down larger molecules to smaller ones and give off energy. A good example of this is the breakdown of blood sugar (glucose) to smaller molecules and adenosine triphosphate (ATP), which is a source of energy for your cells.

TECHNICAL STUFF

An important example of these reactions is called the Krebs cycle. This pathway, along with oxidative phosphorylation, produces cellular energy as ATP in your cells. These metabolic pathways convert proteins, fats, and carbohydrates into energy that your body needs. Vitamins and minerals are essential for many of these enzymatic reactions to catalyze them or speed them up.

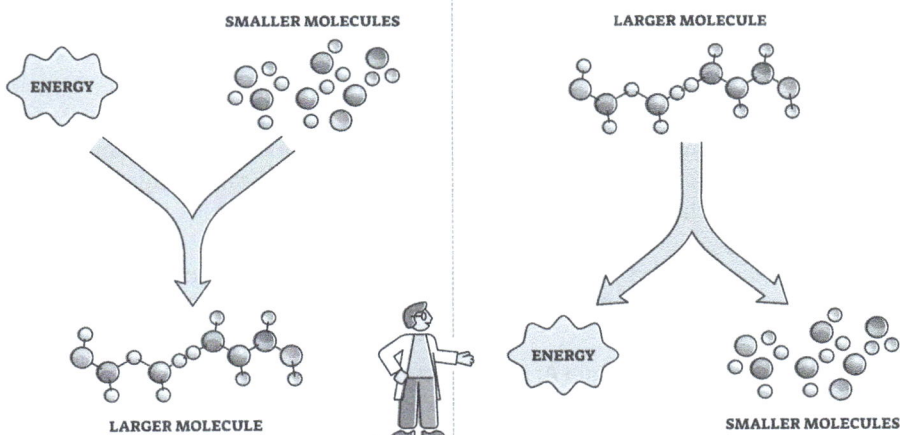

ANABOLIC REACTION   **CATABOLIC** REACTION

SMALLER MOLECULES   LARGER MOLECULE

ENERGY

LARGER MOLECULE   ENERGY   SMALLER MOLECULES

FIGURE 2-1:
Two types of metabolic reactions: anabolic and catabolic.

VectorMine/Adobe Stock Photos

The following are some common types of biochemical reactions:

>> **Group transfer:** Making new amino acids that can be used for protein synthesis.

>> **Formation of carbon double bonds:** For example, hydrogenation of oils to make margarine.

>> **Hydrolysis reactions:** Either adding water or taking it away (dehydrating) to make macromolecules like proteins, carbs, lipids, DNA/RNA.

>> **Oxidation reactions:** Transferring electrons between two substances.

TIP

You may have heard of antioxidants, which help reduce oxidation in your body to lower inflammation. I cover supplements that are antioxidants and how to use antioxidants to lower inflammation throughout this book.

Examining the function of vitamins and minerals in enzymatic reactions

Vitamins (or molecules derived from vitamins) and minerals are nonprotein "helper molecules" that are essential for enzymes to properly function. They are called cofactors or coenzymes, and there are many examples of these in metabolism in all living organisms, but my focus is on humans, of course!

Two types of cofactors:

>> Inorganic ions such as zinc, iron, or copper

>> Organic molecules (called coenzymes) that are mostly vitamins or products derived from vitamins

Cofactors or coenzymes are essential for enzyme functioning and maintaining metabolic health. This is a major reason why vitamin and mineral intake is crucial to metabolism. An absence of a vitamin can change a biochemical reaction, and that in turn can affect overall metabolism.

Here, I list vitamins and the biochemical reactions you need them for. They're needed in small or trace amounts for normal growth and health.

>> **Vitamin A:** Forming vision pigments and the functioning of epithelial cells, which form a thin protective layer on many internal and external surfaces of your body

>> **Vitamin D:** Increases the body's absorption of calcium and phosphorous

>> **Vitamin E:** Acts as antioxidant

>> **Vitamin K:** Forming the prothrombin enzyme that's responsible for blood clotting

>> **Vitamin B1:** Forming the thiamine pyrophosphate coenzyme involved in carbohydrate metabolism

>> **Vitamin B2:** Forming the FAD (flavin adenine dinucleotide) coenzyme for oxidation-reduction reactions in the Krebs cycle and other metabolic pathways that form energy (ATP); important for fat, carbohydrate, and protein metabolism

>> **Vitamin B3:** Forming the NAD (nicotinamide adenine dinucleotide) and NADP (nicotinamide adenine dinucleotide phosphate coenzymes for oxidation-reduction reactions critical to pathways that form energy (ATP)

>> **Vitamin B5 (pantothenic acid):** Forming coenzyme A (CoA) that's essential for fatty acid metabolism, the Krebs cycle, and energy production

>> **Vitamin B6:** Forming pyridoxal phosphate coenzyme for transferring amino acids in amino acid metabolism; transforming glycogen in the liver to glucose when needed for energy

>> **Vitamin B12:** Forming methylcobalamin coenzyme for intramolecular rearrangements essential for fatty acid metabolism and homocysteine metabolism

>> **Biotin:** Facilitating carboxylation reactions, forming fatty acids and glucose that are used for energy, and helping in amino acid and carbohydrate metabolism

>> **Vitamin B9 (folic acid):** Forming tetrahydrofolate coenzyme for carrier of one-carbon units

>> **Vitamin C:** Acting as an antioxidant and aiding in the formation of collagen

>> **Choline:** Acting as a precursor to neurotransmitter formation and providing methyl groups for DNA synthesis and cell growth

And here are some examples of the roles of minerals in biochemical reactions:

>> **Iron:** A component of various enzymes involved in the Krebs cycle, it is integral to the formation of hemoglobin and helps in the proliferation and maturation of immune cells.

>> **Zinc:** It's a cofactor for more than 300 enzymes that catalyze many reactions, including DNA and protein synthesis.

>> **Selenium:** This cofactor in thyroid hormone metabolism acts as an antioxidant that protects cells from oxidative damage and is important in immune cell function.

>> **Copper:** This cofactor for antioxidant enzymes has a role in synthesizing collagen and elastin and is involved in iron metabolism and red blood cell formation.

>> **Iodine:** It has a role in thyroid hormone synthesis.

Digging into other roles of vitamins and minerals

In this section, I give some examples of other important functions served by vitamins and minerals.

Body fluid balance is important in health and disease and is critical to homeostasis (self-regulation of an organism to maintain stability and survive) of your body. It involves not only the total water in your body but also the water inside and outside of your cells. Drinking water is clearly part of maintaining fluid balance, but the way your body controls the fluid intracellularly (inside cells) and extracellularly (outside cells) in your body involves minerals, including sodium, potassium, chloride, and magnesium:

>> Sodium is a positively charged electrolyte that's mostly in the extracellular fluid. It helps regulate blood volume and blood pressure.

>> Potassium is a positively charged electrolyte that's mostly inside the cell. It works closely with sodium to balance and regulate blood pressure.

>> Magnesium is a positively charged electrolyte that helps by aiding the transport of potassium and sodium across cell membranes.

>> Chloride is a negatively charged electrolyte that helps with the electrolyte balance inside and outside of the cell.

Proper fluid balance is essential and supports cellular hydration, nerve function, and muscle contractions.

Vitamins and minerals also play a role in immune response. Vitamins A, D, C, and E and the minerals zinc, iron, and copper all support immune function in different ways. Each of these will be discussed throughout the book, specifically in Part 3.

Vitamin K is responsible for making 4 of the 13 proteins that are needed for blood clotting. Blood clotting is important when you get wounded and are bleeding. Calcium also works together with fibrinogen, a protein, in the clotting process. There are a series of reactions in the clotting "cascade" that involve the breakdown of platelets in your blood that react with fibrinogen to create a mass called fibrin. When this mass is outside the body, it hardens to form a scab.

Red blood cell (RBC) production takes place in the bone marrow. The hormone that controls this is called erythropoietin, which is made by the kidney. Iron, vitamin B12, and folate are essential to the production of RBCs.

Vitamin D, calcium, phosphorous, and protein are important for bone formation. Protein acts as the scaffold upon which calcium and phosphorous form and harden. Vitamin D helps your body absorb calcium in the gut and into the bloodstream.

Appreciating Your Metabolism and Metabolic Health

You may feel like your metabolism is slow, fast, or just right. How do you know? And what happens to your metabolism as you age or as you go through hormonal changes. How much of your metabolism can you control?

Good metabolic health is what you experience when thousands and thousands of biochemical reactions in your body are working well. It's when your body is correctly processing food into energy for all of its uses, including creating the building blocks necessary for bodily functions of all kinds. This sounds like a daunting task, and it is; living organisms are truly remarkable. Metabolic health is important for your health and daily functioning and avoiding chronic diseases. Vitamins and minerals from foods and supplements are essential for maintaining good metabolic health.

You need a minimum amount of energy just to carry out your basic processes. This is called your basal metabolic rate (BMR). It might also be called your resting metabolic rate (RMR), but the two things are actually a little different. BMR is the minimal energy needed just to exist, whereas RMR is the sum of the amount of energy required to keep your body functioning. (See Figure 2-2.)

BMR can be calculated using your height, weight, age, and sex. There are many online calculators that you can use to calculate your BMR, which gives you a number in calories per day that you need to support your basic bodily functions. I happen to like the MyFitnessPal app, which many of my clients use. Noom, Lose It!, and other apps also have BMR calculators.

The online calculators can also help you determine your daily caloric needs for supporting your body. This number is the combination of your BMR plus the energy used for daily activities and physical exercise, and it's known as your total energy expenditure(TEE).

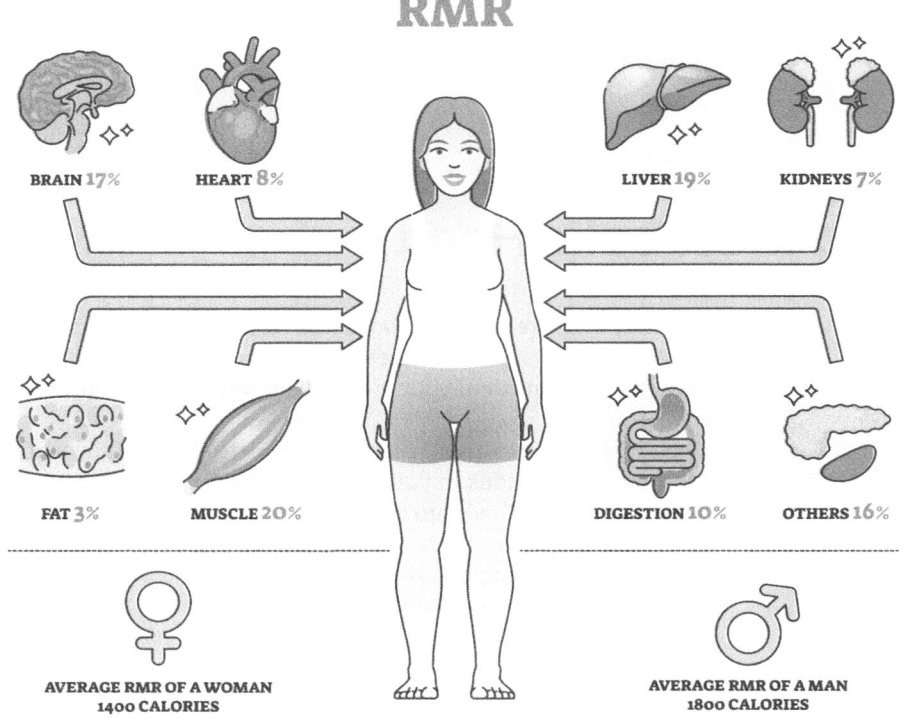

RESTING METABOLIC RATE
RMR

BRAIN 17%   HEART 8%   LIVER 19%   KIDNEYS 7%

FAT 3%   MUSCLE 20%   DIGESTION 10%   OTHERS 16%

AVERAGE RMR OF A WOMAN
1400 CALORIES

AVERAGE RMR OF A MAN
1800 CALORIES

FIGURE 2-2: The breakdown of RMR by different organs and tissues that use energy.

olenka758/Adobe Stock Photos

Influencers of metabolic health

Healthy metabolism is when you can digest the food you eat and metabolize efficiently so that you avoid spikes in insulin or glucose, unhealthy amount of lipids in your blood, and inflammation, to name a few things. You can control some things that affect your metabolism, such as whether you get enough vitamins and other nutrients from your food and supplements. But you can't control all things. Uncontrollable influencers of metabolism include the following things:

>> **Inborn errors of metabolism:** There are hundreds of inherited metabolic disorders caused by changes in specific genes that affect metabolism. They're passed down from one or both parents and are handled medically. Examples include familial hypercholesterolemia, Gaucher disease, phenylketonuria (PKU), Tay-Sachs disease, or Wilson's disease. People with these or other genetic disorders should be followed by their medical team.

>> **Age:** As we age, metabolism can change. In a recent study published in *Science*, researchers found that metabolism doesn't significantly slow down

until about age 60 — which is later than most people think. So blaming weight gain on metabolism at an earlier age isn't supported here! After 60 or so, TEE and RMR decline about 0.7 per year, which can influence weight in older adults. I always recommend a multivitamin supplement in people older than 50 to ensure adequate intake of essential vitamins and minerals.

>> **Sex:** Metabolic differences exist between biological men and women. More muscle burns more calories. Female bodies are predisposed to storing energy for pregnancy and breastfeeding. They often have less lean muscle and burn less fat than men. As testosterone decreases with age, men are less metabolically active, make less lean muscle, burn less fat, and potentially gain weight. There are supplements to help men and women address these different situations.

Here are some examples of controllable influencers of metabolism:

>> **Diet:** A diet high in fruits, vegetables, whole grains, and lean protein and low in sugar and saturated fats optimizes your nutrient intake and is good for your metabolism. Diets high in fast foods, sugar, and fat can lead to vitamin deficiencies, insulin resistance, weight gain, and chronic diseases.

>> **Sleep:** Studies show that getting less than the seven to nine hours of sleep can lead to weight gain. Sleep duration is linked to the body's production of the appetite-regulating hormones: ghrelin and leptin. Insufficient sleep is associated with high levels of ghrelin, which increases appetite, and lower levels of leptin, which leads to feeling less full. In addition, if you sleep less, you may spend some of the time eating.

>> **Exercise:** Regular exercise regulates insulin sensitivity and overall metabolism and therefore reduces the risk for chronic metabolic diseases, such as obesity, type 2 diabetes, and non-alcoholic fatty liver disease. Exercise also increases muscle mass, which improves metabolism. The more muscle mass, the better your metabolism, which is one reason that some men may find it easier to lose weight than women.

>> **Hormones:** Hormones play a key role in tissue and metabolism homeostasis (self-regulation and balance). Those hormones include the following:

- *Insulin:* Produced by the pancreas to regulate sugar and fat metabolism.

- *Estrogen:* A sex hormone that fine-tunes protein turnover and mitochondrial metabolism.

- *Leptin:* The fullness hormone produced by abdominal and other fat cells and signals the brain.

- *Ghrelin:* The hunger hormone produced in the intestines to signal the brain when hungry.

- *Thyroid hormones:.* T3 (triiodothyronine) and T4 (thyroxine) regulate metabolism, growth and development, and energy level.

- *Cortisol:* Made by adrenal glands and triggered during times of stress. It can increase heart rate and energy levels.

- *Neuropeptide (NYP):* Produced in the nervous system and activated in fat tissue to stimulate appetite and decrease energy expenditure in response to fasting or stress. NPY is associated with abdominal obesity and weight gain.

- *Glucagon-like peptide-1 (GLP-1):* Produced in your gut. It keeps blood sugar levels stable and makes you feel full. Some people with obesity have impaired GLP-1 functioning. GLP-1 medications can help people with this problem lose weight.

- *Cholecystokinin (CCK):* Another fullness hormone produced by gut cells after a meal that's important for many bodily functions. It can also increase leptin release.

- *Peptide YY:* A gut hormone that decreases appetite.

- *Progesterone:* A sex hormone that regulates fat distribution.

- *Testosterone:* A sex hormone that affects metabolism.

Sugar/carbohydrate metabolism

Carbohydrates are essentially long chains of sugar molecules bound together. You get carbohydrates from many sources, including fruits, vegetables, grains, and dairy. Your body starts to digest carbohydrates in the mouth. (See Figure 2-3.) Complex carbohydrates (chains of glucose and other sugars) are broken down into smaller pieces in the mouth by a salivary enzyme called amylase. (See Figure 2-4.). The food travels down the esophagus to the stomach and then to the small intestine, where pancreatic amylase — another digestive enzyme — breaks the carbohydrates down more to be single sugar molecules called monosaccharides. These are then absorbed through the intestinal wall into the blood, which then travels to the liver.

In the liver, the monosaccharides are converted to glucose, which is what your body uses to create energy in the form of ATP (a process called glycolysis). Alternatively, it can get stored as glycogen (a chain of glucose molecules) and used at another time for energy. The uptake of glucose by cells is controlled by insulin and another hormone called glucagon.

Human Digestive System

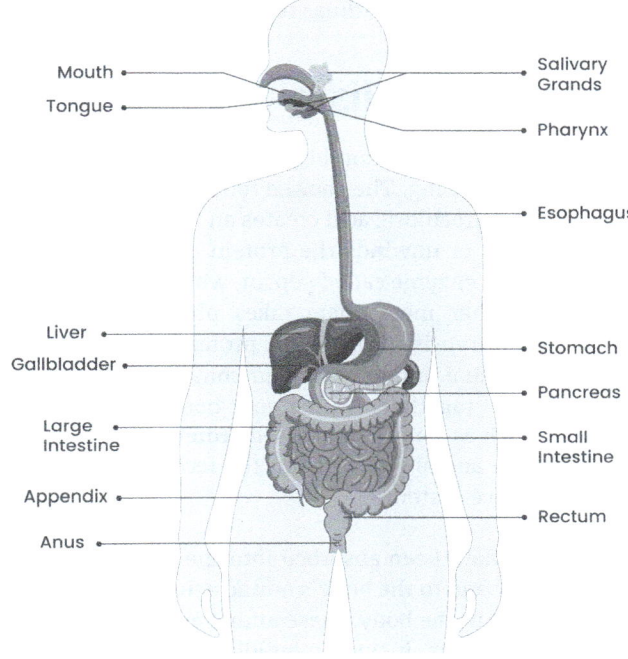

FIGURE 2-3: Sugar, fat, and protein breakdown by enzymes to smaller molecules. These then feed into metabolic pathways and are used for energy or as building blocks for molecules in your cells.

Mouth
Tongue
Salivary Grands
Pharynx
Esophagus
Liver
Gallbladder
Stomach
Pancreas
Large Intestine
Small Intestine
Appendix
Rectum
Anus

VectorMine/Adobe Stock Photos

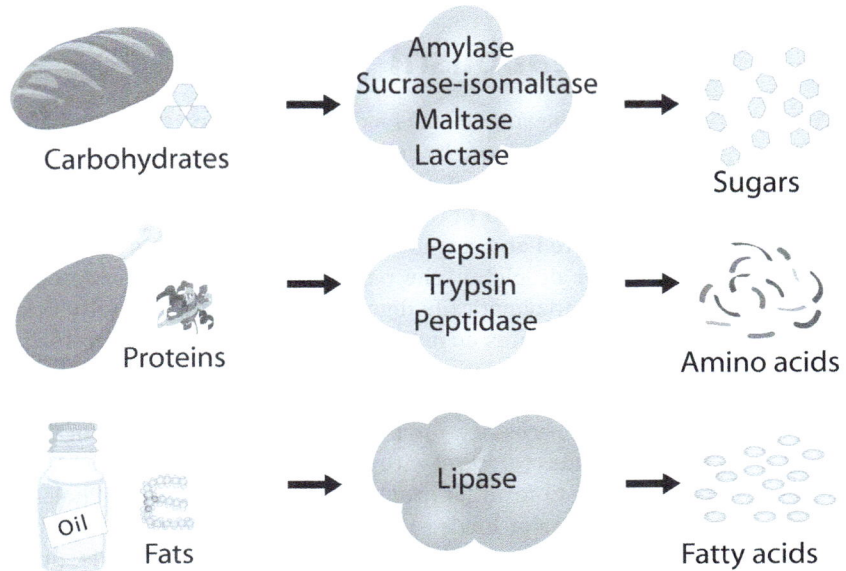

Carbohydrates → Amylase Sucrase-isomaltase Maltase Lactase → Sugars

Proteins → Pepsin Trypsin Peptidase → Amino acids

Fats → Lipase → Fatty acids

FIGURE 2-4: Digestion takes place in the mouth, stomach, and intestines.

Once absorbed into your body, your cells use glucose to make cellular energy (ATP) via the Krebs cycle and other metabolic pathways. Vitamins and minerals are crucial for all of these complex cellular reactions.

Protein metabolism

When you eat protein, digestion begins in the mouth as you mechanically break down the food by chewing. The chewed food travels through the esophagus to the stomach, where hydrochloric acid creates an acidic environment. The acidic environment denatures or unwinds the protein and opens it up to be broken down more by a digestive enzyme called pepsin, which is produced by the cells that line the stomach. Further metabolism takes place in the small intestine. There, enzymes — chymotrypsin, trypsin, and proteases — continue to break down proteins to the individual amino acids and some di- and tripeptides (two or more amino acids bound together), which your body can absorb. Proteins that aren't fully digested (such as some plant-based proteins) in the small intestine pass into the large intestine and are excreted in the feces. Refer to Figure 2-4 for the full path of the digestive system.

Amino acids that have been absorbed into the blood are transported to the liver. These amino acids add to the body's amino acid pool. If there's enough glucose to be used for energy in the body, these amino acids are used as building blocks for various bodily functions, including building and repairing tissues, creating proteins (for example, collagen), forming antibodies, and synthesizing enzymes and hormones.

Fat metabolism

Mechanical chewing breaks food into smaller particles, and an enzyme called lingual lipase is produced by cells on the tongue to break down triglycerides (molecules of fatty acids and glycerol). Gastric lipase in the stomach digests the fats somewhat, but most of the digestion occurs in the small intestine. Bile from the liver and stored and secreted by the gallbladder acts to emulsify the fat (break it into smaller droplets). The pancreas secretes pancreatic lipases into the small intestine to enzymatically digest fats into individual fatty acids. Cholesterol and fat-soluble vitamins do not need to be digested to be absorbed.

Absorbed fats can enter the blood or the lymph and are transported throughout the body as necessary for bodily function. Larger chain fats, cholesterol, and monoglycerides (glycerol with one fatty acid attached) combine with proteins and triglycerides to form fat droplets called chylomicrons. Cholesterol and triglycerides are the major lipids that circulate in blood plasma and form droplets called lipoproteins. These are large structures of phospholipids, proteins (called apolipoproteins), and cholesterol.

The liver and the gut package cholesterol, triglycerides, and fat-soluble vitamins into these lipoprotein structures to deliver contents to other bodily tissues. Chylomicrons get metabolized quickly into smaller particles and go to the liver. In the liver they are broken down to free cholesterol, fatty acids, and protein and combined with glucose and other fatty acids to form other lipoproteins, such as low-density lipoprotein (LDL) that delivers cholesterol to other tissues in your body. High-density lipoprotein (HDL), or the "good" cholesterol, are the lipoprotein globules that transport the cholesterol from other tissues in the body back to the liver, where it is broken down to its parts.

REMEMBER

LDL is the fat globule in the blood that transports cholesterol from the liver to the other organs and tissues in the body. It contains high amounts of cholesterol. HDL is the blood lipid globule that removes the cholesterol from the other tissues and organs back to the liver. The more HDL you have circulating and removing cholesterol from organs and arteries, the better for you!

Understanding Metabolic Disease and Metabolic Syndrome

Metabolic disease is when your biochemical reactions are not working well for some reason, and you have too much or too little of the life-sustaining substances you need. Your body may not be able to efficiently break down your food and use it for energy or for building up substances in your body.

When your metabolism isn't working correctly or efficiently, you may be more at risk for certain health issues, such as weight gain or obesity, high blood pressure, type 2 diabetes, high cholesterol, cardiovascular disease, and stroke.

Metabolic syndrome is when you have three or more of these 5 metabolic factors, as illustrated in Figure 2-5:

>> **Abdominal obesity:** More than 35 inches for women and 40 inches for men

>> **High blood pressure:** A reading of 130/85 mmHg or higher

>> **High fasting blood glucose:** Greater than 100 mg/dl

>> **High triglycerides:** More than 150 mg/dl.

>> **Low HDL cholesterol:** Less than 40 mg/dl for men and less than 50 mg/dl for women

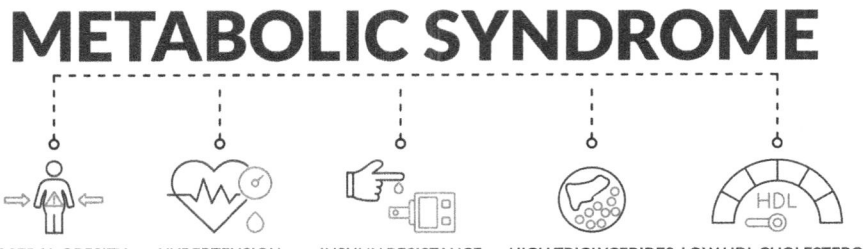

METABOLIC SYNDROME

FIGURE 2-5:
The symptoms of metabolic syndrome.

VISCERAL OBESITY HYPERTENSION INSULIN RESISTANCE HIGH TRIGLYCERIDES LOW HDL CHOLESTEROL

Zero_wing/Adobe Stock Photos

Insulin resistance is often observed in people with metabolic syndrome. Your pancreas makes insulin, which helps sugar get into cells so that it can be metabolized to energy in the form of ATP. If the body doesn't respond well to insulin, sugar accumulates in the blood, and that can lead to the development of type 2 diabetes.

The causes of metabolic syndrome are not completely understood, but obesity and sedentary lifestyle may contribute. Chronic stress and hormone changes may also be contributors.

The risk for metabolic disease goes up with age. BMI greater than 25 puts you at risk. Family history of diabetes or high cholesterol can put you at risk. Also smoking, heavy drinking, stress, and, for women, being post-menopausal. Studies also show that ethnicity and sex can contribute to increase risk.

Metabolic syndrome can also lead to other health problems like polycystic ovarian syndrome (PCOS), fatty liver, sleep problems, some cancers, and gallstones.

The good news is that you can often reverse metabolic diseases with diet and lifestyle change. Dietary changes include eating a well-balanced food plan like the mostly plant-based Mediterranean or DASH diets and getting away from the SAD (Standard American Diet). You may also supplement with vitamins and minerals if you aren't getting enough through your meals.

Chapter **3**

Discovering the Everyday Role of Vitamins and Supplements

I n the United States and many other countries, guidelines for normal daily intake of essential nutrients exist. In the United States, the guidelines come from the Food and Nutrition Board of the National Academy of Medicine (NAM, formerly the Institute of Medicine or IOM). You've probably heard them referred to as the RDA (recommended daily allowances). They're updated every five years in the Dietary Guidelines for Americans.

Once you know what's recommended, you can plan your food and supplement intake. Taking supplements can be important to make sure you meet the recommended daily amounts of nutrients if you're not getting enough from your food. Having the necessary amounts is critical for your metabolism and bodily functions.

In this chapter, you discover more about the science-backed, government recommendations for nutrient intake and how to determine if you're getting enough nutrients from the foods that you eat. This will help you decide which supplements you may need and what to expect from upping your nutrition through supplements.

Exploring the Supplements You Need Every Day

Around the time of World War II came a burst of understanding of what vitamins were and how to synthesize them and put them in pill form. Between then and now, we have slowly become a society obsessed with not just getting the essential necessary vitamins and minerals but also with taking myriad supplements in addition to the ones we actually need.

To be clear, there are 13 essential vitamins and 15 essential minerals. However, hundreds of thousands of supplements are available on the market, contributing to a $77 billion-dollar business globally (2022 estimate).

You probably don't even need every vitamin and mineral every day in exact amounts! What you do want is to eat a variety of foods consistently so you get close to the right amount of this good stuff every day. The best way to get what you need is from a variety of foods.

REMEMBER

This is important because although individual nutrients are important, there are benefits to all the other stuff in foods. For example, it's known that people who eat diets high in vitamin A may have a lower rate of cancer. However, in studies of people using vitamin A supplements as a source, the evidence did not show a benefit in cancer prevention.

Deciding whether to supplement every day

When you go to the doctor for your yearly visit, they usually take blood to measure several routine things, such as levels of iron, vitamins A, B12, and D, folate, calcium, potassium, magnesium, and sodium. Other things may be measured if a deficiency is suspected, but your doctor doesn't routinely check your levels of all vitamins and minerals.

If you're interested in more in-depth information, you can have labs done with companies that measure a more complete panel of micronutrients, antioxidants, and other compounds in white blood cells (WBCs). The reason white blood cells are used may be that they provide a more reliable indication of how well your body is using nutrients at a cellular level rather than getting a snapshot as you would from current blood plasma levels.

Your doctor may make certain recommendations based on your yearly blood test or exam results. For example, your doctor may determine you need to address deficiencies in nutrients by making lifestyle and food choice changes or taking medications. Here are some common nutrition-related issues a blood test can uncover:

>> Low vitamin D

>> Low B12

>> Low iron

>> High BMR (basal metabolic rate)

>> High fasting blood sugar

>> High HbA1C (hemoglobin A1c)

>> High LDL cholesterol

>> Low HDL cholesterol

>> High total cholesterol

>> High triglycerides

You probably do not need a supplement every day if you eat well. Even if you mostly eat the Standard American Diet (SAD), you may be getting vitamins and minerals from foods that are fortified. Food fortification is when vitamins and minerals are added to a food or condiment to improve its nutrition. For example, cereals, grains, salt, and milk are often fortified. Grains often have added B vitamins and iron. Salt is fortified with iodine. Milk is often fortified with vitamins A and D. Eating at least five servings of fruits and vegetables, some whole grains, lean protein, and healthy fats can most likely provide you with most of your essential nutrients.

TIP

Some situations when you may need supplemental nutrients include when you're pregnant, lactating, or want to become pregnant; if you have chronic health conditions, or if you are older. As you age, you may eat less and absorb nutrients from your gut less efficiently. Any of these situations may require taking more of some nutrient to have adequate body amounts.

REMEMBER

The term *supplement* can mean many things. If you're low in iron, you may need an iron supplement. If you're a vegan, you may need vitamin B12 and omega-3 supplements daily. If you're older than 50, you may need a multivitamin every day. Whether you need a supplement every day is a very individual decision based on a personal analysis of your health and needs.

Waiting to see or feel a difference

If you decide to take a supplement to bolster levels of certain vitamins and minerals, whether you see or feel a difference will depend on what you take and your current health or level of deficiency, if any. More than 80 percent of Americans take vitamin supplements, but only 21 percent have vitamin deficiencies!

Generally, if you are deficient in a vitamin and are experiencing some side effects from that deficiency, you may feel the difference. For example, if you're deficient in iron, you may feel tired and possibly be anemic. If levels are sub-optimal, your doctor may prescribe iron supplements that you may need to take for three months to bring your blood iron levels up to a stable level. Along the way you may start to feel less tired, and other symptoms may subside.

WARNING

It is important to note that supplements are not regulated like medicines and that companies don't have to prove that they actually work. For more on the regulation of supplements see Chapter 4.

Knowing how long to take them

We use the term *supplements* because they're meant to *supplement* your diet, not necessarily to prevent or treat disease. What you take is dependent on what your normal diet is and what your current health situation is.

Age, health status, eating habits, and environment may all affect what supplements you need to take, if any. How long you need to take a supplement depends on your nutritional status and the individual nutrient. It also depends on your diet. It's very hard to determine cause and effect in humans! Vitamins and minerals get absorbed differently into the body, and the amount of time needed before effects are noticeable can vary. For example, if you're iron deficient and have anemia, it may take three months of taking an iron supplement to notice the benefits. Similarly, it may take several weeks to months before you see improvements in vitamin D blood levels. On the other hand, you may feel the effects of a B supplement just hours after taking it, but it may take longer to replenish bodily stores of some of these. Also, the effects of any supplements will vary depending on your level of deficiency when you start taking the supplement.

For example, vitamin D, which is fat-soluble, can accumulate in your body fat and be slowly released. The more fat you have, the more the vitamin D you may have in reserve. So, if you are vitamin D deficient and start taking a D supplement, 50,000 IU (international units) one day a week, the absorption rate may be different than if you take 2,000 IU per day. Overall, either works to bring up your blood D levels. Other factors can also affect how long you need to take a supplement. In the case of vitamin D, the following things may have an influence on your absorption rate:

>> Where you live and the seasonal changes in production of vitamin D from sunlight

>> The amount of air pollution where you live can interfere with the UV radiation from the sun

>> Use of sunscreen, which protects your skin from damaging sunrays but also decreases production of vitamin D in your skin

>> The color of your skin

>> The temperature of your skin

>> Your weight

>> Your age

>> The health of your gut because some conditions like celiac, Crohn's, pancreatitis and cystic fibrosis affect vitamin D absorption

>> The health of your liver and kidneys

Another example is vitamin B12. If you become deficient, you may experience symptoms such as

>> Mild fatigue during exercise or daily activities

>> Heart palpitations

>> Skin paleness or hyperpigmentation

>> Glossitis (tongue inflammation)

>> Neurological symptoms such as loss of reflexes, loss of proprioception (knowing where your limbs are without looking at them), forgetfulness

If your B12 level is very low, you may experience a type of anemia called megaloblastic anemia and experience more severe neurological effects.

There are two ways to get B12 supplementation: oral or intramuscular injection. The sooner the B12 levels in your blood increase, the sooner you will feel better. Injections deliver B12 by bypassing the GI tract, so it gets into your system more efficiently. Oral B12 may or may not be absorbed efficiently depending on your health. If you're mildly deficient, you may feel beneficial effects in just a couple days. Otherwise, it may take longer.

TIP

A good way to determine your needs for a particular vitamin or mineral is to keep a food record. There are many apps and websites available to do this. Some can analyze your foods for macronutrients (protein, fat, and carbohydrates) and micronutrients (vitamins and minerals). If you're wondering if your needs are being met, the best thing to do is keep a food record for one week and then evaluate your weekly intake of nutrients. Then compare your intake to the RDA.

For macronutrients, you need to fall within a range. Good protein intake is 10 percent to 30 percent of your caloric intake. Carbohydrate intake should be between 40 percent and 60 percent (understanding that carbohydrates come from dairy, fruits, vegetables, whole grains). Fat intake should be 25 percent to 30 percent of calories and less than 10 percent should be from saturated fats.

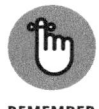

REMEMBER

When you compare your approximate vitamin and mineral intake levels to the RDA, be mindful of your stage of life and sex. If you observe a discrepancy, you can decide whether to take a supplement to bring your intake up to optimal levels.

Understanding U.S. Government Recommendations

The first nutritional recommendations — the Recommended Dietary Allowance (RDA) — were published by the U.S. government in 1941 by the Food and Nutrition Board of the National Research Council. These guidelines aimed to address nutrient deficiencies and health-related consequences including:

>> Vitamin C: Scurvy

>> Vitamin B1: Beri-beri,

>> Vitamin D: Rickets

>> Iodine: Goiter

>> Vitamin B3: Pellagra (symptoms include dermatitis, diarrhea, and dementia)

>> Vitamin A: Xerophthalmia (eye dryness)

>> Vitamins B6, B12, and iron: Nutritional anemias

Since that time, the attention and focus given to nutritional recommendations and research have shifted as more information has come to light:

>> In the 1950s, the major vitamins had been isolated and synthesized.

>> In the 1960s, nutrition policy and agriculture technology focused on calorie content and some vitamins. Food fortification became a way to deliver certain nutrients using food as the vehicle.

>> In the 1980s, government recommendations shifted to address nutrient deficiencies and chronic diseases. The U.S. Senate Select Committee on Nutrition and Human Needs released the "Dietary Goals for the United States," promoting a shift towards a more balanced diet.

>> In the 1990s, the guidelines began to emphasize the importance of food choices, physical activity, and lifestyle factors.

>> By the 2000s, obesity was on the rise and more diet-related and complicated risk pathways studied, including high blood pressure, oxidation, inflammation, glycemic control, muscle health, and fat metabolism.

>> In 2010, the focus shifted to emphasize whole foods, plant-based diets, and less sugar, salt, and saturated fats.

Today, the complexity of nutrition and health includes gut health and interactions with specific foods, brain health, quality of foods, personalized nutrition, epigenetics (how environmental factors and behaviors modify genes without changing your DNA), social determinants, and more focus on chronic diseases. Responsibility for nutrition, food, and supplement recommendations has expanded to several government agencies:

>> **Food and Drug Administration (FDA):** The FDA regulates dietary supplements under the Dietary Supplement Health and Education Act (DSHEA) of 1994. The FDA does not regulate supplements before they are marketed. Its function is to monitor them for safety and labeling compliance once they're on the market.

>> **United States Department of Agriculture (USDA):** The USDA updates the Dietary Guidelines for Americans every five years and oversees MyPlate, a guide for healthy eating used to educate. It oversees the Supplemental Nutrition Assistance Program (SNAP) and WIC (Women, Infants, and Children) supplemental nutrition plan. The USDA also oversees labeling for meat, poultry, and eggs.

>> **Centers for Disease Control (CDC):** This department is focused on public health nutrition and disease prevention and conducts research on nutrition and its impact on health. The CDC has a great searchable database of supplement information.

>> **National Institutes of Health (NIH):** The NIH conducts and funds research on diet and health. It provides evidence-based information via the National Library of Medicine.

>> **Federal Trade Commission (FTC):** The FTC monitors food and supplement advertising to ensure that health claims are truthful.

Explaining the RDA

According to Food and Nutrition Board of the National Academies of Sciences Engineering, and Medicine, the RDA is defined as "the levels of intake of essential nutrients that, on the basis of scientific knowledge, are judged by the Food and Nutrition Board to be adequate to meet the known nutrient needs of practically all healthy persons." People with specific diseases or other health issues may have needs not covered by the RDA.

The RDA was developed based on the scientific information available at the time they were created. Therefore, as time has moved on, and science has uncovered more information, the RDA has been modified and updated. The latest edition is tenth. You can download it from www.dietaryguidelines.gov/sites/default/files/2020-12/Dietary_Guidelines_for_Americans_2020-2025.pdf.

Understanding dietary reference intakes

Dietary reference intake (DRI) is the general term for a set of reference values that include the RDA. They are mostly used to plan and assess nutrient intakes of healthy people. Values differ due to sex and stage of life of a person. DRIs are generally not used by nonscientists or nonprofessionals, but it's good to know what they mean, especially because they're used in the Dietary Guide for Americans to reference how the recommendations for each nutrient were determined:

>> Recommended Dietary Allowance (RDA) is the average intake sufficient for the nutrient requirements of most healthy people. These are the values that you can use to assess your needs and intake. They differ with sex, age, and stage of life. Figures 3-1 and 3-2 give the RDA for macro and micronutrients.

>> Adequate Intake (AI) is the amount of intake generally considered to ensure nutritional adequacy when there is no RDA.

>> Estimated Average Requirement (EAR) is the average level of intake assumed to meet the requirements of half of healthy people. This value is used for planning diets for groups of people, such as school lunch programs or nursing homes.

>> Tolerable Upper Intake Level (UL): This is the largest amount that's unlikely to cause negative health effects. An example of exceeding the UL is that too much iron can cause liver, heart, or pancreas damage.

TIP

You can find more information at the Office of Dietary Supplements at the NIH by visiting https://ods.od.nih.gov/HealthInformation/nutrientrecommen dations.aspx.

Age	11 – 14	15 – 18	19 – 24	25 – 50	+ 51	Pregnant	Lactating (First 6 months)	Lactating (Second 6 months)
Calories (kCal)	2200	2200	2200	2200	1900	+ 300	+ 500	+ 500
Protein (g)	46	44	46	50	50	60	65	62
Vitamin A (ug)	800	800	800	800	800	800	1300	1200
Vitamin D (ug)	10	10	10	5	5	10	10	10
Vitamin E (mg)	8	8	8	8	8	10	12	11
Vitamin K (ug)	45	55	60	60	60	65	65	65
Vitamin C (mg)	50	60	60	60	60	70	95	90
Thiamin (mg)	1.1	1.1	1.1	1.1	1	1.5	1.6	1.6
Riboflavin (mg)	1.3	1.3	1.3	1.3	1.2	1.6	1.8	1.7
Niacin (mg)	15	15 – 18	15	15	13	17	20	20
Vitamin B6 (ug)	1.4	1.5	1.6	1.6	1.6	2.2	2.1	2.1
Folate (ug)	150	180	180	180	180	400	280	260
Vitamin B12 (mg)	2.0	2.0	2.0	2.0	2.0	2.2	2.6	2.6
Calcium (mg)	1200	1200	1200	800	800	1200	1200	1200
Phosphorous (mg)	1200	1200	1200	800	800	1200	1200	1200
Magnesium (mg)	280	300	280	280	280	320	355	340
Iron (mg)	15	15	15	15	10	30	15	15
Zinc (ug)	12	12	12	12	12	15	19	16
Iodine (ug)	150	150	150	150	150	175	200	200
Selenium (ug)	45	50	55	55	55	65	75	75

FIGURE 3-1:
RDA for females.

Age	11 – 14	15 – 18	19 – 24	25 – 50	+ 51
Calories (kCal)	2500	3000	2900	2900	3000
Protein (g)	45	59	58	63	63
Vitamin A (ug)	1000	1000	1000	1000	1000
Vitamin D (ug)	10	10	10	5	5
Vitamin E (mg)	10	10	10	10	10
Vitamin K (ug)	45	65	70	80	80
Vitamin C (mg)	50	60	60	60	60
Thiamin (mg)	1.3	1.5	1.5	1.5	1.2
Riboflavin (mg)	1.5	1.8	1.7	1.7	1.4
Niacin (mg)	17	20	19	19	15
Vitamin B6 (ug)	1.7	2	2	2	2
Folate (ug)	150	200	200	200	200
Vitamin B12 (mg)	2.0	2.0	2.0	2.0	2.0
Calcium (mg)	1200	1200	1200	800	800
Phosphorous (mg)	1200	1200	1200	800	800
Magnesium (mg)	270	400	350	350	350
Iron (mg)	12	12	10	10	10
Zinc (ug)	15	15 – 18	15	15	15
Iodine (ug)	150	150	150	150	150
Selenium (ug)	40	50	70	70	70

FIGURE 3-2: RDA for males.

The Dietary Guidelines for Americans

Since the release of the tenth edition of the RDA, updates have been made in the *Dietary Guidelines for Americans.* In each edition published by the department of Health and Human Services (HHS) and the USDA, new data is considered by a panel of scientists. The newest version will be published in late 2025 as the 2025–2030 edition. The 2020–2025 version is available at www.dietaryguidelines.gov/resources/2020–2025–dietary–guidelines–online–materials.

The recommendations in the *Dietary Guidelines for Americans* are developed and written for policymakers, healthcare providers, and nutrition educators and to provide guidelines used by federal nutrition program operators. It also includes a lot of useful information for laypeople and can be downloaded for free. Its aim is to provide recommendations for what to eat and drink to meet nutrient needs, promote health, and prevent disease. It's a large document with appendixes with many tables on the nutritional goals organized by age and sex. It includes recommendations for macro and micronutrients based on the latest research.

Looking at the Big Picture: General Health and Longevity

The U.S. government offers detailed recommendations based on the latest research, which are available to anyone who wants to read them. However, the majority of Americans don't follow these guidelines!

When you look at the ten top causes of death in the United States, the CDC list based on statistics from 2022 is

>> Heart disease*

>> Cancer*

>> Accidents (unintentional injuries)

>> COVID-19

>> Stroke (cerebrovascular diseases)*

>> Chronic lower respiratory diseases

>> Alzheimer's disease*

>> Diabetes*

>> Nephritis, nephrotic syndrome, and nephrosis

>> Chronic liver disease and cirrhosis*

Items in the list marked with an asterisk (*) are considered chronic diseases or are related to obesity and may be preventable by better lifestyle and diet. An estimated 129 million people in the United States have at least one major chronic disease — heart disease, cancer, diabetes, obesity, or hypertension — as defined by the U.S. Department of Health and Human Services. Sadly, this number is rising.

Getting your essential vitamins and minerals daily and eating a well-balanced diet is very important to help control weight and prevent metabolic issues and chronic diseases. In this section, I cover how supplements may help increase longevity and improve some health issues.

Longevity — living a long life — is a complicated subject! You probably want to lead a long, active, and healthy life. About 25 percent of longevity is influenced by genetics. If your parents, grandparents, and others in your family have lived long lives, then you have a good chance of doing so as well. The other contributing factors to longevity are mostly attributed to how well you take care of yourself.

Studies confirm that nutrition, exercise, and other healthy life choices contribute to longevity. Before I talk about nutrition and supplements specifically, here are some basic lifestyle choices that will improve your chances of living a long life:

>> **Get plenty of sleep.** The recommendation is seven to nine hours per night.

>> **Keep your weight in check.** Obesity is correlated with other chronic diseases.

>> **Don't smoke.** Smoking increases the risk of cancer and is bad for your lung function, heart, skin, and oral health.

>> **Stay social.** Strong and supportive social interactions are correlated to increasing odds of longevity. Frequent interactions with family and friends and reducing loneliness show health benefits and longevity.

>> **Hydrate.** The general rule is to drink about half your body weight in ounces (of water) per day. Results from a study of 11,000 people suggest that staying hydrated improves your heart and lung health and longevity.

>> **Think positive.** Two recent studies support the notion that optimism leads to your health and longevity!

Beyond those general wellness guidelines, nutrition and exercise are key to longevity. A healthy diet provides nutrients that fuel your cells and body. The essential vitamins and nutrients keep your metabolism functioning, support cellular energy production, and promote health and longevity.

One other lifestyle factor that can contribute to longevity is exercise. The U.S. government recommendation for exercise for your health is a minimum of 150 minutes of moderate activity or 75 minutes of vigorous activity a week for adults. This should include both cardio and muscle- and bone-strengthening exercises. Note that this is a minimum and benefits have been shown for between 150 and 300 minutes a week of exercise. Some studies show that even less time has some benefits, and obviously, it makes sense that any exercise is better than none. Being physically active, including walking and doing other types of movement in addition to intentional exercise, is good for many things including weight control or loss.

If you don't get the RDA of vitamins and minerals from your daily food intake, then supplements can help to bring you up to normal levels. Will taking more than the RDA improve longevity? Most likely not. Whether taking supplements will improve health issues is also a complicated question. I get into these topics more in later chapters.

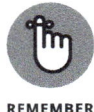

REMEMBER

How much supplements help you depends on your current nutritional status, any health conditions, and your eating habits. If you're low in a nutrient, a supplement may bring your levels up to normal and improve your status and perhaps your health. Several situations may affect your body nutrient levels. Being a vegan or vegetarian may mean you need additional nutrients, such as B12, omega-3, or calcium. If you're ill, you may be eating less and need supplemental nutrition. If you are running a marathon, you may need extra electrolytes. When it comes to supplements, there isn't a one-size-fits-all solution.

Getting What You Need from Foods

A theme I repeat throughout this book is that it's best to get nutrients from whole foods. The reason is that foods are complex and have many components to them in addition to the vitamins or minerals. For example, carrots are a great source of beta-carotene but also have fiber, water, potassium, and other antioxidants. In other words, a carrot has much more to offer than a vitamin A supplement! Nutrition studies have been done to look at overall dietary patterns as well as specific nutrients. Many large clinical studies such as the Framingham study, the Nurses' Health Study, NHANES, or PREDICT collect data on the diets of tens of thousands of people and how they correlate to disease over many years. Some results of these studies support positive outcomes of healthier foods choices. Studies looking at a specific nutrient or vitamin is much harder to do and often have inconclusive results.

Experts agree that the Mediterranean diet and the DASH (Dietary Approach to Stop Hypertension) diet are the best ways to eat for weight loss or weight control; reduce hypertension, risk of cardiovascular disease, and inflammation; and possibly lower risk for osteoporosis, cancer, heart disease, stroke, and diabetes. In addition, the DGA lists the HUSS (Healthy U.S.-style), Mediterranean, and vegetarian dietary patterns as healthy ways to eat.

All of these diets are similar in that they are mostly plant based and stress whole foods, fruits, vegetables, whole grains, low-fat dairy, and good fats (omega-3s). (See Figure 3-3.) The Mediterranean diet encompasses lifestyle factors as well as food, and stressing less beef and more fish, olive oil, and nuts. The vegetarian diet excludes meat and fish and sometimes eggs and dairy. For most people, any of these ways of eating is an improvement on the Standard American Diet (SAD diet).

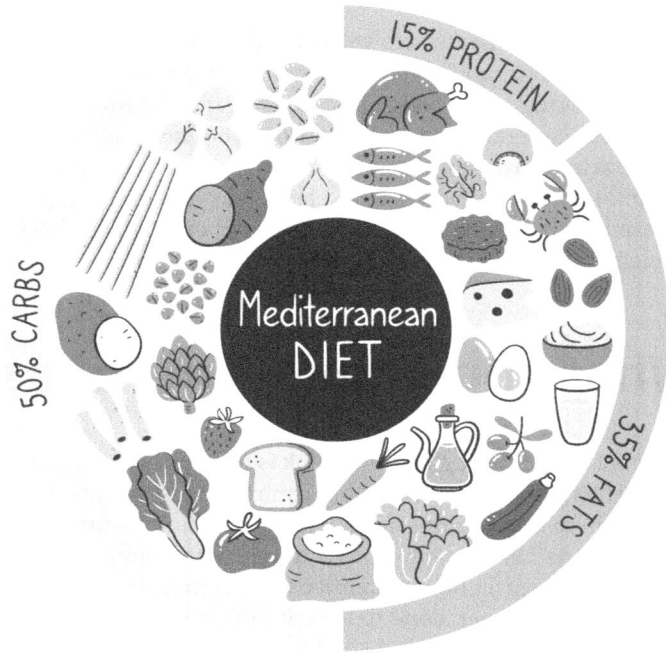

FIGURE 3-3:
General guidelines for what to eat and how to size portions for the Mediterranean diet.

Not only does what you eat make a difference, but how you prepare it can sometimes affect its nutritional value. Some foods are healthier raw, whereas others aren't. Mostly, the best preparation for a food depends on the specific food and your individual health and goals. The raw food trend comes and goes, but because there are benefits to both cooked and raw foods, it's doubtful that a completely raw diet is beneficial. For the most part, eating raw or cooked foods is a personal choice.

Raw foods may retain some vitamins that are sensitive to heat and lose their potency when cooked, including vitamins C, A, and the Bs. The raw form of some foods has more fiber than their cooked version because the heat breaks the fiber down. (In some cases, this breakdown is a benefit that makes some cooked foods easier to digest.)

On the other hand, cooked foods may increase the bioavailability of some nutrients, particularly some polyphenols. For example, the polyphenol lycopene in tomatoes is more available when cooked than in raw tomatoes. Another example is spinach, in which cooking increases its iron bioavailability. Cooking spinach also reduces the oxalic acid content of the spinach (oxalic acid is a compound that contributes to a type of kidney stone).

COMPARING THE SAD AND MEDITERRANEAN DIETS

The SAD generally includes processed foods, refined grains, fast foods, and sugary snacks and beverages. The "refined grains" refers to foods made with white flour and white rice. This diet may include red meats, deli meats, processed meats, and fried meats and chicken. It tends to be high in the unhealthy saturated and trans fats. The SAD usually doesn't include enough fruits and vegetables and can be very high in sodium. Because so many of the foods are highly processed, the SAD often is low in vitamins and essential minerals and fiber. Clinical studies show a direct correlation between the SAD and chronic diseases such as heart disease, stroke, diabetes, obesity, and some cancers. This diet high in fats, sugar, and salt can also lead to inflammation, which contributes to disease. Lastly, a low-fiber diet such as this one is bad for gut health and can lead to constipation. It's also low in vitamins C and E, which are important antioxidants and help prevent inflammation.

The Mediterranean diet is very different than the SAD, and studies show that it's good for both health and weight control. It emphasizes whole foods, including fruits, vegetables, whole grains, legumes, nuts, olive oil, and lean protein (chicken, fish, and eggs). It limits red meat and whole-fat dairy, such as butter and cheese. It is mostly plant based and includes healthy mono- and polyunsaturated fats — from fish, nuts, seeds, and olive oil — which is linked to lower risk of cardiovascular disease. It contains a lot of fiber, which is good for feeding your microbiota and reducing risk of chronic disease. Fiber can also lower your cholesterol by binding to the cholesterol and excreting it from the body. The Mediterranean diet also encourages the use of good fresh herbs, spices, and garlic, which all have health benefits. It's low in sugar and keeps your blood sugar more stable so you experience fewer sugar spikes and place less demand on your pancreas for insulin. The foods in the Mediterranean diet are high in antioxidants, especially C and E, that work to reduce cell damage and lower risk of inflammation–related diseases.

Studies have shown that the Mediterranean diet is correlated to a longer and healthier life, with less chronic disease than in people who eat the SAD. On a broader scale, it's also less damaging environmentally than the SAD because it uses less resources and processing and produces less waste. Unfortunately, in the United States, following the SAD can be less expensive than eating the Mediterranean diet, especially if you go to restaurants or get a lot of takeout. However, it is very possible to eat well on a budget by buying foods in bulk, using frozen fruits and vegetables, and cooking at home.

Furthermore, cooking foods kills bacteria, parasites, and pathogens found in some foods like meat, fish, and eggs. Some foods, such as beans and grains, cannot be eaten unless they're cooked, and cooking enhances the nutrients, palatability, and water content. Some people may find certain cruciferous vegetables, such as broccoli, Brussels sprouts, kale, and cauliflower, to be easier to digest when cooked.

Fermented foods may have health benefits by increasing the bioavailability of some micronutrients such as calcium, iron, and magnesium. The International Scientific Association for Probiotics and Prebiotics (ISAPP) defines fermented foods and beverages as "foods made through desired microbial growth and enzymatic conversions of food components." Some fermented foods include yogurt, kefir, kombucha, and sometimes sauerkraut (depending how it's made). Some, but not all, fermented foods may also have probiotics, which are good for gut health.

REMEMBER

When it comes to choosing whether to eat your foods raw or cooked, keep it balanced! Mixing it up is the best way to go for the best taste, nutrition, gut health, and safety.

Chapter **4**

Understanding the Vitamin and Supplement Marketplace

When you're determining what supplements you would like to take, I recommend you check into whether there is scientific evidence backing its use. In this chapter, I hope to give you an understanding behind animal and clinical studies to help you do online research. You will learn about the roles of these studies, how they are designed, their strengths and limitations, and how they help to aide in diet and supplement recommendations.

Examining Nutritional Science Basics

Nutritional science is the field of science in which scientists work to understand the complexities of how foods we eat impact our health. The field has been evolving from when essential nutrients were first discovered in the 1800s. In the first half of the 1900s, scientists started to understand many of them and how they are metabolized and function. As scientists learned more, they discovered interactions between nutrients and the complexities of how specific dietary components influence metabolic health, chronic diseases, mental health, and longevity. A major focus today is on dietary patterns and metabolism — the chemical processes that occur within a living organism to maintain life.

The study of nutrition explores the macronutrients — carbohydrates, fats, and proteins— that fuel your body and the micronutrients that support cell and organ function. Although much is already known, the quest for understanding continues to make advances in the field. There are still many questions about how individual nutrients interact with each other, affect metabolic health, longevity, and disease.

Nutrition studies are difficult to do because there are so many variables to control. To address the many questions, scientists use a variety of research methods. Two of the most common are animal studies and human clinical trials. Animal studies are useful because researchers can conduct a study in a very controlled environment. For example, specific diets can be fed in exact amounts to a group of animals. Researchers can also control other environmental factors so that all the subjects experience the same surroundings, and other variables can be manipulated as necessary. Human clinical studies provide real-world insights into how food or specific nutrients may impact health outcomes in subjects. These studies are published in peer-reviewed scientific journals and build the evidence-based information used to shape clinical practice and everyday life.

Animal studies

Animal studies allow researchers to investigate biochemical and physical effects of vitamins and other supplements before testing on humans. It also is helpful because they can control the environment and diet of animals in a way that isn't possible in human studies. Researchers can explore mechanisms of action, interactions between nutrients, and long-term effects.

There are different types of studies:

>> **Dose-response studies:** The aim is to determine the best dose of a substance needed for the optimal effect being studied. The animals are divided into groups and given different doses, and then the outcome is measured. One example of this was a study done with rats to determine the effect of different doses of vitamin D on bone health, calcium absorption, and immune function.

>> **Longitudinal studies:** These studies follow animals for a period of time to look at the long-term effects of a supplement. This is especially useful for investigating disease prevention, aging, and toxicity. An example of this might

be a study looking at the long-term effect on omega-3 fatty acids in mice to understand the effects on heart disease or aging biomarkers.

>> **Toxicology studies:** To help identify whether there are any bad effects of high doses of supplements, researchers can do a toxicology study. In animals, they can give high doses and check for organ damage, oxidative stress, or other long-term issues. An example of this is a study looking at high levels of vitamin D on liver function in rats.

>> **Mechanistic studies:** These studies specifically look at the biological and biochemical actions of supplements and how they exert their effect. For example, do they affect enzyme activity or gene expression or binding to receptors. A study may examine how zinc affects the immune system by looking specifically at certain cell types, like T-cells.

>> **Behavioral studies:** Some studies investigate the effects of supplements on behavior or cognitive function. This can be done using animal models — such as running a rodent through a maze to assess memory and learning. Overall neurological health, including mood and neurodegenerative diseases, can also be investigated using animal models.

Human studies

Human clinical studies are important for determining any health benefits or safety issues of diets or supplements. They are designed to test hypotheses about how nutrients, diets, or supplements impact human health and wellness.

The types of clinical studies include the following:

>> **Randomized controlled trials (RCTs):** This type of study is considered the gold standard of clinical research studies. In these studies, subjects are randomly assigned to a study group (receiving the treatment) or the control group (placebo group). The investigators and subjects are "blinded" to which treatment they are given. Once the study is completed, the data are analyzed, and test group versus control group results are compared and statistically evaluated.

>> **Intervention trials:** This type of RCT involves the subjects' diet being changed to test the impact of a specific intervention. An example could be studying the effect of a Mediterranean diet on cardiovascular disease in overweight people.

>> **Randomized crossover trials:** When each participant in a study receives both arms of the study — both the intervention and the control treatment — at separate times during the study, it's a randomized crossover trial. Essentially,

each subject is their own control. This method reduces variability and improves the statistical power of the study. It can be part of an RCT.

>> **Blinded studies:** In blinded studies, the treatment allocation is concealed from the study participants or researchers (single blind) or both (double blind). This is a key component of RCTs.

>> **Cohort studies:** Sometimes, researchers follow a group of people — a cohort — over a period of time to observe how their nutrient intake affects specific health outcomes. Researchers track the subject's intake or supplement use and observe any changes. A famous cohort study is The Framingham Study that started in 1948 (and is still going on) to investigate the risk factors for cardiovascular disease.

>> **Cross-sectional studies:** These studies determine the relationship between dietary patterns, nutritional status, and health outcomes in a specific population at a single point in time. These observational studies can help determine correlations between a number of variables such as nutrient intake, exercise, and health conditions.

>> **Dose-response studies:** Some studies investigate how different doses of a supplement affect health outcomes. For example, there have been studies looking at different doses of vitamin D on blood calcium levels and bone density in healthy women.

>> **Placebo-controlled trial:** When the intervention group is given the treatment supplement and a control group receives a placebo that looks identical to the treatment supplement, the study is called a placebo-controlled trial. Researchers pay attention to the type of placebo to be sure that any observed effect is due to the intervention and not to other variables.

>> **Meta-analysis and systematic reviews:** When researchers aggregate data from multiple studies to assess the evidence about a supplement or intervention, it's this form of study. For example, a meta-analysis could evaluate the data from all studies on the use of CoQ10 supplements on muscle issues in people taking statins. This type of review usually takes into consideration what type of study was conducted and how significant the data is and presents a detailed discussion and conclusions.

>> **Longitudinal studies:** These nutrition studies follow individuals to observe long-term effects of specific supplements or nutrients on health outcomes, such as chronic diseases, aging, risk of cancer, or wellness. These studies involve collecting detailed diet and lifestyle data over a long period of time — sometimes decades. A good example of this is the Nurses' Health Study, which started in 1978, has a total of 280,000 subjects, and on its third generation of volunteer subjects.

Epidemiological studies

Epidemiological studies are done to help understand the patterns, causes, and effects of conditions in populations. These are widely used in the nutrition and public health fields. Nutrition-related epidemiologic studies may provide evidence for individual health recommendations, clinical guidelines, and public health policies.

Specifically, epidemiological studies can identify connections between dietary habits and risk of developing certain chronic diseases like diabetes, heart disease, and some cancers because the studies help identify patterns. For example, studies have shown that increasing fruit and vegetable consumption helps to reduce the risk of cardiovascular disease.

Results from epidemiological studies have helped to design nutrition guidelines for the U.S. government and medical organizations such as the American Pediatric Association. These types of studies are helpful in addressing public policy issues, such as health disparities and how age, sex, geographic location, or socioeconomics affects health outcomes. They are also useful in understanding cultural trends.

Here are some examples of epidemiological studies and use of their outcomes:

>> Providing evidence-based recommendations for reducing sugar intake to reduce risk of obesity and type 2 diabetes

>> Establishing a connection between diet, physical activity, and long-term health outcomes, as in the Nurses' Health Study

>> Aiding health organizations such as the World Health Organization (WHO) or governments on food fortification intervention programs, such as fortifying salt with iodine and sometimes iron (in other countries) to address deficiencies. Another example is the fortification of breakfast cereals with iron and B vitamins in the United States.

>> Helping to determine what areas of studies might be worth further investigation, such as what people living in Blue Zone areas do to experience greater than normal longevity

>> Understanding dietary patterns globally and the impact of health — for example, how the Mediterranean diet contributes to better cardiovascular health

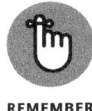

REMEMBER

It's important to note that epidemiological studies identify correlation but not necessarily causation. This means that they cannot prove that the intervention causes the outcome. An example is that a study may show that people who eat a diet high in fruits and vegetables helps reduce cancer rates. However, you cannot conclude or prove that more fruits and vegetables or any of the nutrients in them caused the decrease in cancer without further studies. In addition, lifestyle interventions, such as smoking or exercise, cannot always be controlled in these studies or analyses. And if the study is a survey of subjects, they may inadvertently introduce inaccuracies when they self-report, which may introduce bias into the study.

There are different types of epidemiological studies in nutrition:

REMEMBER

- >> **Descriptive epidemiology:** This type of study examines diseases and health outcomes within a population for patterns based on things like location, time, age, sex, ethnicity, and lifestyle. This could include a study looking into the prevalence of obesity in a certain region of the world and correlation with diet and lifestyle.

  Correlation describes a relationship between something like diet and obesity but not necessarily cause and effect.

- >> **Analytical epidemiology:** This study tries to determine cause-and-effect relationships between diet or nutrients and health outcomes. An example might be a cohort study that tracks the relationship between saturated fat intake and markers of cardiovascular disease over a time period.

- >> **Cross-sectional studies:** These studies examine the relationship between a dietary pattern or nutrient intake and a health outcome at a single time-point. This could also be a study surveying dietary habits and correlating with a specific factor — such as cholesterol levels — at a specific time-point.

- >> **Cohort study:** In epidemiology, these studies are similar to studies done in a clinical trial. They follow a group of people over time to see how supplements or diet or some specific intervention affects health outcomes. This can be a prospective study where people are followed going forward in time. If they're retrospective, the investigators look back in time at existing data to determine cause and effects of interventions.

- >> **Case-controlled studies:** These studies compare individuals with specific diseases to those without the disease to see if an intervention helps. These studies usually compare people with a specific disease, such as a cancer, to someone without the disease to see if a nutrient or diet intervention is helpful.

- >> **Randomized-controlled trials:** RCTs are considered the gold standard of epidemiological studies because they provide the highest quality causal information for an exposure to a diet or nutrient and a health outcome. RCTs are intervention studies in which researchers control the exposure and randomize the subjects into groups so as to control confounding factors. An example might be to test whether increasing fiber intake reduces the incidence of colon cancer in a specific population.

Seeking Out Evidence-Based Information

When you're perusing the internet for information, it's challenging to know which vitamins and supplements have scientific evidence to recommend their usage or dose. If you like to dig deep and find information, then searching for scientific studies is the best thing to do. If that kind of digging isn't your cup of tea, there are other ways to navigate through all the information and access trustworthy, evidence-based information.

TIP

Consulting with a doctor, nutritionist, or dietitian is a reliable way to get personalized, evidence-based advice for vitamin and supplement use. These people are trained to evaluate your needs through blood tests, lifestyle, and other factors affecting your needs for interventions. It's always best to discuss need and to list your medications and supplements when speaking to your healthcare providers so they can also determine if there may be any negative interactions between them.

If you're doing your own research, be sure to check scientific sources. Here's a list of some reliable sources:

>> **PubMed:** This is a free database of scientific research articles.

>> **Cochrane Library:** This nonprofit organization produces systematic reviews to help people make informed health decisions.

>> **National Institutes of Health (NIH) Office of Dietary Supplements (ODS):** This site provides comprehensive information on most vitamins, minerals, and supplements. There are fact sheets for both consumers and professionals, so you can determine what level of information you want. The ODS website includes benefits, recommended doses, safety issues, mechanism of action, and scientific evidence for each of the supplement fact sheets.

>> **ConsumerLab:** This independent testing organization evaluates supplements and offers detailed reports and ratings for many of them. It also offers a lot of scientific information on supplements. It is a paid service (about $5 per month).

>> **The American Journal of Clinical Nutrition:** This well-respected journal features studies on diet, nutrition, and supplementation.

>> **The European Food Safety Authority:** This organization evaluates the safety and efficacy of supplements and health claims in the European Union.

>> **The Linus Pauling Institute:** The research programs at this institute provide data on vitamins, minerals, and other dietary compounds.

- >> **Examine.com:** This independent, research-driven website analyzes scientific studies on supplements, nutrition, and health. They follow a rigorous science-based approach.

- >> **Google Scholar:** This component of the Google search engine provides academic articles related to your search.

- >> **ClinicalTrials.gov:** This government website enables you to view both completed and ongoing clinical studies about the safety and effectiveness of supplements.

Some professional organizations that have information on their website include the following:

- >> American Society for Nutrition (ASN)

- >> American Nutrition Association

- >> The Academy of Nutrition and Dietetics

WARNING

Be skeptical of claims on supplement labels. Always look for third-party certification by NSF International (NSF), ConsumerLab (CL), and United States Pharmacopeia (USP). Their mark should be visible on the label. (Read more in Chapter 13.) Be sure to check the supplement facts label and the other ingredients list to be sure the supplement has what you are specifically looking for. Especially watch out for marketing claims. For example, "all natural" does not necessarily mean that the ingredients are safe and effective. Also remember there are no "miracle cures" or quick fixes.

TIP

Read more about the laws regarding the claims that manufacturers can put on their labels later in the chapter in the "Regulating Supplements (Enter the FDA)" section.

Getting a Glimpse into Manufacturing

In this section, I share specifics about how supplements are made. The details vary from type to type, but this general overview can help you make informed choices.

Ingredients

The ingredients in vitamins and supplements can be natural and from a variety of sources, or they can be synthetic.

Natural ingredients include the following:

» **Herbs and botanicals that are directly derived from plants:** Often these have been used throughout history for their medicinal properties. Examples of these are echinacea, turmeric, and ginger.

» **Whole food sources, or food-based supplements are made from concentrated fruits, vegetables and other plants:** A couple of examples are wheatgrass or spirulina. The idea is that these nutrient forms are closer to what is found in nature and are therefore more bioavailable (being absorbed from the gut and then entering the bloodstream). In addition, if these are concentrated from real foods, they will have all the other healthy stuff found in foods in addition to the specific vitamin or nutrient. These other compounds found in food-based supplements may act together to benefit you.

» **Marine ingredients:** One example is omega-3 fatty acid supplements, which come from fish or algae.

» **Animal-derived ingredients:** Some supplements come from shellfish or shark cartilage (glucosamine).

Synthetic ingredients may include vitamins, minerals, enzymes, or amino acids supplements that are synthesized by a chemical process. They may also be derived from a natural source and then chemically processed. Examples include synthesized vitamin C, calcium carbonate (derived from limestone and altered), or synthesized amino acids used for protein supplements.

Synthetic ingredients may be the same as what you find in the natural form. In this case, they're called *bioidentical*. However, some may be other forms or derivatives, which may or may not be as effective as the natural form. For example, folic acid is often used in supplements and is actually considered more bioavailable than the natural form, folate.

Synthetic ingredients in some supplements may have the advantage of being more concentrated than in natural products, which may mean that you can get a higher dose. This is important if you have a therapeutic need for a product. They're also often less expensive. Sometimes choosing a supplement may come down to cost, so I recommend you do a cost/benefit analysis for yourself. Is it better for you to spend more money for a natural product with fewer fillers and other ingredients or go for a store brand that tends to be lower cost but may be synthetic while still being a perfectly acceptable (and often third-party certified) product. This is a personal decision with no right or wrong answer.

TIP

Determining which ingredients are good may require you exert some effort. Always check to see that there is scientific evidence that supports the use of the supplement. Look for third-party certification to assure the quality, safety, and dose of the supplement. Read the ingredients labels so you can try to avoid fillers artificial colors, flavorings, sugar, and any other ingredients that may be unnecessary or perhaps even allergens.

Some supplements are more bioavailable or absorbed well by the body than others. For example, magnesium citrate is more bioavailable than magnesium oxide. Or when you take a CoQ10 supplement, only 5 percent to 10 percent may be absorbed. So, it's important to choose the best form for your needs.

TIP

If you're concerned about the source of your food and supplements and want to know if the products you use are sustainably and ethically sourced, make sure to check the label for this information. Some labels indicate what the company's practices are in this regard.

Assessing the quality

Many things determine the quality of the supplements that you choose to take. Third-party certification helps you to verify quality, safety, and purity.

The three main third-party certifications for vitamin and supplement quality, safety, and purity are

>> **NSF International (NSF):** NSF tests supplements for potency, purity, and contaminants. It determines that the supplement includes what it claims on its label that it contains. It ensures that there are no harmful substances like heavy metals, pesticides, and microbes.

>> **USP (United States Pharmacopeia):** USP certifies that the product meets standards for identity, strength, purity, and consistency and checks for contaminants.

>> **ConsumerLab:** This organization also conducts independent tests on supplements for safety, quality, and potency and verifies that the product contains what the label claims it does. It also checks for contaminants. ConsumerLab has a website with reviews that you can access.

Other certifying organizations include

>> **Informed Sport:** This is a global testing and third-party certification company specifically for sports and nutritional supplements.

>> **Informed Choice:** This program is a global standard in sports nutrition that has a retail monitoring and <u>quality assurance program</u> to help reduce the risk of impurities and banned substances.

>> **BSCG:** This is a third-party tester and certifier of dietary supplements and natural ingredients for safety, quality, GMP manufacturing. It also verifies that supplements are free of contaminants, including substances banned from sports.

Regulating Supplements (Enter the FDA)

In the United States, dietary supplements and vitamins are regulated primarily by the FDA. They're regulated differently than pharmaceutical drugs and sometimes differently than other countries in the world regulate supplements. The FDA guidelines involve laws concerning manufacturing, sales, and marketing.

The law

The Dietary Supplement Health and Education Act (DHSEA) of 1994 is a law that defines dietary supplements "as products intended to supplement the diet, containing one or more dietary ingredients (vitamins, minerals, herbs, amino acids, etc.)." This law does not require supplement manufacturers to have FDA approval or inspection before supplements are marketed. It's the manufacturers' responsibility to ensure the safety and proper labeling of their products. They cannot make misleading or fraudulent claims or therapeutic claims. They also must follow Good Manufacturing Practices (GMP). A manufacturer can get in trouble with the FDA for any noncompliance after a product is on the market, but only after consumers have complained or the product has been proven unsafe.

Supplements can only have certain types of claims on their label. They cannot make therapeutic claims. The FDA Modernization Act of 1997 (FDAMA) Health and Nutrient Content Claims page lists the different types of health claims for foods and supplements with details about how companies can file for them and what is acceptable. The following list is a shortened version of this information; you can check out the FDA website if you'd like more information on how companies file for these and to get a more comprehensive list of the acceptable claims.

The three types of claims that you may see on a food or dietary label are:

>> **Health claims that meet significant scientific agreement (SSA):** These must be supported by good scientific evidence. Disease or health claims must show a link between a substance or a food and a disease or health-related

condition. Here are some you may see on a food or supplement label that are acceptable:

- Calcium, vitamin D, and decreased risk osteoporosis

- Dietary saturated fat and cholesterol and risk of coronary heart disease

- Folic acid and decreased risk of neural tube defects

- Fruits and vegetables and decrease risk of cancer

- Fruits, vegetables, and grain products that contain fiber, particularly soluble fiber, and decreased risk of coronary heart disease

- Sodium and hypertension

- Soy protein and decreased risk of coronary heart disease

>> **Nutrient content claims:** These describe the amount of a nutrient in a food or dietary supplement according to the Nutrition Labeling and Education Act of 1990 (NLEA). This permits the use of words like "free," "low," or "high" when referring to a nutrient in foods or a supplement. An example is a product may be "high in calcium" or "low in saturated fats."

>> **Structure/function claims for dietary supplements and conventional foods:** Structure and function claims pertain to general well-being and nutrient-deficiency disease. Here are some examples:

- Vitamin C supports immune function.

- Calcium builds strong bones.

- Antioxidants maintain cell integrity.

- Fiber maintains bowel regularity.

Additional requirements or regulations include the following:

>> Products must be labeled with a supplement facts panel that contains ingredients, serving size, and active ingredients. (You can find more details on this in Chapter 13).

>> Products must be manufactured with GMP, which ensures the quality of the supplement. This applies to the materials and equipment used.

>> Consumers can report any adverse reaction to the FDA, which can then investigate a potentially unsafe product. The MedWatch can also be used to make a complaint.

>> The Federal Trade Commission (FTC) regulates the marketing and advertising of supplements to be sure that claims aren't deceptive. Claims like "cures," "prevents," or "treats" are not allowed unless the product has gone through the rigorous approval process for a drug.

Taking responsibility for safety

Ultimately, you're responsible for taking your safety into account when incorporating vitamins and other supplements into your routine. Laws are there to protect you, but they're more of a safety net than a shield. Until someone reports an issue or makes a complaint, the manufacturers are responsible for the safety and efficacy of their product and can put it on the market without FDA approval. Know why you think you need a particular supplement and do your own research. When I ask my clients about this, they often say that someone told them to take something, that they read about it somewhere, that they've already been doing it for a long time, or that their doctor told them to take a supplement. In other words, they don't truly know why they're taking it.

Obviously, if your doctor tells you to take something for your health, it is probably a good idea. But as a consumer and advocate for your own health, you have a part in the solution.

WARNING

Always research whether a supplement has interactions with other supplements you're taking. Some combinations are helpful, like taking vitamin C to enhance iron absorption. Others may interfere with each other, like calcium interferes with iron absorption.

WARNING

Also beware of any supplement interactions with medications. Let your doctor know everything that you are taking to be sure to avoid any bad interactions. For example, taking licorice or ginseng with blood pressure medications can lead to dangerously high or low blood pressure, respectively.

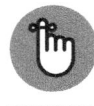

REMEMBER

Always speak to your doctor, nutritionist, or pharmacist about supplements that you are taking. Stick to your recommended dosages or RDA and avoid megadoses — especially of A, D, E, K, and iron. More is not always better!

Understanding the Multibillion Dollar Supplement Industry

The supplement industry is expected to grow to over $200 billion by 2029. This expected growth is largely driven by the aging population, having more understanding of the benefits of dietary supplements, and increasing health consciousness. People want to age well, stay or become fit, enhance mood, improve immunity, and have overall holistic wellness. Personalized nutrition is also driving the supplement industry.

The dietary supplement market is diverse in the types of products it includes and how and where you can purchase them. The top largest categories of supplement sales globally are the following:

>> **Vitamins:** These account for about 20 percent to 25 percent of sales. Vitamins D, C, and E, the B vitamins, and multivitamins are the key products. This is especially true for vitamins D and C in the post-COVID world. Many people take multivitamins for overall health and metabolism.

>> **Minerals:** Minerals are about 15 percent of the market share, with calcium, magnesium, iron, zinc, potassium, and selenium being key products. The drivers are general concern for health, muscle function, and immune support.

>> **Herbal and botanicals:** These represent 12 percent to 15 percent of the market, with turmeric, ashwagandha, ginseng, echinacea, garlic, and ginkgo biloba being some of the common products. Many people like to use natural remedies when possible.

>> **Protein supplements:** These are about 10 percent to 12 percent of the global market (although the number is probably higher in the United States). These include whey protein, collagen, casein, and plant-based protein from pea and hemp. If you're an athlete, vegetarian or vegan, or perhaps older, you may be supplementing your protein intake with these products.

>> **Omega-3 fatty acids:** These are about 7 percent to 9 percent of the market. Fish oil and algal oil are two examples. They have heart and brain benefits and reduce inflammation. If you eat fish two or three times a week and use olive oil, you're probably getting enough omega-3s from foods and may not need supplements.

>> **Probiotics and digestive health supplements:** This category includes probiotics, prebiotics and digestive enzymes. It makes up 6 percent to 8 percent of the market. These have increased in popularity because of the understanding of how gut health affects mental health, skin health, immunity and overall health and well-being.

>> **Weight-loss supplements:** These contribute 6 percent to 7 percent of the market and include green tea extract, conjugated linoleic acid, glucomannan (Konjac root), garcinia cambogia, berberine, and ketones. Because of the increase in people with obesity in the world, these products are sought after as a quick fix. Weight loss is usually more complicated and requires food and lifestyle changes.

>> **Joint and bone health:** About 5 percent to 6 percent of the market is this category, which includes glucosamine, chondroitin sulfate, collagen, calcium, and vitamin D. This segment is growing because of an aging population and concern with bone and muscle health and strength.

>> **Sports and fitness supplements:** These supplements are 4 percent to 6 percent of the market and include creatine, branched-chain amino acids, and electrolytes. There also seems to be a surging popularity in electrolyte powders and pre-/post-workout products.

>> **Cognitive and mental health supplements:** A growing segment of the market is for cognitive and mental health supplements, which is 3 percent to 5 percent of the market. These include nootropics, ginseng, St. John's wort, theanine, and rhodiola. These may reduce stress and enhance focus and memory.

Getting to the message through the hype

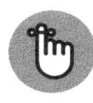

REMEMBER

You're responsible for weeding through all the hype about supplements to get to the truth to make the right choices for you. Advice from your doctor, nutritionist, pharmacist, or other healthcare professional is always helpful in determining your needs. Be sure to understand why you may need a certain vitamin or mineral so that you can understand the effect, the dose, duration, and any interactions with other supplements or medications you take.

WARNING

Be wary of media hype, social media advertisements, celebrity and influencers endorsements, before and after pictures, and other things that try to convince you that a certain product will address your concerns. Advertisements that offer quick fixes or immediate results — such as weight-loss supplements or wrinkle creams — are especially suspicious.

Distinguishing science and marketing

Distinguishing between science-based claims and marketing hype is one way to get to the truth. It isn't easy and requires a critical eye and knowing what to look for amid advertisements, celebrity endorsements, and misleading claims or labels. Supplements must be marketed truthfully, so be aware and do your research. As defined by the law and regulations covered in this chapter, a company cannot make claims unless those claims are supported by science. Even with those precautions in place, online marketers and influencers can be misleading about their products.

TIP

Some things that you can do is to find evidence-based sources that might include clinical trials, peer-reviewed scientific studies, and systematic reviews or meta-analyses. Other good sources are reliable websites of health organizations such the NIH, WHO, or the American Heart Association. It isn't easy to read scientific articles and understand results, but looking at the abstract (or summary) can be helpful. The kinds of things to look for include the number of people in a study, the results, and conclusions from the study. Also pay attention to any limitations of a study because sometimes this may apply to your situation. Information pours out of research labs and companies, so you may want to try to stay abreast of new information on a regular basis.

Look for products that say things like "may support," that provide the proper dose, or that suggest consulting your physician. An honest company may say something like "the scientific evidence is mixed" or "a preliminary study showed promising results."

Marketing information may quote studies, but they may not include the scientific references. Companies may also exaggerate claims or use only studies that support their product, disregarding other nonsupportive (but valid) evidence. Always read websites and labels carefully to avoid erroneous claims that sound too good to be true. Check references by going to the NIH ODS website, PubMed, or other scientific sources. Beware of over-the-top claims like "this supplement cures baldness" or "lose 10 pounds in 10 days."

Always look at the ingredient list. You may want products that have fewer fillers, are food-based vitamins, or have no artificial ingredients. If you're a vegan or vegetarian, you can look for a certification on the product label. Beware of products that promote a "proprietary blend" because it isn't broken into broken down to its specific components. That isn't to say that there aren't good, reliable brands that contain their own proprietary mixes, but it's worth being cautious. Just do your best to discern between the better and reliable brands and the less reliable sources.

Look at the dose recommendations on the label or marketing material. Remember that more is not always better. Megadoses aren't necessarily more effective and may not be safe. Marketing words like *superfoods* may not have any real significance, so read carefully.

The best test for safety, purity, and efficacy of a product is to look on the packaging for the third-party certifications mentioned earlier in this chapter in the "Assessing the quality" section. Don't accept other claims of purity or safety. If you don't see the logo on the bottle, go to the manufacturer's website and check for information to indicate testing or independent lab results.

Be wary of false promises, quick results, luxury brands, slick marketing, and before and after pictures. These are often just marketing tricks. Also, "limited time offer" or "2 for 1 offers" may just be sales tricks to get you to buy.

Making a checklist for identifying the right supplements

Choosing the right supplements for you involves several factors to ensure you're making informed, safe, and effective decisions. Follow this checklist to help guide you through the process.

» Identify your health goals.

- ☐ Overall wellness
- ☐ Healthy aging
- ☐ Preparing for pregnancy
- ☐ Preventing chronic disease
- ☐ Increasing energy
- ☐ Enhancing immunity
- ☐ Improving athletic ability
- ☐ Addressing specific problems
  - ☐ Weight control or weight loss
  - ☐ Digestive issues
  - ☐ Type 2 diabetes
  - ☐ Elevated lipids and cardiovascular disease
  - ☐ Other metabolic or hormonal disorders

» Evaluate your current diet.

- ☐ Consider your diet, especially if you're vegan, vegetarian, or limited in your dietary intake.
- ☐ Eat at least five servings of fruits and vegetables each day as well as whole grains.
- ☐ Speak to a nutritionist to determine any reason you might need a supplement.
- ☐ Use an app (MyFitnessPal, Lose It!, Chronometer, or other apps) to look at macro and micronutrient intake or deficiencies.
- ☐ Identify any potential nutrient gaps that need to be supplemented — like vitamin D, Ca, omega-3's.

>> **Consult a healthcare professional.**

- ☐ Always check with your healthcare provider (dietitian, doctor, nutritionist) to get a personalized approach to your needs.

- ☐ Have routine blood work or other necessary blood tests at least yearly.

- ☐ Consider any medications you take.

- ☐ Consider diagnosed medical issues.

- ☐ Check for any side effects from supplements or interactions with your medications.

>> **Research products and effectiveness.**

- ☐ Look for the scientific evidence that supports the use of the supplement and any other ingredients in the supplement.

- ☐ Choose the right form of the ingredient best for your needs. For example, do you need magnesium citrate, which may be more bioavailable?

- ☐ Look at other ingredients in the product that add to the effectiveness or that you may want to avoid.

>> **Check dose and potency.**

- ☐ Make sure the dose matches the RDA or is a therapeutic dose based on science.

- ☐ Verify the potency is correct for you. For example, vitamin D comes in many strengths, so you must determine the correct dose for your needs. Be sure not to get too much of certain nutrients — especially A,D,E,K, and iron.

>> **Assess the quality and safety of the supplement.**

- ☐ Check for third party certifier's logo.

- ☐ Consider whether the brand uses GMP

- ☐ Verify the supplement is free of fillers, preservatives, pesticides, or other contaminants to avoid.

>> **Your lifestyle and preferences.**

- ☐ Think about what form you like: pills, powders, or gummies.

- ☐ Consider your preference for plant- or food-based supplements.

- ☐ Consider your activity level.

>> **Review the brands and evaluate cost.**

- ❑ Be sure the brand is reputable by reading reviews.
- ❑ Consider whether health experts trust the brand.
- ❑ Consider how long the brand has been in business.
- ❑ Check into whether the brand has transparency about sourcing, ingredients, and manufacturing.

SOME RELIABLE BRANDS OF SUPPLEMENTS

Note that there are an overwhelming number of supplement brands and products and more coming to market all the time. There are also several websites and magazines that can offer advice. The "best" brands depend on what you define as "best." Here, I include reputable brands, but you still need to do your research for your particular needs.

There are good drugstore brands that are third-party certified, including Garden of Life, Nature Made, Nature's Bounty, and Nordic Naturals. Also, Costco, CVS, and Walgreens may have their own brands that are good quality. Always check each supplement label for the certifications you want, additives, and the other information on there to help you choose.

Some brands are available only online or in specialty shops. They may be more expensive but more appealing to you. If you're looking for products with more food-based ingredients and fewer fillers or those that are gluten free, these brands may be for you. Some of these brands are Country Life, Klean Athlete, MegaFoods, Metagenics, New Chapter, NOW, Pure Encapsulations, Ritual, Standard Process, Thorne, and True Grace.

If you plan to take a food-based or whole-foods multivitamin, watch for USDA Organic, Non-GMO Project verified, Certified Gluten-Free, and Certified Vegan verifications. These types of products may also use sustainable agriculture and be transparent with their ingredients.

2

Exploring Specific Vitamins, Minerals, and Supplements

Understand why vitamins and minerals are essential.

Deal with the danger of deficiencies and power up your immunity, energy, and mood.

Distinguish among the myriad supplements on the shelves and understand the functions of a variety of herbs and botanicals.

Get enough amino acids and protein.

Chapter **5**

Finding Out about Essential Vitamins

There are 13 essential vitamins that are found in a variety of foods, and they're either fat-soluble or water soluble. The fat-soluble vitamins are A,D,E, and K; excess amounts of these vitamins can be stored in your body fat. The water-soluble vitamins are the eight B vitamins and vitamin C. Excess amounts of water-soluble vitamins are excreted in your urine. You can become deficient in a vitamin if you don't get enough of them and sometimes a deficiency can lead to mild to severe side effects. All of the vitamins are available in foods, but supplements can help fill a need if you don't consume a sufficient amount in your diet.

In this chapter, I describe each vitamin, its many functions, how much you need, and the best food sources for it.

Envisioning Vitamin A: Your Vision and Beyond

Vitamin A is a fat-soluble vitamin critical for your body to develop and function properly. It's involved in immune functions, cellular communication, growth, development, and reproduction. It plays a critical role in the formation and maintenance of your organs, including your heart, lungs, and eyes, and in skin and bone health.

There are two types of vitamin A, which come from different sources:

>> **Preformed vitamin A** (retinoids that include retinol or retinyl esters): This form is readily metabolized by the body and is found in in eggs, fish, milk, and liver.

>> **Provitamin A** (carotenoids): This form is found in plant-based foods. Beta-carotene, which is the most common carotenoid, is responsible for the color in orange and red foods such as carrots, sweet potatoes, and peppers. Your body converts carotenoids from foods to retinol, the usable and active form of vitamin A.

Table 5-1 lists the recommended daily allowances for vitamin A. The quantity depends on your sex, age, and status of being pregnant or lactating. This is true for many of the essential vitamins and minerals in this chapter and Chapter 6. I've included the tables for the more critical vitamins and minerals.

TABLE 5-1   Recommended Dietary Allowances (RDA) for Vitamin A

Age	Male	Female	Pregnancy	Lactation
Birth to 6 months	400 mcg RAE	400 mcg RAE		
7–12 months	500 mcg RAE	500 mcg RAE		
1–3 years	300 mcg RAE	300 mcg RAE		
4–8 years	400 mcg RAE	400 mcg RAE		
9–13 years	600 mcg RAE	600 mcg RAE		
14–18 years	900 mcg RAE	700 mcg RAE	750 mcg RAE	1,200 mcg RAE
19–50 years	900 mcg RAE	700 mcg RAE	770 mcg RAE	1,300 mcg RAE
51+ years	900 mcg RAE	700 mcg RAE		

TIP

RAE (retinol activity equivalent) is now the measure of the content and activity of vitamin A in foods. Here are the conversions:

>> 1 IU (international unit) retinol = 0.3 micrograms (mcg) RAE

>> 1 IU supplemental beta-carotene = 0.3 mcg RAE

>> 1 IU dietary beta-carotene = 0.05 mcg RAE

>> 1 IU dietary alpha-carotene or beta-cryptoxanthin = 0.025 mcg RAE

Vitamin A deficiency is rare in the United States. However, in low- and middle-income countries (such as some countries in Asia and sub-Saharan Africa), the incidence of vitamin A deficiency is high. This is because of limited access to food and a high level of poverty. Vitamin A deficiency is especially significant in pregnant women, infants, and children younger than 5 years of age.

Chronic vitamin A deficiency is associated with blindness, abnormal lung development, respiratory diseases, and an increased risk of anemia and death. There is also an increased risk of severity and mortality from infections (such as measles) in children who are vitamin A deficient.

Retinoids can be found in animal products, such as salmon and other fish, beef liver, dairy products, eggs, cod liver oil, and shrimp. Carotenoids are in some vegetables and fruits, such as these:

>> Carrots

>> Tomatoes

>> Sweet potatoes

>> Leafy green vegetables

>> Fruits, including mangoes, apricots, and plums

Keeping your eye on your sight

Vitamin A is important for your vision because it helps to form the pigments needed in your retina to see. Vitamin A combines with a protein in your eye called opsin to form rhodopsin, which absorbs light and is essential for your color vision and ability to see in dim light. It's also important in the normal function of conjunctival membranes that lubricate and protect your eyes.

The World Health Organization (WHO) reports that an estimated 250,000 to 500,000 vitamin A–deficient children become blind every year, and half of them die within 12 months of losing their sight.

Deficiency of vitamin A can also contribute to the development of age-related macular degeneration in older people. Vitamin A is one of the vitamins that acts as an antioxidant to protect the eyes against the damaging effects of oxidants (molecules that speed up cellular degeneration).

Upping your immunity

Immunity is dependent on your cellular response to a challenge such as a virus. These cellular responses include cell differentiation and proliferation and maintaining good levels of natural killer cells that have antiviral and antitumor activity. Vitamin A is important in these cellular processes and in increasing other important mediators of inflammation, which is also important in immunity.

Reducing your cancer risk

Studies show that people who eat diets high in beta-carotene or vitamin A from mostly plant foods may be protected against certain types of cancer. However, other research shows that high doses of vitamin A may increase the risk of cancer in people who smoke (or even used to smoke). As with many nutrition studies done on people, more research is needed to know if vitamin A reduces cancer risk. However, it is still a good idea to eat foods rich in vitamin A to get the RDA. Getting more than the RDA does not necessarily do anything to improve your health.

Supporting your reproductive health

In over half of all countries, mostly in Africa and Southeast Asia, vitamin A deficiency is a public health problem. According to the WHO, vitamin A deficiency contributes to maternal death and other poor pregnancy and lactation outcomes. It contributes to childhood blindness and mortality. Vitamin A deficiency is rare in the developed world, but deficiency can cause infertility, so it is important to get enough.

WARNING

On the other hand, too much vitamin A during pregnancy can be harmful to the fetus. It is recommended to avoid some foods high in vitamin A, such as liver. In the United States, pregnant women are prescribed a prenatal vitamin that has everything they need in terms of supplemental nutrition.

Healthy skin in and out

Topical vitamin A stimulates collagen production and therefore may work to reduce fine lines and wrinkles. Retinol also helps remove damaged elastin fibers and promote the formation of new blood vessels, which may improve skin elasticity and prevent sagging as well. Topical retinoids are also used to treat acne. They work by exfoliating skin on the surface to prevent pimples. Their absorption into the skin stimulates collagen and elastin production, which helps further to improve your skin appearance and acne scarring.

Oral vitamin A and carotenoids (beta-carotene) can protect your skin from pollution and UV radiation from the sun and help prevent cell damage, skin aging, and skin diseases. Topical retinol promotes skin turnover, which also improves age spots and sunspots and promotes even skin tone.

The combination of oral and topical vitamin A is sometimes used to treat other skin diseases such as psoriasis. This inside/out approach is also big in the beauty business. Some companies promote the idea of using moisturizers with "anti-aging vitamins" in combination with oral vitamin supplements to support skin health.

Maintaining your bones and teeth

Vitamin A is important in mediating bone cell functions resulting in the forming of healthy bones. However, it's also been shown that too much vitamin A can result in a decrease in bone mass, resulting in skeletal fragility, fractures, and osteoporosis. It's important to be sure you're getting enough but not too much to maintain healthy bones.

Vitamin A helps your body absorb calcium, which is necessary to form tooth enamel. It's also important in production of saliva, which helps to protect your teeth against decay.

Banking Up on the B Vitamins and Choline

There are eight B vitamins, which are all essential to your metabolism. Table 5-2 lists these B vitamins with their chemical name, the RDA for adult women and men, and good food sources. Choline is not a B vitamin but is an essential nutrient that is grouped with the B vitamins because of its similarities.

TABLE 5-2 RDA and Food Sources for the B Vitamins for Adults

Vitamin	RDA (Adult Women/Men)	Food Sources
B1, Thiamin	1.1/1.2 mg	Fortified cereals, whole grains, oatmeal, and other foods, pork chops, trout, black beans, mussels
B2, riboflavin	1.1/1.3 mg	Fortified cereals, plain yogurt, milk, beef, pork and lamb, clams, almonds, cheese, leafy vegetables like spinach and kale
B3, niacin	14/16 mg	Beef liver, chicken breast, marinara sauce, turkey, salmon, tuna, pork, beef, brown rice, peanuts, fortified cereals
B5, pantothenic acid	5 mg	Beef liver, fortified cereals, shitake mushrooms, sunflower seeds, chicken breast, tuna, avocado, milk, white mushrooms
B6, pyridoxine	1.3–1.5/1.3–1.7 mg	Chickpeas, beef liver, tuna, salmon, chicken breast, fortified cereals, turkey, potatoes (with skin), banana
B7, biotin	30 mg	Chicken liver, egg yolk salmon, avocado, pork, sweet potato, nuts and seeds like almonds and sunflowers seeds, legumes (soybeans, lentils), whole grains
B9, folate and folic acid	400 mg	Beef liver, spinach, asparagus, Brussels sprouts, dark leafy vegetables, broccoli, avocado, oranges, bananas, peanuts, black-eyed peas, kidney beans, fortified breakfast cereal
B12, cobalamin	2.4 mcg	Beef liver, clams, oysters, nutritional yeast, salmon, tuna, beef, chicken, egg yolks, dairy products (milk, yogurt, cheese) fortified cereals
Choline	425/550 mg	Liver, eggs, cod, salmon, cauliflower, broccoli, and soybean oil

Powering up your mitochondria with ATP

The mitochondria is the powerhouse of the cell where chemical energy in the form of ATP (adenosine triphosphate) is created and powers the biochemical reactions in all the cells in your body. This is called cellular respiration and involves the breakdown of food to blood sugar (or glucose) that feeds into metabolic pathways called glycolysis, the Krebs cycle, and oxidative phosphorylation — a series of biochemical reactions catalyzed by numerous enzymes to create ATP. Figure 5-1 represents these processes and shows the production of ATP. The B vitamins are involved in many of these reactions as well as other biochemical pathways that release energy from fat, break down amino acids, and transport oxygen and energy-containing nutrients throughout the body. More details on some of these are in Chapter 2.

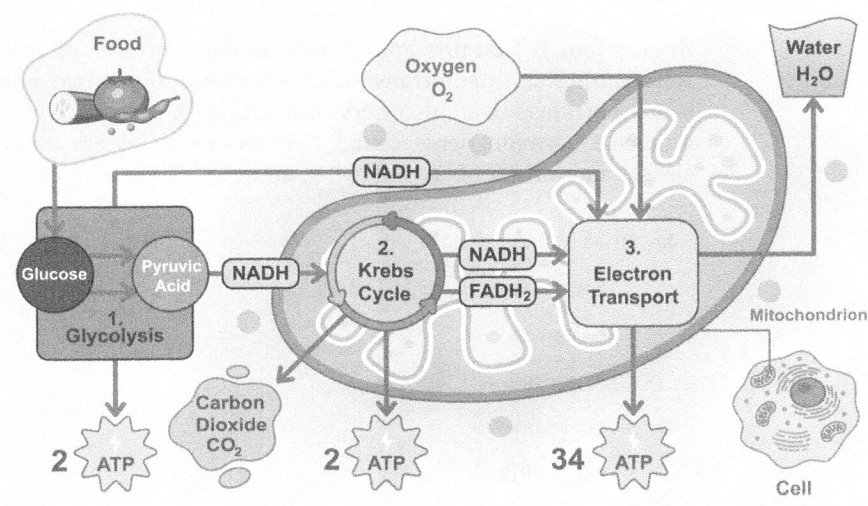

CELLULAR RESPIRATION

FIGURE 5-1:
ATP production.

Rudzhan/Adobe Stock Photos

Breaking down homocysteine

Homocysteine is an amino acid that helps create proteins in your body. Vitamins B6, B12, and B9 break down homocysteine to form other necessary amino acids, methionine, and cysteine. If your homocysteine is too high, it can be harmful to your arterial walls and can cause blockages leading to heart attack or stroke. High blood homocysteine is also linked to dementia and osteoporosis. Some studies show that B6, B12, and folate lower homocysteine (via something called the methionine cycle), which is potentially a good thing. They do this by catalyzing biochemical reactions that metabolize homocysteine. Although homocysteine may be lower because of these B vitamins, so far, studies have not shown the risk for these diseases to be reduced. More studies with larger numbers of subjects are needed to show that the lowering effect of homocysteine helps reduce the risk of certain diseases.

Working together for brain health

A 2016 review of the B vitamins and the brain published by David O. Kennedy in *Nutrients* describes how important all the B vitamins are for brain health. The Bs are involved in myriad enzymatic reactions involved in all cells, including brain cells. Many of the Bs are involved in ATP production, and deficiency in any one of them has negative consequences for this process. In addition to providing energy in the form of ATP, the Krebs cycle produces compounds important in the synthesis of many other important compounds in all cells including amino acids, fatty acids, and pyrimidines (important for RNA and DNA synthesis).

In addition, B vitamins are critical for the synthesis of important brain neurotransmitters. A neurotransmitter is a chemical released from a nerve cell that sends a message to another nerve cell. (Figure 5-2 shows how these work to communicate between nerve cells.) Neurotransmitters are divided into two main classes and consist of the following, all of which are all critical for brain function:

>> Small amino acids

- Y aminobutyric acid [GABA]

- Glutamate

- Aspartate

>> Biogenic amines

- Dopamine

- Epinephrine

- Norepinephrine

- Serotonin

- Histamine

- Acetylcholine

Too much or too little of these neurotransmitters can affect mood, energy, anxiety, and depression, so making sure you have enough of these vitamins can help keep your brain functioning well and stabilize your mood.

A meta-analysis of effects of B vitamin supplements on mood, depression, anxiety, and stress in both healthy and "at-risk" people (those who have poor nutrient intake or poor mood status) supported B supplement use for mood and stress. The data did not support use for anxiety and depression. During stressful times or for mild mood swings, supplementing your diet with B vitamins may help you feel better. B vitamins, especially B12 and folate, are available in their methylated forms, which are the active forms and are more readily used by your body. This form of B vitamins may be easier for some people to absorb and utilize, especially for mood, lowering homocysteine, and if you have the MTHFR genetic mutation. This genetic mutation makes it difficult for converting folate into its active form.

NEUROTRANSMITTER

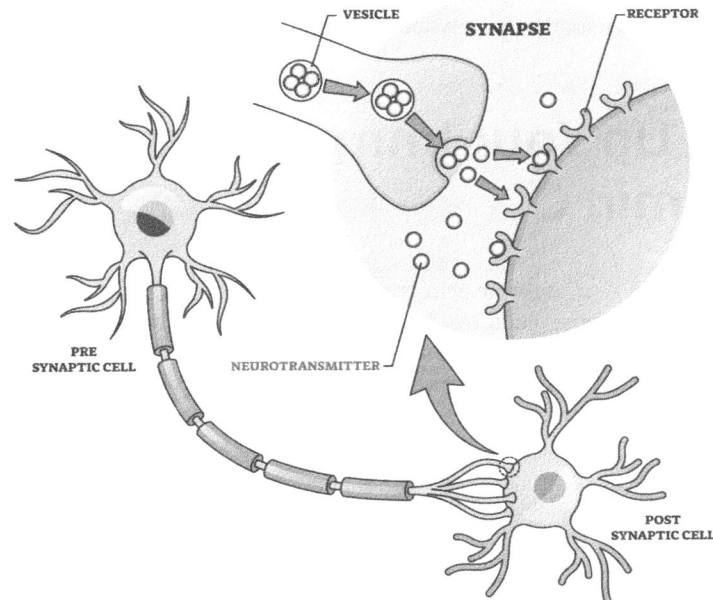

FIGURE 5-2:
Neurotransmitters
are synthesized in
the brain from
amino acids and
function to send
signals from one
neuron to other
neurons in
the brain.

Building strong hair, nails, and skin

As described earlier in this chapter, B vitamins are very important in cellular energy production; glucose, fat, and protein metabolism; and a plethora of biochemical reactions. Specifically, biotin (B7) strengthens hair and increases its density. In addition, some B vitamins may lower precancerous skin growth, and pantothenic acid (B5) may help hair and scalp hydration.

Numerous vitamin supplements and products with added B vitamins are on the market for hair, nails, and skin. Unfortunately, there's little scientific evidence to support the claims that supplements make a difference when you're getting enough of the vitamins from your food intake. In other words, if you eat well and aren't deficient in these vitamins (in addition to vitamins A, C, and E), taking more than you need should not make a difference in your hair nails, or skin.

Preventing birth defects

Women of childbearing age should be consuming 0.4 mg of folic acid daily. Folic acid reduces the risk of spina bifida and anencephaly — two very serious birth defects called neural tube defects (NTD). If you're planning to conceive, it's important to take folic acid for three months before conception because NTDs develop very early in pregnancy often before the pregnancy is confirmed. Prenatal vitamins usually contain about 0.8 mg of folate.

Charging Up Your Immune System with Vitamin C

Vitamin C or ascorbic acid is a water-soluble vitamin that acts as an antioxidant to protect your cells inside and out against the damage caused by free radicals. Free radicals are molecules that are naturally produced in your bodies that have an uneven number of electrons, which makes them very reactive. They can then take electrons from other molecules, causing oxidative stress and cell damage. Vitamin C absorbs and deactivates free radicals, making it a good antioxidant.

Vitamin C is also essential for forming blood vessels, cartilage, and collagen in bones. It's important for healing and enhances iron absorption and storage.

The RDA for vitamin C is 90 mg for adult men and 75 mg for women. Deficiency in vitamin C can cause bleeding gums, frequent bruising, poor wound healing, anemia, and, in extreme cases, scurvy. (Scurvy is defined as a deficiency of vitamin C and characterized by spongy gums, loosening of the teeth, and a bleeding into the skin and mucous membranes.) Vitamin C deficiency is uncommon worldwide except in areas of food scarcity. Good food sources for vitamin C are

>> Orange juice and other citrus

>> Bell peppers (red, green, yellow)

>> Strawberries

>> Kiwifruit

>> Tomatoes and tomato juice

>> Cruciferous vegetables (broccoli, Brussels sprouts, cabbage, cauliflower)

>> Potatoes

>> Spinach

>> Kakadu plums

>> Acerola cherries

>> Rose hips

>> Chili peppers

Preventing colds or reducing symptoms

Much research has been done over the years to determine whether vitamin C helps prevent colds or reduce symptoms. According to the Linus Pauling Institute at Oregon State University, regular intake of vitamin C *will* reduce the severity of cold symptoms but *will not* reduce your chance of getting sick in the first place. Most people get enough vitamin C from their diet, and supplements aren't necessary. If you still want to take large doses of vitamin C, there are many products on the market with extra C in them. Luckily, there's no scientific evidence that large amounts of vitamin C will be toxic; however, you may experience GI side effects. The bottom line is that many products claim to enhance immunity with high doses of vitamin C, but this is not backed by science.

Linus Pauling and megadoses of vitamin c

Linus Pauling was a brilliant scientist with varied interests who won the Nobel Prize twice. His first was the 1954 Nobel Prize in Chemistry for "for his research into the nature of the chemical bond and its application to the elucidation of the structure of complex substances." His second was the 1962 Nobel Peace Prize "for his fight against the nuclear arms race between East and West."

He was very interested in the idea that megadoses of vitamins could prevent or treat diseases — in particular that vitamin C might prevent the common cold and also treat cancer. Later in his career, he started the Linus Pauling Institute and wrote books about these beliefs. Some of the science at the time supported his theories, but his more recent research doesn't support them. As a result, the institute's website says this about the benefits of and recommended doses for vitamin C: "Therefore, the Linus Pauling Institute's intake recommendation of 400 mg/day of vitamin C for generally healthy adults takes into account the currently available epidemiological, biochemical, and clinical evidence, while acknowledging the extremely low toxicity of vitamin C and the incomplete information regarding optimum intake."

Healing wounds

Vitamin C is a cofactor in enzymes that synthesize collagen, carnitine, and substances that act as hormones or neurotransmitters. It seems logical that vitamin C would therefore be helpful for healing processes. As I repeat very often in this book, the problem is that the number, design, and quality of the studies on this (and other nutrition topics) are not sufficient to prove effect. A 2022 review of 22 vitamin C studies concludes that if you're deficient in vitamin C or don't eat fruits and vegetables, then vitamin C supplementation is beneficial to wound healing. If you're not deficient, there isn't evidence to support taking more to support wound treatment except in the case of treating pressure ulcers or bedsores.

Providing protection from free radicals

Vitamin C is an antioxidant and works by protecting your cells by reacting with harmful (naturally produced) free radicals. Consuming normal amounts of vitamin C along with other antioxidants found in foods may help reduce damage caused by free radicals, which is helpful because studies have connected free radical oxidative damage to a number of diseases — for example, neurodegenerative diseases, cancer, and cardiovascular disease (CVD) — and aging.

There are many animal and small human studies demonstrating the importance of sufficient vitamin C for reducing blood pressure, uric acid (involved in gout), CVD, and dementia and boosting immunity. Vitamin C helps absorb iron from the gut, so consuming vitamin C may help reduce iron deficiency.

Catching Some Rays with Vitamin D

Vitamin D (calciferol) is a fat-soluble vitamin essential for building and maintaining your bones because it facilitates the absorption of calcium. (Read more in Chapter 6.) Vitamin D is also important for other anti-inflammatory, antioxidant, and neuroprotective functions. Vitamin D has really been the "it" vitamin the last several years because it's important in so many cellular functions that promote immunity and support muscle and brain function.

The RDA for vitamin D is 15 mcg (600 IU) in people aged 1 through 70 and goes up to 20 mcg (800 IU) after age 70. As you get older, you absorb less vitamin D and calcium and therefore need to supplement more. The National Academy of Medicine (formerly the Institute of Medicine) and the current European guidelines recommend a level between 20 ng/mL and 50 ng/mL However, some professional societies in the United States recommend a level of at least 30 ng/ml for optimal skeletal health. The blood levels of 25-hydroxyvitamin D that your doctor measures will tell you whether you're deficient.

You get vitamin D from exposure to the sun, certain foods, and supplements. Of course, you know that too much sun exposure isn't good for your skin because it can cause skin cancer. However, short exposure converts pre-vitamin D in skin to usable vitamin D. It's hard to know how much sun exposure is appropriate, but research suggests that 5 to 30 minutes of sun between 10:00 a.m. and 4:00 p.m. on exposed arms, face, hands, and legs without sunscreen two to seven times per week will give you enough vitamin D. Where you live makes a difference, as does the time of year, the clouds in the sky, or the shade of your skin. If you live in the south or in California, then you might get enough vitamin D all year long. If you live in the northeast United States, you may want to supplement in the winter.

It's hard to get enough vitamin D from food because there aren't many that naturally contain vitamin D. Fortified foods like milk, plant-based milks, some juice, yogurt, margarine, and some cereals provide much of the vitamin D in the United States and Canada. Other food sources include yeast, mushrooms, fatty fish, beef liver, eggs, and cheese.

According to the National Institutes of Health (NIH), the only research that is conclusive about vitamin D supplements and health outcomes is the work related to bone health. However, research is being done in several other areas, which I cover in the following sections.

Strengthening bones

Most of the studies on vitamin D and bone strength also include use of calcium, so it's difficult to isolate the effect of only vitamin D. Both are essential to build bone, which is constantly changing — that is, being broken down and rebuilt.

Vitamin D is vital for the absorption of calcium from the intestines. Without adequate vitamin D, the body can't absorb enough calcium, even if dietary intake is sufficient. Vitamin D helps regulate calcium and phosphate in the body, which are necessary for the bone remodeling process, where old bone tissue is replaced with new bone tissue.

Fighting certain diseases

According to the Mayo Clinic and NIH and many research papers, there isn't enough evidence to claim that vitamin D prevents or treats any diseases except for promoting bone-related health. However, there is much research being done for several diseases including osteoporosis, cancer, CVD, depression, multiple sclerosis (MS), type 2 diabetes, and weight loss. At this point, despite all the research, no conclusions have been made to link vitamin D to disease prevention. Specifically, in the studies on many types of cancers, vitamin D with or without calcium supplementation doesn't reduce the incidence of cancer, although adequate or higher 25-hydroxyvitamin D levels might reduce cancer mortality rates.

Regulating mood

Low levels of vitamin D have been correlated with anxiety and depression. Vitamin D can cross the blood-brain barrier, and some parts of the brain (prefrontal cortex, hippocampus, cingulate gyrus, thalamus, hypothalamus, and substantia nigra) include receptors for vitamin D. Although cause and effect have not been proven definitively, there is good reason to believe that being deficient in vitamin D could affect mood.

Boosting anti-inflammation and immunity

Vitamin D receptors and enzymes involved in vitamin D metabolism are found in immune cells that support involvement in anti-inflammatory processes. Some epidemiological data link vitamin D deficiency to a poorly functioning immune system, an increased risk of infections, and a predisposition to autoimmune diseases. This indicates that you need adequate vitamin D levels to boost your immunity. But is that the case?

Animal studies done with doses of almost toxic levels of vitamin D have shown some improvement of some diseases, but there were side effects to these high doses. Studies in people with higher-than-normal amounts of vitamin D have not shown an improvement in immunity or infectious or autoimmune disease.

Managing your muscle function

Vitamin D receptors (VDR) are found in muscles, which means that vitamin D binds to these receptors and then has effects on the muscle tissue. Vitamin D is important to maintain muscle strength, regeneration, and recovery after an athletic event. If you're deficient in D, you may experience muscle pain, bone pain (since vitamin D helps with calcium absorption), or muscle weakness. Having adequate circulating vitamin D is helpful in muscle recovery after exercise; however, clinical studies do not support that vitamin D supplementation has an effect in post-exercise muscle recovery.

Exploiting Vitamin E

Vitamin E, a fat-soluble antioxidant, is important for immunity and many cellular processes. It's important for vision, reproduction, and blood, brain, and skin health. The RDA for vitamin E for adult women and men is 15 mg. Vitamin E deficiency in the United States is rare. Naturally occurring vitamin E exists in eight chemical forms that have varying levels of biological activity, but alpha-tocopherol is the most biologically active and the only form that meets human requirements. Naturally occurring vitamin E includes alpha, beta, gamma, and delta-tocopherol and alpha, beta, gamma, and delta-tocotrienol, but supplements usually just include the alpha form. Getting vitamin E from foods may therefore provide other forms of E that have health benefits. These other forms have not been studied as much as the alpha form.

Nuts, seeds, and vegetable oils (for example, canola, corn, soybean) are loaded with vitamin E. Other good sources include wheat germ oil, spinach, broccoli, tomatoes, mango, kiwifruit, and fortified cereals.

Antioxidant properties

Vitamin E is an antioxidant that protects cells, tissues, and organs from damage caused by free radicals. Free radicals play a role in aging and the development of cancer, arthritis, and cataracts. Vitamin E protects cell membranes from free radical damage (see Figure 5-3), which means it also protects the overall health and stability of the cell.

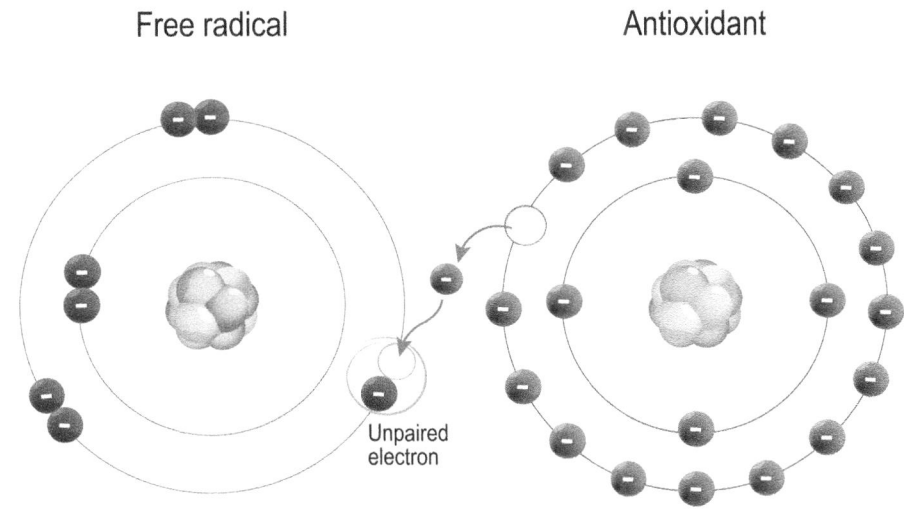

Free radical   Antioxidant

Unpaired electron

FIGURE 5-3: Antioxidants can react with the free radical and deactivate its ability to react with biomolecules.

Proper organ function and heart disease

Vitamin E may help organ function because of its antioxidant and anti-inflammatory processes, inhibition of platelet aggregation, and immune enhancement. Vitamin E helps protect cells from oxidative stress caused by free radicals, which is particularly important for organs like the heart and liver because they're most susceptible to oxidative damage.

Vitamin E can help maintain the health of blood vessels and may prevent the oxidation of low-density lipoprotein (LDL) cholesterol (the "bad" cholesterol) which may lead to atherosclerosis and heart disease. Vitamin E might also help prevent the formation of blood clots that could lead to a heart attack or venous thrombo-embolism. However, clinical trials haven't provided strong evidence that routinely using vitamin E supplements prevents cardiovascular disease. In one study in 40,000 women taking vitamin E, observations included a 24 percent reduction in cardiovascular death rates, and in those ≥65 years of age, a 26 percent decrease in nonfatal heart attack and a 49 percent decrease in cardiovascular death rates. In a more recent study in 15,000 men over 50 years old, vitamin E supplementation had no effect on the incidence of major cardiovascular events, myocardial infarction, stroke, or cardiovascular morality. And there was some increased risk of stroke in these men.

Vitamin E, which has moisturizing properties, is often used in skin care products. It also may protect against UV damage. Your healthy skin is vital for overall body health and protecting your organs.

Some evidence shows that vitamin E may support cognitive function and help protect against neurodegenerative diseases by reducing oxidative stress in the brain. Lastly, vitamin E influences hormone balance and supports overall organ function related to reproduction.

Supports immune function

In both animal and human studies, Vitamin E has been shown to enhance immune responses and help protect against several infectious diseases, such as respiratory infections, allergies, and asthma. Although the mechanism for this protection isn't clear, it may have to do with vitamin E's antioxidant properties as a free radical scavenger, which reduces oxidative stress that can weaken immune responses. It may also reduce inflammation. Research demonstrates that vitamin E supports the proliferation and function of important immune cells called T cells and B cells. These cells help the body respond to pathogens.

Staying Strong with Vitamin K

Vitamin K is a fat-soluble vitamin that plays a significant role in synthesizing proteins important for blood clotting and strengthening your bones. Vitamin K is involved in making four proteins needed for clotting. The RDA for adults is 120 mcg which is fairly easy to get if you like fruits and vegetables.

There are two types of Vitamin K:

>> K1 (phylloquinone) is in green leafy vegetables. Gut bacteria convert it into menaquinones (vitamin K2).

>> K2 (menaquinone) is found in animal foods and fermented foods but is also produced by gut bacteria. Foods that are good sources of K2 are natto, chicken, and kimchi. Salami, beef, butter, and cheese also include K2, but they're not as healthy for you.

Most people get enough vitamin K from their diets. The best sources for K1 include spinach, collard and other leafy greens, Brussels sprouts, broccoli, asparagus, soybeans, cabbage/sauerkraut, pumpkin, pine nuts, and blueberries.

Blood clotting and bone strengthening

Perhaps the most important role of vitamin K is in the synthesis of proteins needed for blood clotting. The K in this vitamin's identifier comes from the Danish and German word *Koagulation*, which in English means coagulation. You may be more familiar with the term *clotting*, the important process that stops the bleeding from injuries or wounds.

Because of its function as a coagulating agent, vitamin K can interfere with blood thinner or anticoagulant medications. If you're on a blood thinner such as warfarin, it's not advisable to take vitamin K supplements; take it only in consultation with your healthcare professional.

Vitamin K participates in synthesis of a protein called osteocalcin, which is made in the bones and binds calcium. This protein prevents bone demineralization and therefore loss of bone density. This then contributes to increasing bone strength.

Improving your brain and heart

A limited number of human studies suggest that low vitamin K may be correlated with decline in cognition (brain function). Some studies suggest that deficits in vitamin K levels may negatively influence visual memory, verbal fluency, and brain volume. More recently, osteocalcin (mentioned earlier in the "Blood clotting and bone strengthening" section) has been shown to be involved in the regulation of metabolism, reproduction, and cognition.

A recent study tracked 53,000 Danish adults for 21 years to examine cardiovascular disease outcomes in people eating a diet high in vitamin K–containing foods. They distinguished between vitamin K1 and K2 intake and found a 21 percent or 14 percent lower risk in hospitalizations due to clogged arteries in people with high K1 and K2 levels, respectively.

These studies aren't conclusive, but they seem promising. It's wise to eat foods high in vitamin K to help to protect against cardiovascular disease and brain function decline.

Chapter 6

Meeting the Essential Minerals

Essential minerals are inorganic components that are important for many physiological and biochemical processes in human cells and tissues. These processes include catalyzing enzymatic reactions that synthesize and break down proteins, DNA, fats, and carbohydrates. Your organ systems also use essential minerals for growth, development, movement, energy production, and maintenance of internal physiological balance.

In this chapter, you will learn about each of the 13 essential minerals and why they are important. It will also cover how much you need, and the best food sources.

Getting to Know the 13 Essential Minerals

The essential minerals are minerals your body needs to function properly. They're either macrominerals or trace minerals, depending on the amount you need for normal bodily function. Your body can't produce essential minerals, so you need to get them from your food. As with essential vitamins, most people get the required amounts from a well-balanced and diverse diet. If your diet includes an inadequate amount of a mineral or you're deficient for some other reason, you may need to take a supplement.

Here are the 13 essential minerals and their important functions:

>> **Calcium:** Building strong bones and teeth, regulating metabolism, blood clotting, enabling communication between cells, and cell signaling

>> **Iron:** Forming hemoglobin which transports oxygen in the blood

>> **Magnesium:** Participating in many enzymatic reactions, including those that synthesize DNA.

>> **Zinc:** Supporting cell division, supporting immunity, and aiding in wound healing

>> **Phosphorus:** Building and repairing bones and teeth, supporting nerve function and muscle contraction

>> **Potassium:** Balancing fluids, supporting muscle contraction and nerve function

>> **Selenium:** Helping fight oxidative damage to cells, aiding metabolism of thyroid hormone

>> **Iodine:** Participates in thyroid hormone production, supporting metabolism and physical and mental development

>> **Sodium:** Aiding in muscle contractions, conducting nerve impulses, maintaining fluid balance

>> **Chloride:** Maintaining fluid balance (in conjunction with sodium), forming hydrochloric acid in the stomach for digestion, sustaining electrical neutrality

>> **Phosphorus:** Building and repairing bones and teeth, supporting nerve function and muscle contraction

>> **Copper:** Producing energy, taking up iron from the gastrointestinal (GI) tract

>> **Manganese:** Supporting cell division; breaking down protein, carbohydrate, and cholesterol; blood clotting (in conjunction with vitamin K)

>> **Sulfur:** Repairing DNA damage, fighting acne-causing bacteria in the skin

Capitalizing on Calcium

Calcium is the main structural component in bones and teeth, and getting the recommended amount helps keep your bones strong and functioning. Calcium also helps keep tissues flexible and strong. About 1 percent to 2 percent of the body's calcium circulates in the blood and is important for blood vessel contraction and dilation, muscle function, blood clotting, transmission of nerve impulses, and hormonal secretion.

Table 6-1 shows the recommended daily allowances (RDA) for calcium. The required amount changes depending on where you are in your life cycle. As with other nutrients, you can reach the RDA with a combination of foods and supplements, if needed.

TABLE 6-1 **Recommended Dietary Allowances (RDA) for Calcium**

Age	Male	Female	Pregnant	Lactating
0–6 months*	200 milligrams (mg)	200 mg		
7–12 months*	260 mg	260 mg		
1–3 years	700 mg	700 mg		
4–8 years	1,000 mg	1,000 mg		
9–13 years	1,300 mg	1,300 mg		
14–18 years	1,300 mg	1,300 mg	1,300 mg	1,300 mg
19–50 years	1,000 mg	1,000 mg	1,000 mg	1,000 mg
51–70 years	1,000 mg	1,200 mg		
70+ years	1,200 mg	1,200 mg		

Adequate Intake

Source: National Institutes of Health Office of Dietary Supplements (NIH ODS)

TIP

The biggest source of calcium is dairy. In the United States, dairy products account for approximately 70 percent of calcium intake. The rest can come from certain vegetables such as kale, broccoli, and bok choy. You can also get calcium from canned sardines and salmon with bones. If you do not get enough calcium in your food plus supplements, then your body draws calcium from your bones. If you don't replace the calcium in the bone or if the deficiency goes on for too long, your bones can weaken.

Maintaining strong bones

Ninety-nine percent of the calcium in your body is in the bones as hydroxyapatite. Calcium is constantly turning over in the bones as they're formed and strengthened. Bone is constantly being built up and broken down or remodeling, and both calcium and vitamin D are critical to this process.

As you age, bone metabolism changes, and the balance may shift so that bone loss is greater than bone formation. As you age, you also absorb less calcium from your food and supplements. At all ages, it's important to get enough calcium to ensure that loss isn't slowly occurring over time.

REMEMBER

Bone loss becomes more important in postmenopausal women because of lower intestinal absorption and hormonal changes that can result in a decrease in bone density and lead to bone fractures. This is why the RDA goes up for older women. If bone density decreases, osteopenia and then osteoporosis can develop. Eating calcium-rich foods and getting enough vitamin D are both important for bone health; however, studies are mixed as to whether taking supplements will lower the risk of developing osteoporosis. The jury may be out but getting the RDA of both calcium and D, and no more than the Tolerable Upper Intake Level (UL) from food and supplements is recommended.

WARNING

A 2018 review of randomized controlled trials in normal healthy postmenopausal women found that taking calcium and vitamin D supplements for seven years did *not* reduce the incident in fractures. This feels confusing and contradictory, but the bottom line is to continue taking enough vitamin D and calcium.

Maintaining important daily bodily functions

The other 1 percent of calcium in the body is found in blood, muscle, and tissue. The body uses hormonal regulation to maintain the proper balance of calcium in the blood to perform necessary functions. If calcium levels get too low in the blood, a hormone called parathyroid hormone (PTH) activates the release of calcium from your bones. If calcium is too high, then another hormone called calcitonin stops the release from the bone and facilitates excretion of calcium through the kidneys and out of your body via the urine.

Keeping an eye on your cardiovascular health

Recent research has indicated that too much calcium might cause hypercalcemia (toxic calcium in the blood). Getting too much calcium from supplements or food — more than the UL of 2,000 to 2,500 mg — might cause blood clotting or blockages in the arteries, leading to cardiovascular disease. The research is not conclusive however, but it's still best to get the RDA amounts and not to take any more than that in the form of supplements.

Avoiding kidney stones

A common type of kidney stone is formed when calcium combines with oxalates to form calcium-oxalate stones. The best way to avoid kidney stones is *not* by reducing your calcium–rich foods. Three large studies, the Nurses' Health Study, the Women's Initiative, and a large men's cohort of over 46,000 men, found that eating a diet that included normal daily intake of calcium-rich foods decreased the risk of kidney stones.

TIP

Taking calcium supplements more than the RDA can cause kidney stones. It's important if you are low in calcium to eat calcium–rich foods. The best dairy to eat for overall health and to reduce kidney stones is low-fat or skim dairy such as milk, yogurt, or cottage cheese. You should take supplements to bring your daily intake up to the RDA level for your age group or medical needs, but don't go beyond that amount.

NERVOUS SYSTEM AND BRAIN FUNCTION

Calcium helps to precisely regulate the nervous system and brain function by assisting in neurotransmitter release from one neuron and uptake by another. This is how neurons communicate with each other. This function of calcium results in neurotransmitter release in the body and brain. The brain neurotransmitters are important for mood, memory, and sleep. Calcium is also important for nerve transmission to muscles in the body for proper functioning.

Too little calcium can result in reduced nervous system function, which affects the brain and your musculature. These might include memory issues, brain fog, irritability, anxiety, depression, or seizures. Symptoms can include muscle cramps and spasms, tingling in the fingers and toes, or stiffness of muscles.

Too much calcium is also bad and can cause mood changes, irritability, fatigue, and difficulty concentrating. High calcium can also cause muscle weakness, digestive issues such as loss of appetite and nausea, vomiting, and constipation. Too much can also affect kidneys, increase risk of kidney stones, and also cause heart palpitations or high blood pressure.

Protecting yourself from colon cancer

Epidemiological studies and some cohort and clinical studies suggest that calcium may be protective against colon cancer. A review by the World Cancer Research Fund and the American Institute for Cancer Research reported evidence that more than 200 mg daily of calcium (which is less than the RDA) via a combination of high-calcium dairy foods and supplements may decrease risk of colorectal cancer. They noted that this may be because the calcium binds to toxic substances to prevent growth of tumor cells or that the bacteria in dairy may offer some protection.

Keeping an Eye on Iron

Most of the iron in your body — about 3 to 4 grams — is in hemoglobin, a protein that carries oxygen from your lungs to the rest of your tissues and organs. Myoglobin, a protein in your muscles and tissues that stores and transports oxygen within muscle cells, also contains some iron. The rest is stored as ferritin or hemosiderin in your liver, spleen, and bone marrow. Iron is also important in processes such as physical growth, neurological development, cellular functioning, and synthesis of some hormones.

The recommended amount changes with age. Table 6-2 lists the different amounts based on age.

TABLE 6-2   RDA for Iron

Age	Male	Female	Pregnancy	Lactation
Birth to 6 months	0.27 mg*	0.27 mg*		
7–12 months	11 mg	11 mg		
1–3 years	7 mg	7 mg		
4–8 years	10 mg	10 mg		
9–13 years	8 mg	8 mg		
14–18 years	11 mg	15 mg	27 mg	10 mg
19–50 years	8 mg	18 mg	27 mg	9 mg
51+ years	8 mg	8 mg		

* Adequate Intake

Source: National Institutes of Health Office of Dietary Supplements (NIH ODS)

There are two kinds of dietary iron: heme and non-heme. Heme iron is found in meat, seafood, and poultry. Non-heme iron is found in plants and iron-fortified foods, such as cereals. The foods highest in iron include the following:

TIP

>> Fortified cereals

>> Shellfish

>> Spinach and other leafy greens (including parsley)

>> Liver and other organ meats

>> Legumes such as chickpeas, lentils, peas, beans, soybeans

>> Red meat

>> Pumpkin seeds

>> Turkey and chicken

>> Tofu

>> Broccoli

Transporting oxygen and avoiding anemia

Iron is essential in forming hemoglobin, which transports oxygen in your body. It is also critical for forming myoglobin, which provides oxygen to your muscles. Hemoglobin is in red blood cells, and a lack of it creates smaller red cells and less efficient transport of oxygen to tissues.

A deficiency in iron leads to decreased hemoglobin and smaller red cells, which can result in iron-deficiency anemia (IDA). The symptoms of IDA include fatigue and light headedness. If you suffer from this IDA, you may need supplements. It's best to speak with your healthcare provider to decide how much to take.

Boosting immunity

The metabolic mechanisms related to iron function and immunity are complex and subject of many scientific papers. Here's a summary of how iron is important for various immune cell types that are essential in addressing pathogens in the body. The immune response of cells is either innate (immediate and nonspecific) or adaptive (slower, targets specific antigens, may produce antibodies, and remembers specific pathogens to fight next time you are exposed).

>> **Neutrophils:** These white cells are important in immunity as a first line of defense for fighting bacteria and other infections and healing wounds. Iron is essential to the functioning of neutrophils.

>> **Eosinophils:** Another white cell that is important in immune responses for fighting parasites and allergies. Adequate amounts of iron to support this immune response.

>> **Macrophages:** Macrophages are scavenger cells that clear pathogens from the circulation. They also take up old or damaged red blood cells and recycle the iron in them as part of the constant daily turnover of RBCs.

>> **T-cells:** These cells are part of the immune system and are either cytotoxic T cells (CD8+) or helper T cells (CD4+). Iron is necessary for their development. CD8+ cells kill cells infected with viruses or bacteria and destroy tumor cells. CD4+ cells send signals to tell other cells in the immune system to do the attacking!

>> **B cells:** These cells are part of the immune system and make infection-fighting antibodies. Iron is essential for their proliferation and function.

>> **Natural killer (NK) cells:** These need iron to be activated. They're immune cells that kill infected or cancerous cells.

Iron is also important for the overall function of the immune system, which includes the production of red blood cells and transporting of oxygen. Iron needs to be regulated because too much or too little can affect the immune system. We also have proteins in our bodies that can deprive pathogens of iron, thus reducing their survival and function.

Making Inroads with Magnesium

Magnesium is everywhere! It's abundant in foods as well as in our cells and tissues. It's an important cofactor in more than 300 enzyme systems that regulate biochemical reactions in your body.

The RDA for adult women and men is 310 to 320 mg and 400 to 420 mg per day, respectively. There are slight differences for teens, people who are pregnant, and people who are lactating. See Table 6-3 for details.

TABLE 6-3

RDA for Magnesium

Age	Male	Female	Pregnancy	Lactation
Birth to 6 months	30 mg*	30 mg*		
7–12 months	75 mg*	75 mg*		
1–3 years	80 mg	80 mg		
4–8 years	130 mg	130 mg		
9–13 years	240 mg	240 mg		
14–18 years	410 mg	360 mg	400 mg	360 mg
19–30 years	400 mg	310 mg	350 mg	310 mg
31–50 years	420 mg	320 mg	360 mg	320 mg
51+ years	420 mg	320 mg		

* Adequate Intake

Source: National Institutes of Health Office of Dietary Supplements (NIH ODS)

Recent data from large health studies show that about half of Americans don't get enough magnesium from food intake. Magnesium is not routinely measured as part of a typical annual checkup with your physician, but it can be ordered separately if a deficiency is suspected. The more accurate test for deficiency is a RBC magnesium test rather than a serum magnesium level.

Magnesium deficiency can occur for a number of reasons, including decreased intake, drug-induced deficiency, endocrine issues, stress, chronic alcoholism, excessive lactation, heat, prolonged exercise, or severe burns.

WARNING

Magnesium is found in many foods and beverages, and if you eat a healthy diet, you probably get enough. However, if your diet is the Standard American Diet (SAD), you may not be getting enough magnesium, and a chronic lack of enough of it can lead to health issues. As with other minerals and vitamins, it's best to get your magnesium from foods. Getting too much from supplements can result in side effects.

Here are some high-magnesium foods:

TIP

>> Nuts and seeds (almonds, cashews, peanuts, flaxseed, pumpkin seeds, and chia seed)

>> Fatty fish, mackerel, halibut, and salmon

>> Legumes (black beans, edamame, lima beans)

>> Whole grains (quinoa, brown rice, fortified foods like cereals)

>> Dairy (milk, low-fat yogurt)

>> Dark leafy greens (spinach, Swiss chard, collard greens, kale)

>> Fruit (avocados, bananas, papaya, blackberries)

>> Vegetables (green peas, sweet corn, potatoes)

>> Mineral water and hard water, depending on the source

TIP

Some waters are rich in magnesium because it's found in Earth's crust and oceans and rivers!

>> Dark chocolate (70 percent to 80 percent cocoa)

Catalyzing enzymatic reactions

Magnesium is required in relatively large amounts and is a cofactor in more than 300 enzymatic reactions, making it crucial for your physiological functioning. Some of these essential functions are heart rhythm, vascular tone, nerve function, muscle contraction and relaxation, and bone formation.

Magnesium is important for synthesizing protein, DNA, RNA, and glutathione (an important antioxidant). It's also critical in the breakdown of glucose and oxidative phosphorylation for energy (ATP production) and for blood glucose control and blood pressure regulation. Magnesium helps with muscle and nerve function and building and maintaining bone structure. As if all those functions aren't enough, magnesium helps calcium and phosphorous ions cross cell membranes which is important in nerve function, muscle contraction, and normal heart rhythm.

Muscle contractions

Magnesium is required for normal muscle function in your body. Magnesium blocks calcium and allows muscles to relax. This is part of the natural mechanism of muscle tension and relaxation.

A number of companies sell magnesium supplements to address muscle cramps for this reason. There has been much research on the mechanism by which magnesium works. And as with other essential vitamins and nutrients, if you don't have enough in your body, you can get symptoms of deficiency such as muscle weakness. But will supplements of magnesium stop muscle cramping?

In a 2012 Cochrane Review and a 2019 update by NIH of the literature for using supplements for muscle cramp here are the conclusions:

>> Magnesium supplementation does not provide clinically meaningful cramp prevention to older adults experiencing skeletal muscle cramps.

>> For pregnancy-associated rest cramps, the studies are conflicting, and more research is needed.

>> Surprisingly, there were no randomized controlled trials on the effects of magnesium in exercise- or disease-related muscle cramps

In short, there probably isn't enough evidence to recommend supplements for muscle cramping although there may be plenty of anecdotal information out there (and there's certainly a lot of marketing by supplement companies). In addition, other studies have not demonstrated that magnesium supplements help athletes by supporting muscle metabolism.

Regulating neurotransmitters in the brain and nerves

Whole books have been written on magnesium because of how extensively it's enmeshed in the biochemistry in your body. Magnesium gets into the brain and is a cofactor in many biochemical reactions, including the synthesis of neurotransmitters and to transmit nerve impulses necessary for brain function and messages between nerve cells and the entire body.

Magnesium also functions in a protective role against neuronal cell death and may be a part of multiple neurological disorders, including migraine, chronic pain, epilepsy, Alzheimer's, Parkinson's, stroke, and possibly anxiety and depression. More research is needed in all of these areas. The strongest data suggests a role for magnesium in treating migraine and depression.

WHAT ARE NEUROTRANSMITTERS?

Scientists have discovered more than 100 neurotransmitters, which are chemicals that transmit impulses or messages between nerves cells or between nerves cells and a muscle or gland cell. Your nervous system controls most bodily functions — including heartbeat, blood pressure, breathing, muscles, brain function, sleep, stress, hormone regulation, digestion, and senses — in some way. The most common neurotransmitters are glutamate, gamma-aminobutyric acid (GABA), glycine, serotonin, histamine, dopamine, epinephrine, norepinephrine, endorphins, and acetylcholine.

Helps your mood and sleep

Because magnesium is important for neurotransmitter function, it makes sense that it could help mood and sleep. More research is needed but magnesium may help by regulating GABA in the central nervous system, relaxing muscles, supporting melatonin amounts, or decreasing cortisol, a stress hormone.

Magnesium may improve your mood by decreasing cortisol or regulating neurotransmitters in the brain. A comprehensive look at the studies done in this area support a link between magnesium and depression more than other mood disorders, although there wasn't a clear understanding of the correlation between different levels of blood magnesium and mood disorders.

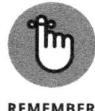

REMEMBER

Magnesium deficiency may lead to a variety of problems, including sleep and mood issues. Be sure to get the correct levels from foods whenever possible to avoid magnesium deficiency.

Repairing your DNA

DNA can be damaged by environmental factors, processes in your cells, or by DNA replication. Your cells have mechanisms for repairing this damage normally with the help of enzymes and cofactors including magnesium. Studies show that magnesium is essential to this repair at normal levels and that low levels may affect repair.

Feeling Zen with Zinc

Zinc is another mineral that catalyzes hundreds of enzymatic reactions and is part of more than 3,000 proteins involving myriad cellular functions. These include enhancing immune function, protein and DNA synthesis, wound healing, and cell signaling and division. Zinc is essential for growth and development throughout pregnancy, infancy, childhood, and adolescence.

The RDA for zinc for adult women and men is 8 mg and 11 mg, respectively, unless a person is pregnant (11 mg)or lactating (12 mg). The best sources of zinc are beef, pork, fish, and seafood. Oysters are highest in zinc per serving of all foods. Other good sources are eggs and dairy products, pumpkin seeds, and fortified cereals. Although whole grains, beans, and nuts naturally have zinc, sometimes they combine with another compound called phytates that make the zinc less bioavailable (available for your body to absorb).

Zinc deficiency is rare in the United States but is more common in low- and middle-income countries, affecting approximately 2 billion people. Deficiencies manifest themselves in these populations as premature birth and low birthweight, child mortality, and maternal morbidity. In addition, zinc deficiency can interfere with the sense of taste and cause delays in wound healing in the elderly. A deficiency can also affect cognition and psychological function.

Growth and development

Zinc participates in several biochemical pathways responsible for cell division and growth, so it's essential for infant and child growth. In a 2018 article, researchers from Tufts University, Boston Children's Hospital, and Harvard University performed a meta-analysis to examine the effects of zinc and zinc deficiency in children younger than 5. The researchers concluded that zinc supplementation in infants and early childhood, but not pregnancy, increases specific growth outcomes and may be even more important after 2 years of age.

A multivitamin that includes zinc is recommended for infants and children under 5 to support growth and development. Worldwide, stunting (defined as if a child's height-for-age is more than two standard deviations below the World Health Organization Child Growth Standards median) effects 165 million children. Many organizations and governments have a mission of getting vitamin and mineral supplements to children in the first 1,000 days of life to try to alleviate this problem.

Cellular communication

Zinc is in cell membranes and is important for enzymes involved in transporting information both within and between cells. There is research on this crucial cell signaling function of zinc and potential molecular pathways linking zinc metabolism to disease progression, possibly including cancer, neurodegenerative diseases, and infectious diseases.

Protecting your immunity

A deficiency in zinc can cause problems specific to your immune system. Because zinc is critical for metabolic processes of your immune system, any deficiency can lead to dysregulation of cell-mediated immune responses. At the microcellular level, it has a significant effect on the normal functioning of macrophages, neutrophils, and natural killer cells, which are important aspects of the immune system.

Zinc deficiency can increase the risk of metabolic and chronic diseases as well as infectious diseases such as respiratory infections, malaria, HIV, or tuberculosis. A deficiency can also produce inflammation and oxidative stress.

You may be wondering whether zinc supplements can prevent or treat infections because you've heard people recommend taking zinc during cold and flu season. Certainly, if your body is low in zinc, then zinc supplements will help bring you up to normal levels and do its job. But if you eat well and get enough zinc in your diet, will taking a supplement prevent colds and flus and other infectious diseases?

The results of research about using zinc to prevent or treat the common cold are mixed. A 2021 systematic review and meta-analysis included 5,446 participants with respiratory viruses. Subjects were given zinc lozenges (45 mg to 300 mg per day) or nasal spray for up to two weeks. In those who took the zinc, symptoms resolved an average of two days earlier than in those who received a placebo. However, the severity of their symptoms did not seem to differ. Another study suggested that you need a dose of more than 75 mg per day to reduce the duration of the common cold. The bottom line is that supplements in lozenges, syrups or nasal sprays may reduce the duration of a cold but not the severity.

WARNING

It's important to know that taking too much zinc can have side effects. The UL of zinc is 40 mg. If you decide to take it when you have a cold, COVID-19, or flu, be careful of exceeding that amount because at high doses, zinc can cause nausea, dizziness, headaches, gastric distress, vomiting, and loss of appetite.

Repairing at the cellular level

Zinc is a catalyst for enzymatic reactions involved in DNA, RNA, and protein synthesis and repair and in processes involved in wound healing. It stabilizes organelles in the cells and the membranes and protects against free radical damage. Zinc is in the skin and keeps it healthy so that it protects you from pathogens.

Investigating Other Important Essential Minerals

These essential minerals are also critical for good health and metabolism. Remember that doctors don't often test for them, so it is up to you to be sure to eat well and get all of your essential nutrients. This section summarizes the rest of the essential minerals and their functions in health and disease.

Phosphorous

Phosphorus combined with calcium makes up hydroxyapatite, the main structural component in bones and tooth enamel. Phosphorous is also in DNA and RNA, part of the cell membrane, phospholipids, and adenosine triphosphate (ATP, where cellular energy is stored). Many proteins and sugars in the body are biochemically activated by phosphorous (a process called phosphorylation) and into forms that are then further used by the body. And there is more! Phosphorus is important in regulation of gene transcription, activation of enzymes, and maintenance of normal pH in extracellular fluid.

The RDA for phosphorous for adults is 700 mg and the UL is 3,000 to 4,000 mg depending on your stage of life. Phosphorous deficiency is rare in the United States, and most people get more than they need from foods. The exceptions can be premature babies or people who are malnourished or have genetic disorders. Getting too much usually doesn't cause any issues unless you have chronic kidney disease or possibly cardiovascular disease.

Plenty of foods contain phosphorous, including dairy such as yogurt, milk, and cheese; grain; bread; tortillas; brown rice; oatmeal; meat; poultry; fish; eggs; nuts and seeds; legumes; and vegetables.

Potassium

Potassium is an electrolyte (meaning it carries a charge). It's in all body tissues and is necessary for normal cell function. It's important in maintaining your cellular fluid volume and cell membrane function. Potassium — along with sodium — is the main regulator of fluid volume outside your cells and in your body.

WARNING

The RDA for adult women and men is 2,600 and 3,400 mg, respectively. Many Americans don't get the daily amount of potassium needed from their food. Many think of bananas first as a good food for potassium. They are because they provide about 9 percent of the daily value. But other foods high in potassium include avocados, dried apricots, orange and vegetable juices, lentils, beans, watermelon, coconut water, acorn squash, sweet potatoes, spinach, tomato paste, milk and yogurt, chicken, salmon, beef, tuna, coffee, and salt substitutes.

Selenium

Selenium is a part of 25 selenoproteins that play critical roles in thyroid hormone metabolism, DNA synthesis, reproduction, and protection from oxidative damage caused by free radicals and infection. RDA for adult women or men is 55 micrograms (mcg) per day.

TIP

Selenium is found in soil. Foods grown in regions where soil selenium is high are a good source of dietary selenium. The best food sources include seafood, meat, poultry, eggs, dairy products, breads, cereals, and other whole grain products. The absolute highest selenium content is in Brazil nuts, which have a whopping 544 mcg in 1 ounce (six to eight nuts). This is ten times the RDA, so eating just one or two is sufficient. The UL for selenium is 400 mcg for adults and chronic high intakes of selenium can cause hair loss, skin rash, nausea, diarrhea, fatigue, irritability, and nervous system abnormalities.

Selenium deficiency is very rare in the United States. Some deficiencies may occur in regions where the soil concentration of selenium is low. Selenium deficiency can cause a type of heart disease (Keshan disease) and male infertility. It might also cause a type of arthritis called Kashin-Beck disease.

Iodine

Iodine is an essential component of thyroid hormones (T3 and T4) that regulate important biochemical reactions critical for controlling metabolism and health. Thyroid hormones regulate protein synthesis enzymatic activity and important metabolic processes. In addition, iodine is essential for skeletal and nervous system development in fetuses and infants.

The RDA for iodine in adult women and men is 150 mcg; people who are pregnant and lactating need more. Iodine is found naturally in ocean water and soil, which means it's in a lot of foods. Most people in the United States get sufficient iodine, although pregnant women may not get enough. Iodine is critical for fetal development. In the United States, it isn't mandatory to include iodine in prenatal vitamins, but the American Thyroid Association (ATA) recommends that if you are pregnant, lactating, or planning to get pregnant that you take supplements containing 150 microgram of iodine per day.

Iodine is found naturally in some foods. You can get the RDA by eating a variety of foods including seaweed (the *best* source), cod, tuna, iodized salt, dairy, oysters and other seafood, eggs, enriched bread, and liver.

REMEMBER

Restaurants may use a lot of salt in their cooking, but often the salt used is *not* iodized. Specialty salts, such as sea salt, kosher salt, Himalayan salt, and fleur de sel, are not usually iodized. Similarly, processed foods, such as canned soups, almost never contain iodized salt.

Worldwide there are 2 billion people who have insufficient iodine intake, mostly in southeast Asia and sub-Saharan Africa. Iodized salt, flour, water, and milk programs all over the world help to address this deficiency, but it's still a problem. Deficiency in iodine can lead to goiter (swelling or excessive growth of the thyroid gland) that can result in developmental delays, intellectual disabilities, and other health problems.

Getting too much iodine is also a danger. It can cause thyroid inflammation and thyroid cancer. The adult UL for iodine is 1,100 mcg.

Sodium

Sodium is the sixth most abundant element in the earth's crust, and it's essential for all animals and some plants. Sodium is one of the body's important electrolytes (it carries a charge), and we can't live without it. Sodium is essential for conducting nerve impulses, contracting and relaxing muscles, and maintaining the proper balance of water and minerals. Interestingly, the human body only needs a small amount (about 500 mg per day) for these important functions.

Salt (sodium chloride) is about 40 percent sodium and 60 percent chloride. Most people easily get their daily needs from table salt or other kinds of salt and foods that contain salt. Although you need only 500 mg per day and the RDA is 1,500 mg, the average American gets about 3,600 mg! Experts with organizations such as the American Heart Association recommend no more than 2,300 mg per day, which is about a teaspoon of salt. When levels are too high, you have an increased risk for high blood pressure and cardiovascular disease.

TIP

The DASH (Dietary Approach to Stop Hypertension) Sodium trial was a large feeding clinical study that observed a two to three times reduction in blood pressure in people on the DASH diet compared to controls. The DASH diet contains about 2,600 mg of sodium daily. (You can find more information at www.nhlbi.nih.gov/education/dash-eating-plan.)

TIP

Most people need to lower their sodium intake rather than find good sources for sodium. To lower your sodium intake, eat fruits, vegetables, whole grains, lean protein sources, and good fats like olive oil. Some foods to avoid are processed foods, hot dogs, deli meats, salted nuts, canned foods, pickles, pretzels and other snack foods, soy sauce, teriyaki sauce, jars of prepared sauces and condiments, and restaurant foods. Read labels because salt is added for taste and as a preservative.

Chloride

Chloride is the other element in salt (sodium chloride). It's an important mineral found in foods, but it's not really available (or necessary) as a supplement. It carries a charge like sodium and potassium, so it's considered an electrolyte. Along with sodium and potassium, it helps regulate fluids and nutrients going in and out of cells. Chloride is also important for stimulating stomach acid for digestion and maintaining proper pH levels in cells. It plays a role in nerve and muscle cell stimulation and helps the flow of oxygen and carbon dioxide within cells.

The amount of chloride you need is correlated to the amount of sodium because they're bound together in your body. The recommended amounts for people ages 14 to 50 and pregnant or lactating people is 2.3 grams daily. For people aged 51 to 70, it's 2 grams daily, and for people older than 71, it's 1.8 grams daily.

In healthy people, deficiency in chloride is rare because salt is such a significant part of most people's diets. Toxicity from chloride is also rare because excess chloride is excreted from the body by the kidneys. Foods high in chloride are salt and salty foods, seaweed, and shrimp.

Copper

Copper is a cofactor for many enzymes (called cuproenzymes) that catalyze reactions that produce ATP and participate in iron metabolism, neuropeptide activation, neurotransmitter synthesis, and connective tissue synthesis. One cuproenzyme that is abundant is called ceruloplasmin; it carries copper in the body and plays a role in iron metabolism. Copper is also involved in immune system functioning and as defense against oxidative damage to cells. It's important for brain development.

The RDA for copper in adults is 900 mcg. It's easy to get what you need from foods such as liver, shellfish, nuts, seeds, whole grain products, potatoes, mushrooms, avocados, chickpeas, and tofu.

WARNING

Deficiency of copper is rare in healthy people, but if you have celiac or Menkes disease or take high doses of zinc, you may have trouble getting enough copper from your diet. Toxicity is also rare in healthy people. The UL is 8,000-10,000 mcg, and getting too much over time can give you some side effects like nausea and diarrhea. Unless you're getting too much in your water from leachy copper pipes or have a genetic disease called Wilson's disease, it is difficult to get too much copper.

Manganese

Manganese is a cofactor in many enzymatic reactions, including those involved in glucose and carbohydrate metabolism, bone formation, the immune system, reproduction, blood clotting, and immune response. The RDA for adult women and men is 1.8 and 2.3 mg, respectively. Most people have no trouble getting enough manganese from their food, so deficiencies are rare in the United States.

The best food sources for manganese are whole grains, clams, oysters and mussels, nuts, legumes, green leafy vegetables, some fruit (especially pineapple and blueberries), tea, black pepper, and other spices.

Sulfur

Your body uses sulfur for various important functions, including cell repair, metabolism, digestion, and growth. It's incorporated into certain biomolecules in the cells and is important for their function. Sulfur is part of the amino acids cysteine and methionine and other important metabolites like homocysteine. It's involved in building and repairing DNA and in protecting your cells via an antioxidant called glutathione. A fun fact is that sulfur bonds in the protein in your hair create kinks and curls! Topical sulfur may act as an antibacterial agent to reduce acne.

There is no RDA established for sulfur. It's the third most abundant mineral in your body, and it is very easy to get from your foods. It's in protein-based foods (because they contain the sulfur-containing amino acids methionine and cysteine) as well as non-protein-based foods that supply other forms of sulfur (sulfides, thiosulfates, and others), including turkey, beef, eggs, fish, chicken, nuts, seeds, whole grains, legumes, chickpeas, couscous, eggs, lentils, oats, allium vegetables (garlic, leeks, onion, scallions, and shallots), and cruciferous vegetables and leafy greens.

EFFECTIVE USE OF ELECTROLYTE SUPPLEMENTS

Electrolyte powders and drinks are a growing segment of the supplement business, and they're quite popular at the moment. Electrolytes are charged (– or +) and include the minerals sodium, chloride, potassium, magnesium, phosphorous, and calcium. All of these electrolytes are readily available in foods, so if you eat a well-balanced diet, you will get what you normally need. The general recommendation is that if you exercise for an hour or less a day, you only need to drink water when exercising and do not need extra electrolytes. However, if you work in the heat, spend a lot of time outdoors, are very physically active, sweat excessively, or have been sick or have certain medical conditions, you may experience dehydration and need extra electrolytes.

Carefully read the labels on sports drinks and electrolyte-enhanced waters. Many of the drinks do not contain adequate amounts of electrolytes to make a difference, and the packets of powders that you add to water may be a better option. Electrolyte products are popular for hangovers, but the clinical studies do not support the purported benefits compared to drinking water. In chronic alcohol abuse, there is the danger of electrolyte imbalance that might warrant supplementation, but for the occasional hangover, staying hydrated with water is the best strategy. When choosing electrolyte products, watch for too much sugar, too much sodium, too little of some of the electrolytes, and artificial ingredients.

Chapter **7**

Navigating the Supplement Aisles

According to a 2024 report by McKinsey and Company, the wellness market is worth $1.8 trillion and growing (https://tinyurl.com/87m988c9). The report authors surveyed people in China, the United Kingdom, and the United States. Younger generations outspend older consumers, but all age groups are making purchases of supplements in support of health, sleep, nutrition, fitness, appearance, and mindfulness.

The report stated that consumers seem to want "effective, data-driven, science-backed health and wellness solutions." When it comes to relevant health products people seem to want clinically proven items. Recommendations from doctors seems to drive consumers to products.

In this chapter, I hope to help you understand the supplement options so you can be an informed consumer. I present the uses of many herbs and botanicals for a variety of health and wellness conditions. Most consumers want to know if a supplement does what it claims and is hopefully backed by clinical evidence, so I want to be clear about many that I've included here. Some botanicals have been used for centuries and their benefits are documented from a historical perspective. Clinical studies have been done on some, but not all, of these. In addition, the clinical studies vary in the number of subjects and other factors that may affect outcomes. With many herbal supplements, it is the combination of historical perspective from other cultures (for example, traditional Chinese medicine or Ayurvedic medicine) and small clinical studies. I recommend doing your own research and speaking with your healthcare provider when weighing the pros and cons of a supplement for your particular needs.

Getting to Know the Market

Supplements are only a portion of this $1.8 trillion market. It represents about $35 billion in the United States. In this section, I introduce you to some of the fastest growing categories and some of the brands that are players in the market.

Fast-growing categories

High-priority healthcare issues relevant to supplement intake include the broad topics listed here. I've provided some examples of available supplements in each category. (These are not complete lists and are not necessarily scientifically backed).

>> **Fitness:** Amino acids, protein powders

>> **Gut health:** Probiotics, glutamine

>> **Mental health:** B vitamins, St. John's wort, folate

>> **Healthy aging:** Magnesium, vitamin D, nicotinamide mononucleotide

>> **Plant-based diets:** vegan and vegetarian vitamin supplements

>> **Sexual health:** Valerian root, ashwagandha, damiana, maca root

>> **Weight management:** Green tea, cocoa, hoodia

>> **Women's health:** Multivitamin, calcium, black cohosh, evening primrose oil

Forty-one percent of consumers are affected by the following conditions and look for supplements to help the following:

>> **Anxiety:** GABA, B6, amino acids, valerian root, passionflower

>> **Cognition improvement:** Omega-3's, coenzyme Q10

>> **Depression:** Vitamin D, omega-3, St. John's wort, B vitamins, folate, S-adenosyl methionine (SAM-E)

>> **Fatigue:** Protein powders, caffeine

>> **Insomnia:** Melatonin, magnesium, L-theanine

>> **Mood enhancer:** GABA, B vitamins, L-theanine, 5-hydroxytrypamine (5HT)

>> **Stress:** B vitamins, magnesium

At the time of this writing, the following were the key trends in supplement sales:

>> Sales of herbs and botanicals made up 19 percent of the supplement market.

>> Sales of medicinal mushrooms had quadrupled since 2018.

>> Magnesium was the fastest growing mineral supplement because of its uses for mood, sleep, and immunity.

>> About 60 percent of adults in the United States were taking a vitamin supplement.

>> Sports nutrition products and various powders continue to increase in sales — especially collagen, and plant-based protein, creatine.

>> CBD products sales continue to rise with the United States leading the world in revenue of about $2.5 billion yearly.

>> Beauty from within market consists of skin, hair, nails, and antiaging supplements and is in addition to the topical product market.

Sifting through the brands

There are three independent labs that analyze supplements: ConsumerLab.com, NSF International, and the United States Pharmacopeia (USP). Each lab measures and certifies that supplements contain the ingredients listed on the label, their amounts, and their contaminants (if any).

TIP

The best brands have one of these symbols on the label so that you can be sure you're getting a quality supplement.

The National Institutes of Health (NIH) and the U.S. Food and Drug Administration (FDA) have websites where you can look for information on herbs and botanicals, such as any ingredient listed on a supplement label. This also helps you to understand what you're ingesting. In addition, Herblist is an NIH app for looking up information about specific herbs. It can help you decide whether a supplement is for you.

On the FDA site, you can look up information about the ingredients listed on your supplement bottle. The information may include links related to the ingredient, such as the FDA's evaluation of any health claims, safety communications, and compliance and enforcement actions.

Looking into Common Herb and Botanical Supplements

Herbal usually refers specifically to plant-based products used for cooking or as a medicine or a therapeutic. *Botanical* is a more general term for any plant-based products used as an additive or supplement. Botanicals include not only herbal products but also plant-based ingredients used in cosmetics, food, or other products or essential oils.

The effectiveness or tendency to produce a result (which is known as *efficacy*), and safety of botanical supplements can vary based on quality, dosage, and individual health conditions. For centuries, plants have been the treatment choice in traditional medicine, and many of our modern drugs came from plants. However, modern scientific research may not always support their use for certain health issues.

Most common herbs and botanical products

The Herbs at a Glance page on the website for the NIH, National Center for Complementary and Integrative Health (NCCIH) includes a list of the most common herbs. You can click one of the herbs to drill down to a page with information, including an introduction, supplement information, evidence of health benefits and risks, interactions with medications, and reference links. Here, I've listed some of the popular botanical supplements:

- » Ashwagandha
- » Bilberry
- » Bromelain
- » Chamomile
- » Cranberry
- » Elderberry
- » Evening primrose oil
- » Flaxseed and flaxseed oil
- » Goldenseal
- » Hawthorn
- » Kava
- » Milk thistle
- » Mugwort
- » Sage
- » Saw palmetto
- » Valerian

- » Asian ginseng
- » Bitter orange
- » Butterbur
- » Chasteberry
- » Dandelion
- » Ephedra
- » Fenugreek
- » Garcinia cambogia
- » Ginger
- » Grape seed extract
- » Hoodia
- » Lavender
- » Noni
- » Peppermint oil
- » Red clover
- » Soy
- » St. John's wort
- » White mulberry leaf

- » Astragalus
- » Black cohosh
- » Cat's claw
- » Cinnamon
- » Echinacea
- » European mistletoe
- » Feverfew
- » Garlic
- » Ginkgo
- » Green tea
- » Horse chestnut
- » Licorice root
- » Passionflower
- » Pomegranate
- » Rhodiola
- » Tea tree oil
- » Thunder god vine
- » Turmeric
- » Yohimbe

The NIH Office of Dietary Supplements (ODS) also has a website (`https://ods.od.nih.gov/factsheets/list-Botanicals/`) with a searchable list of botanicals. Clicking an option takes you to a page with information on the compound, known benefits and risks, interactions with medications, and more health information.

WARNING

Before taking an herbal supplement, consult a healthcare professional to be sure that it is the correct choice for you. Some of these have side effects or may interfere with your medications.

HERBS VERSUS PHARMACEUTICALS: HOW DO YOU DECIDE?

An example of choosing the use of an herb over a pharmaceutical is the current use of a traditional Chinese medicine called red yeast rice extract (RYRE), which is used to lower cholesterol. It contains monacolin K (also known as lovastatin), which is the active ingredient in a prescription statin drug named Mevacor. RYRE seems like a great natural option over a pharmaceutical if you have high cholesterol. Many people use RYRE, and it often works. However, it is important to understand the pros and cons of using the herbal supplement.

Pros of RYRE are that the natural statin in this herb may lower your cholesterol. Clinical studies have been done in people that have demonstrated some strains of RYRE lower total cholesterol and low-density lipoprotein (LDL) cholesterol (the "bad" cholesterol). The doses in these studies varied between 1.2 grams/day and 2.4 grams/day (which is considered a high dosage), and they lowered cholesterol by up to 26 percent in 8 to 12 weeks.

However, you also must consider the cons of RYRE. The FDA considers extracts that contain statins to be illegal. Monacolin K is the same as lovastatin, which is classified as a drug. There are still many RYRE products on the market claiming to have natural statins. The problem is that since the FDA does not regulate or oversee manufacturing, there's is no way to know what's in supplements available to buy. In addition, there may be mild side effects from RYRE extracts such as headaches, heartburn, and upset stomach. RYRE also may have similar side effects as the prescription version, including high liver and muscle enzymes, which can lead to muscle and liver problems. Lastly, since the extracts in the products vary and they aren't being regulated or tested, it's hard to determine the correct dosage.

How do you choose? One clear advantage of a pharmaceutical is that its active ingredient or drug is chemically pure, the dose is exact, and the label includes a package insert with in-depth information. An advantage of an herbal supplement may be that there are other natural ingredients along with the active ingredient that provides some benefit. But your choice is best determined by understanding the pros and cons, researching the supplement brands, and, most importantly, consulting with your doctor or other healthcare provider.

Current medicinal uses of herbs and botanical supplements

This section covers some commonly used herbs and botanicals that are sold as supplements for a variety of issues. Unfortunately, I don't have the space in this book to cover every possibility, so make sure to do your own investigation to find out if there's an herb or botanical supplement that may work for your unique situation.

WARNING

Before taking any supplement, be sure to do your research and note any interactions with medicines you're already taking. Many supplements sold for different health purposes do not have scientific evidence to support their use.

TIP

Many botanical supplements are considered safe but lack enough scientific evidence to support specific uses, so use your best judgment about whether to take a supplement or try to get some of these botanicals from food. For example, you may want to eat grapes for resveratrol, use turmeric in your food for its antioxidant properties, or drink ginger tea for your stomach because it may be helpful or because you like the taste. Taking a supplement in pill form is a different story, so check for dose and safety before taking.

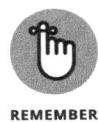

REMEMBER

The supplements I include in this section have been studied for their safety and use. The types of studies, number of participants, and the results sometimes vary, and the evidence to support their use may be weak or strong. In all cases, you should proceed by using your best judgment and consulting with your healthcare provider before choosing to use any supplements.

Immune support

If you're interested in supporting your immune system to help defend yourself from infections and reduce inflammation, you may want to investigate the following options:

>> **Echinacea (*Echinacea purpurea* or purple coneflower):** The chemicals in the plant may have cellular properties that support immunity, such as antibacterial activities including stimulating immune cells, inhibiting virus binding to host cells, and inhibiting inflammation. Echinacea may slightly help prevent these illnesses, but it doesn't appear to shorten the duration.

>> **Elderberry (*Sambucus nigra*):** A small number of studies have been done to evaluate elderberry's effects for cold and flu. Some scientific studies suggest that it may reduce some symptoms.

>> **Astragalus (*Astragalus membranaceus*):** This is used for centuries — often in combination with other herbs — to strengthen the immune system and fight infections.

>> **Turmeric:** Turmeric, which is also known as curcumin, has anti-inflammatory, antibacterial, antiviral, and antiparasitic benefits.

>> **Ginger:** This root has been used for centuries and helps digestion and blood circulation, which supports immunity. It's a potent anti-inflammatory and antioxidant.

>> **Garlic:** Garlic is known for its anti-inflammatory and antioxidant affects.

>> **Oregano:** This herb as well as its oil are natural antibiotics and anti-inflammatories.

>> **Cinnamon:** This offers antifungal, antibacterial, and anti-inflammatory benefits.

>> **Goldenseal:** This has been popular since the nineteenth century as an herb that supports the mucous tissues of the respiratory and GI tracts, which strengthens your body's defense barriers.

>> **Maitake and reishi:** These mushrooms contain beta-glucans, which contribute to supporting the immune system.

Adaptogens

Adaptogens are herbs that help the body adapt to stress. This section covers a few options:

>> **Ashwagandha (Indian ginseng, *Withania somnifera*):** Ashwagandha is known for its stress-reducing and mood-stabilizing effects. Clinical studies support that some ashwagandha preparations may be helpful for insomnia and stress and possibly for anxiety and other health conditions.

>> **Rhodiola (*Rhodiola rosea*):** Theses supplements are often used to increase energy, enhance endurance and mental clarity, resist effects of stress, manage depression, and improve athletic performance.

>> **Holy basil (*Ocimum sanctum*):** This medicinal herb, which is also known as tulsi, is used in Ayurvedic medicine. It is an antioxidant and could have positive effects on metabolism. It may also support stress relief, neurocognition and mood, and immune health.

Anti-inflammatory herbs

Inflammation is a natural process in response to stimuli in our body and may cause pain, heat, redness, and swelling. Uncontrolled inflammation in your body can lead to many disorders, including allergies, cancer, heart, and metabolic dysfunctions. Herbs and dietary supplements may offer a safe and effective alternative treatment for inflammation that can cause pain or chronic diseases.

>> **Turmeric (*Curcuma longa*):** Turmeric contains curcumin, known for its strong anti-inflammatory and antioxidant properties. Its use is promoted for arthritis, digestive disorders, respiratory infections, allergies, liver disease, and depression.

>> **Boswellia (*Boswellia serrata*):** This is used in Ayurvedic medicine for its anti-inflammatory effects, particularly for joint health. It may slightly improve pain in people with osteoarthritis.

>> **Spirulina (*Arthrospira platensis*):** Spirulina is a blue-green algae rich in nutrients and antioxidants. It contains some protein, B vitamins, and phycocyanin, which is an antioxidant.

>> **Nettle (*Urtica dioica*):** This plant is often used for its anti-inflammatory properties, as an aid for arthritis, and to support urinary health. Stinging nettle may also reduce production of histamine to prevent cells from releasing pro-inflammatory mediators. Nettle extract also inhibits the production of pro-inflammatory prostaglandins, reducing pain and inflammation.

>> **Ginger:** This root has been used to help reduce pain in osteoarthritis and reduce chronic inflammation in type 2 diabetics.

>> **Borage seeds:** These seeds contain a lot of omega-6-fatty acids and can help with inflammatory processes in conditions including eczema, psoriasis, arthritis, diabetic nerve pain, and depression.

>> **Evening primrose:** This seed oil contains fatty acids that have anti-inflammatory effects. It's often used for conditions related to menstruation and menopause like PMS, breast pain, and osteoporosis.

>> **Devil's claw:** This can be used orally for pain and in osteoarthritis and rheumatoid arthritis.

>> **Green tea or epigallocatechin gallate (EGCG):** A cup of tea is rich with polyphenols (antioxidants) and caffeine. It has been used for centuries, and benefits include decreasing risk of death from cardiovascular disease, regulating blood sugar, and preventing stroke. It also has anti-inflammatory and anti-cancer benefits for skin and can be used in an ointment for genital warts.

>> **Holy Basil:** This herb contains eucalyptol which is anti-inflammatory.

>> **Chamomile:** Chamomile is known for being calming and anti-inflammatory. This may be helpful for sleep.

>> **Rosemary:** This herb is in the same family as oregano and lavender and may have possible health benefits, including improved concentration, digestion, reduced muscle pain, and boosted immunity.

>> **Peppermint:** This plant has menthol in it and is used topically to relieve inflammation and pain. It is also useful orally for some GI conditions.

Digestive health

Digestive disorders cover a range of issues and symptoms that can include heart-burn, gas, and bloating. The following herbs may help relieve some symptoms associated with diagnosable issues such as gastroesophageal reflux disease (GERD), irritable bowel disease (IBD), gastritis, and colitis:

>> **Peppermint (*Mentha piperita*):** Both the plant leaves and peppermint oil (which is extracted from the flowering parts and leaves of the plant) are often used to relieve digestive discomfort, gas, and bloating and may help with IBS (irritable bowel syndrome). It may calm the stomach muscles and improve the flow of bile. It's not to be used if you have GERD because it acts to relax your sphincter muscle between your stomach and esophagus and will make the symptoms worse.

>> **Ginger (*Zingiber officinale*):** Various forms of ginger are often used to relieve digestive issues and inflammation. It has been used in China for more than 2,500 years. There have been many studies showing that ginger may be helpful for nausea and vomiting during pregnancy and possibly in other cases of nausea. It is considered safe when used as the root or as a supplement.

>> **Slippery elm (*Ulmus rubra*):** Slippery elm is used to soothe the digestive tract and reduce inflammation in conditions like gastritis or irritable bowel syndrome (IBS).

Mood and cognitive support

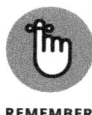

REMEMBER

Mood disorders, including anxiety and depression, can be serious. Sometimes alternative or natural remedies may help alleviate symptoms, but when your condition is serious, be sure to consult with a psychiatrist. Improving your memory, relieving brain fog, or enhancing cognitive performance might be helped with some herbs described here:

>> **St. John's wort (*Hypericum perforatum*):** St. John's wort is widely used for mild to moderate depression and anxiety. Studies show that it might also be helpful for menopausal symptoms. It interacts with many medications, so you shouldn't take it without first seeking your doctor's advice.

>> **Ginkgo biloba (*Ginkgo biloba*):** This one is known for improving cognitive function, memory, and circulation. There is no conclusive scientific evidence that it helps dementia or cognitive decline. It's safe in moderate amounts but may interact with some medications.

>> **Lemon balm (*Melissa officinalis*):** This calming herb is used to reduce anxiety and improve mood. There also is some promising evidence that shows that lemon balm can assist in improving some lipid markers.

Heart and circulatory health

If you're looking to support your cardiovascular health, eating a heart healthy diet and exercising are important. If you want to supplement your healthy lifestyle with herbs, here are a few that may help:

- » **Hawthorn (*Crataegus* species):** Hawthorn is traditionally used to support cardiovascular health and improve circulation. In Germany, this has been used therapeutically for years for certain heart conditions with good results.

- » **Garlic (*Allium sativum*):** Garlic is known for its heart health benefits, including lowering cholesterol and supporting healthy blood pressure. The most reliable data supports that garlic supplements may reduce total cholesterol and LDL cholesterol levels if your levels are high. However, garlic supplements may have no effect on blood pressure, cancer, or common colds.

- » **Cayenne pepper (*Capsicum annuum*):** Cayenne pepper contains capsaicin, which is purported to help blood circulation and heart health. It can be useful as a topical cream or patch for moderate pain relief.

Hormonal support

Hormonal support usually refers to male and female sex hormones and is often helpful for women going through menopause. For men, the support is usually around effects on testosterone levels resulting in improvement in sexual wellness and muscle building. Here are some supplements that may be helpful:

- » **Black cohosh (*Actaea racemosa*):** This may alleviate menopausal symptoms like hot flashes and night sweats. It has been used for decades, and side effects are mild if any. Black cohosh is in a number of over-the-counter products for menopause.

- » **Dong quai (*Angelica sinensis*):** This herb, known as "female ginseng," is commonly used in traditional medicine to support female reproductive health.

- » **Maca root (*Lepidium meyenii*):** Maca root is used to boost energy, balance hormones, and improve sexual health in men and women. It's helpful in men to boost sexual desire.

- » **Fenugreek:** This is a common Indian spice that may help support normal testosterone levels in men.

- » **Korean ginseng:** This root is different than American ginseng and may support stress management and male vitality.

>> **Tribulus terrestris:** This plant, also known as gokshura, is a small leafy plant used traditionally in Ayurvedic and traditional Chinese medicine to enhance male sex drive and maintain a healthy urinary tract. It also contains polyphenols that have general wellness benefits.

>> **Evening primrose oil:** This supplement is used topically for skin and orally for PMS and menopausal symptoms.

Skin and hair health

Some topical products for skin and hair contain herbs and botanicals with proposed benefits. Here, I list several of these that you may see on the labels of your beauty products or on supplements meant for skin and hair health:

>> **Aloe vera (*Aloe barbadensis Miller*):** Aloe vera is applied topically for skin healing, burns, and inflammation. Clinical research supports using it topically for acne, burn healing, herpes simplex, and psoriasis. Evidence for using it orally for IBS or ulcerative colitis is less clear but is hopeful.

>> **Calendula (Calendula officinalis):** Calendula oil is safe to use topically for skin inflammation and wound healing. It's known for its anti-inflammatory and antiseptic properties, and it helps with healing wounds, soothing dry skin, and reducing redness.

>> **Chamomile:** This plant soothes irritated skin, reduces inflammation, and promotes healing. Chamomile also has antioxidants that help protect the skin.

>> **Tea tree oil:** This oil is a powerful antibacterial agent that helps fight acne and other skin infections. It also has antifungal and anti-inflammatory properties.

>> **Green tea:** This tea is rich in antioxidants. It helps protect the skin from premature aging and damage from free radicals. It also has anti-inflammatory properties and can help calm irritated skin.

>> **Rosehip oil:** This oil is high in vitamin C and essential fatty acids, so it helps with skin regeneration, reduces signs of aging, and improves skin texture.

>> **Witch hazel:** This natural astringent helps tighten and tone skin. It's also great for reducing inflammation and treating acne.

>> **Turmeric:** Known for its anti-inflammatory and antioxidant properties, turmeric helps with redness, acne, and brightening the skin.

>> **Rosemary:** Rosemary improves circulation to the scalp, promotes hair growth, and strengthens hair follicles. It's also believed to prevent dandruff and reduce hair thinning.

>> **Peppermint:** This oil may stimulate the scalp, increases circulation, and promotes hair growth. It also has a cooling effect that can help with dandruff and itchiness.

>> **Saw palmetto:** This is often used to prevent hair loss, particularly in cases of male pattern baldness, by blocking the metabolism of testosterone, which can contribute to hair thinning.

>> **Burdock root:** This root can detoxify and purify the scalp and helps reduce dandruff, improve scalp health, and stimulate hair growth.

>> **Amla:** Also known as Indian gooseberry, this plant is rich in vitamin C and antioxidants and strengthens hair, prevents premature graying, and nourishes the scalp.

>> **Fenugreek:** Fenugreek seeds are high in protein and nicotinic acid, which help strengthen the hair, prevent dandruff, and reduce hair loss.

>> **Lavender:** This plant is known for its calming properties, but it also may help with acne, dryness, and irritation. Lavender oil can improve circulation to the scalp and help with hair growth and preventing hair loss.

>> **Nettle:** This is rich in vitamins and minerals like iron, silica, and vitamin A and may promote hair growth and strengthen hair.

>> **Polypodium leucotomos:** This plant is a species of fern that may be good for psoriasis, atopic dermatitis, prevention of sunburn, and squamous cell carcinoma.

Liver and detox support

Your body is very efficient at detoxing and cleansing itself. Herbs marketed for detox and liver support tend to be rich in antioxidants to protect the liver against free radical damage and inflammation.

>> **Milk thistle (*Silybum marianum*):** This plant is known for supporting liver detoxification and regeneration. Milk thistle is a strong antioxidant that supports healthy liver function by defending against oxidative stress. Studies are promising, and milk thistle is well tolerated. Small studies also show some benefits for diabetes and hepatitis C.

>> **Dandelion root (*Taraxacum officinale*):** Dandelion root is often used as a liver tonic and diuretic for detoxification. Some laboratory studies also show it has some anti-inflammatory, antioxidant, and antiviral properties. It may also support the production of bile, which aids in digestion of fats and rids them from the liver.

>> **Artichoke leaf extract:** This extract contains silymarin similar to milk thistle and promotes liver function. The leaf extracts are richer than the stem and root in flavonoids that protect the liver.

Sleep and relaxation

If you experience insomnia, there are some herbal remedies that are very effective for some people:

>> **Valerian root (*Valeriana officinalis*):** Valerian root is commonly used to promote relaxation and help with insomnia. Research is limited and inconsistent, and the American Academy of Sleep Medicine recommended against its use in 2017.

>> **Chamomile (*Matricaria chamomilla*):** Known for its calming effects, chamomile is often used as a mild sedative to promote sleep. Some research shows chamomile may benefit anxiety, but there's little other evidence to support its usefulness.

>> **Lavender (*Lavandula angustifolia*):** You likely already know that lavender is used in aromatherapy and teas for relaxation and sleep support. Oral use is believed to be safe. Topical and aromatherapeutic use or use of soaps and cosmetics has not been studied enough to know if evidence supports use for anxiety, relaxation, or sleep. However, it certainly smells good and isn't harmful, so it's worth a try.

>> **Cannabidiol (CBD):** CBD is a nonpsychoactive substance that works on natural receptors in your body to potentially reduce anxiety and promote sleep. It does not make you high and is legal in 47 states (except for Idaho, Nebraska, and South Dakota).

Weight management

Weight loss and maintenance can be difficult, and there is no magic pill or herb for them. Healthy eating and a good lifestyle are the best ways to address weight control, but these herbs may assist you in your overall plan to control and manage your weight:

>> **Garcinia cambogia (*Garcinia gummi-gutta*):** This is used in weight-loss supplements due to its potential appetite-suppressing effects.

>> **Green tea extract (*Camellia sinensis*):** This extract contains antioxidants like epigallocatechin gallate (EGCG) that may help with fat burning and metabolism. It may increase metabolism, which may help in weight loss. Some studies show that green tea and ginger and possibly with capsaicin (the spicy component of chili peppers) may promote weight loss.

Antioxidant and antiaging

In addition to the herbs mentioned throughout the other sections that have anti-inflammatory effects, the following herbs are rich in antioxidants:

TIP

>> **Green tea and green tea extract (*Camellia sinensis*):** Green tea is rich in polyphenols, especially EGCG, and has powerful antioxidant effects. Many studies on green and other teas with caffeine and/or EGCG show some benefits on metabolism, mental alertness, heart disease, blood pressure, and cholesterol management.

    Read more about polyphenols later in this chapter in the "Using plant polyphenols" section.

>> **Acai berry (*Euterpe oleracea*):** This fruit is known for its high antioxidant content, which may support antiaging and immune function.

>> **Resveratrol:** Resveratrol is a polyphenol found in red grapes, berries, and certain plants. It has antioxidant properties and is believed to support cardiovascular and longevity benefits. It's a sirtuin activator; sirtuin is a family of enzymes that are involved in metabolic regulation. Activating the enzyme SIRT1 in particular may slow down the aging process of cells.

Explaining Botanical Compounds

Botanicals are plants or plant parts that have been used for medical purposes throughout history. Herbs are a subgroup of botanicals in that they are plants with leaves, seeds, or flowers. It's estimated that there may be more than 10,000 types of phytochemicals — plant based bioactive compounds — thousands of which may have health-related effects. Figure 7-1 shows the types of phytochemicals.

In this section, I discuss some of the possible benefits of common phytochemicals, including caffeine, turmeric and polyphenols

Benefitting from caffeine

Caffeine is an alkaloid found in coffee, tea, chocolate and as an additive in some foods, beverages, and supplements. Much of the world and an estimated 90 percent of the U.S. population uses caffeine in one form or the other. Much research has been done on its use; it's considered safe in quantities up to 400 mg (or 4 cups a day of coffee or tea) if you do not experience any side effects. Side effects can include gut distress, feeling jittery or anxious, and insomnia.

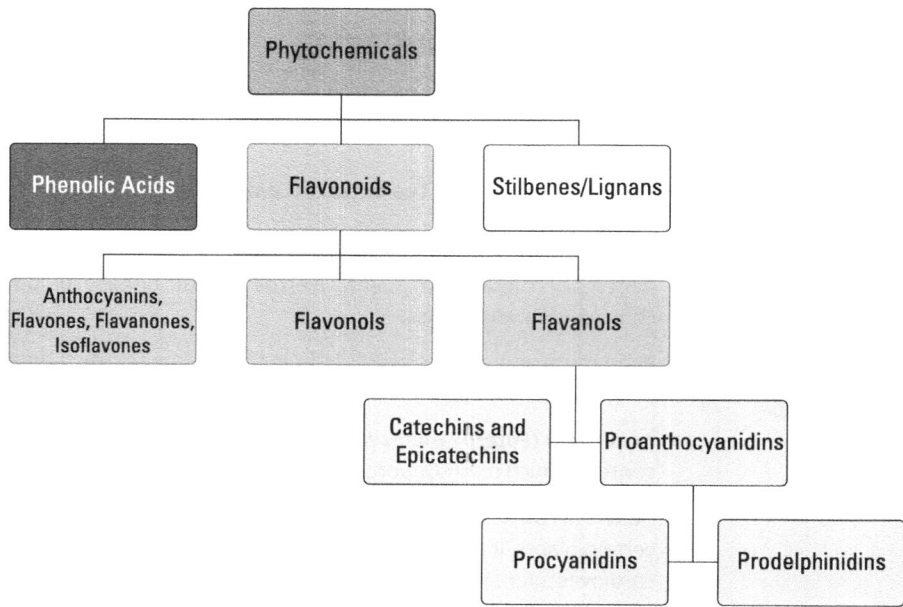

FIGURE 7-1:
The different
categories of
phytochemicals.

Many studies look at coffee consumption but not necessarily isolated caffeine consumption. Coffee contains more than 100 bioactive compounds aside from caffeine, such as phenolic compounds, chlorogenic acids, tannin, thiamin, spermidine, trigonelline, lignans, and minerals like potassium and magnesium. Any or all of these could also be contributing to benefits from coffee.

Caffeine is rapidly absorbed into your blood, and blood levels can last for three to four hours. Caffeine is a central nervous system (CNS) stimulant that acts at the neurotransmitter level in the brain. It can boost dopamine and serotonin, both of which are involved in mood regulation. It blocks the action of adenosine, which is an inhibitory neurotransmitter that depresses the CNS to promote sleep and relaxation. If caffeine interferes with this, you will feel more awake. You may have experienced this increase in mental alertness that helps to focus better. You also may have noticed that coffee enhances your mood as well. A large study in more than 50,000 women who were part of the Nurses' Health Study found that women coffee drinkers were at a lower risk of becoming depressed. They also found that as the number of cups per day increased, the risk of depression was lower.

Some studies have shown that caffeine can improve athletic performance, which may be because it improves focus and energy. It may increase adrenaline, which can increase performance. Another possible reason is that caffeine increases your ability to burn fat, which can then be used as energy. It may also improve muscle performance.

Epidemiological studies have shown that moderate coffee consumption of two to five cups is associated with a lower risk of cardiovascular disease, lower blood pressure, and improved metabolism. In a recent 2024 review of health supplements of caffeine, it was found that drinking coffee (which contains other antioxidants and neuroprotective properties) prevents progressive neurodegenerative diseases, such as Alzheimer's and Parkinson's diseases.

Spicing up with curcumin

Curcumin is in turmeric, a plant in the ginger family; it's what gives turmeric its yellow color. The rhizome (underground stem) is used as a spice and a traditional medicine.

According to the NCCIH, there has been much research on turmeric and curcumin, and they have many interesting biological activities. However, the understanding of the health effects is inconclusive. For one thing, it's challenging to study the effects in animals and people because curcumin is unstable chemically and has a low bioavailability (how well a substance is absorbed into the blood after ingestion). Also, curcumin products have many other substances in them and products differ greatly from each other. It's hard to isolate what happens as a result of curcumin, and it's difficult to interpret results.

Although there isn't a lot of scientific proof that curcumin use has health effects, there is some history of its use. For example, turmeric is used in Ayurveda and other traditional medicines. It may act as an antioxidant but may require very high doses. Cell and animal studies show it may block reactive oxygen species (ROS). Several studies show that curcumin may act as an antioxidant and reduce inflammation and reduce risk of cardiovascular disease. It is possible that curcumin helps reduce pain in people with osteoarthritis.

TECHNICAL
STUFF

Many antioxidants work by blocking the damaging effects of reactive oxygen species or ROS. ROS are molecules that have an oxygen molecule and one unpaired electron. They are produced naturally in the cells and are a part of normal cellular metabolism, but they can also cause damage if there are too many of them. Your body has natural antioxidants that mitigate the damage ROS do to cells, but if ROS are out of balance, they can contribute to the development of free radical–mediated diseases. This oxidative stress can contribute to circulatory, respiratory, and nervous system conditions.

Using plant polyphenols

A variety of plant phytochemicals called polyphenols are found in foods we eat and in supplements. There are more than 8,000 types of polyphenols, so I can't even begin to cover all of them here!

Most are considered antioxidants and therefore are anti-inflammatory. They may reduce the risk of chronic diseases including cardiovascular disease, diabetes, neurodegenerative diseases, and certain cancers. Good scientific studies show that eating fruits, vegetables, whole grains, seeds, and nuts is healthy, and people who do this may not suffer as much from chronic diseases. Studies also show that people who have diets rich in polyphenols have lower death risks than those who don't.

The recommendation is that you get these plant nutrients from the plants themselves by eating whole foods as much as possible. But if you're like many people who don't get enough plant-based foods, then supplements may be necessary.

Here, I've listed some types of polyphenols:

>> **Flavonoids** come from quercetin and catechins in fruits. Quercetin is found in fruits, vegetables and tea and may increase energy production in muscles and improve blood flow throughout your body. It's mostly been studied in athletes in small studies, and the limited available data show no benefit. Flavonoids are also found in wine and dark chocolate. Anthocyanidins are also flavonoids found in red, purple, and blue fruits and vegetables.

>> **Luteolin** is a biologically active flavonoid found in plants like lettuce, celery, and green pepper. Studies continue to support health benefits that have been used as natural remedies throughout history, such as anti-inflammatory-related chronic disease. It can also support memory and the nervous system with its antioxidant abilities.

>> **Polyphenolic amides** come from capsaicin in chili peppers. Supplements of capsaicin are purported to increase energy use, burn fat, and decrease appetite. It has also been studied for weight loss. Too much can cause gastrointestinal (GI) issues, and the long-term safety isn't known.

>> **Phenolic acids** are widely distributed in plants and foods including cereals, legumes, oils, seeds, dried fruits, fruits, vegetables, coffee, and herbs. They are antioxidants and can alter cell signaling pathways.

» **Catechins** include ECGC, which is a polyphenol found in green tea. It has antioxidant and anti-inflammatory properties and may increase metabolism.

» **Polyphenol stilbene** comes from resveratrol, which is a plant-based antioxidant that helps plants under stress or injury and may have antiaging effects in people. A lot of research has been done on resveratrol, which is found in grapes, red wine, and grape juice. It is an anti-inflammatory and may have neuroprotective effects. It may help brain function and be a preventative for heart disease and stroke. It may increase levels of high-density lipoprotein (HDL) cholesterol (the "good" cholesterol) and lower LDL (the "bad" cholesterol). It's purported to be an antiaging supplement, but more research is needed.

WARNING

Red wine contains about 12 mg of resveratrol per liter. You may need about between 40 and 500 mg per day to see benefit. This means that you would need to drink at least 3 liters of red wine for the benefit of the resveratrol — which is too much for anyone! A supplement is a better option.

Chapter **8**

Discovering Amino Acids and Protein Supplements

Adequate intake of amino acids and protein is essential for human health. Amino acids are the building blocks of proteins, like the beads on a strand of pearls, that are strung together in different patterns to create different types of proteins. Each gene (strand of DNA) that you have in your body gets translated into protein. After that, each protein can be further modified. Scientists who study this field estimate that there are between 10,000 to billions of different proteins.

You need the building blocks of the proteins — amino acids — so that proteins are naturally formed in the body. The pool of amino acids come from your food intake as well as the constant turnover of proteins in your cells.

In this chapter, I present information first on protein and supplement needs and uses. Then I discuss essential amino acids, their importance in metabolism, and the use of supplementation.

Protein Powders and Drinks

Protein is made up of amino acids, the basic building block of all proteins. In your body, protein is synthesized from a pool of amino acids in all cells. When you eat protein, it gets broken down into amino acids, which then join the animo acid pool in your body. They're transported via your blood to all your tissues and organs, including muscle cells, where they are used to synthesize proteins. (See Figure 8-1.)

Schematic of protein breakdown and synthesis

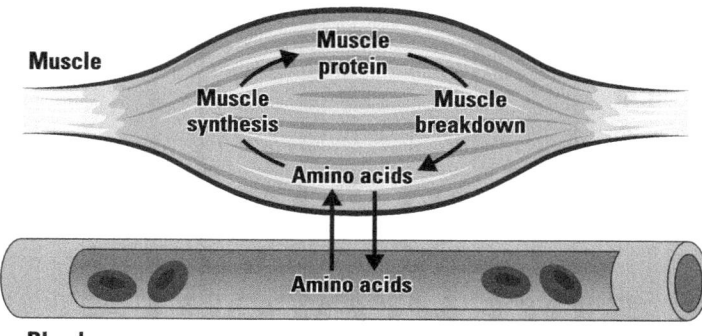

FIGURE 8-1: Amino acids from the blood and from protein breakdown are used to make protein in the muscle tissue.

There are at least 10,000 proteins in your body that have a variety of functions, including enzymes that catalyze biochemical reactions, components of your muscles, and hemoglobin that carries oxygen.

Protein intake is very important, and research in many studies with tens of thousands of subjects show that the quality of the protein and the "protein package" is more important than the amount of protein intake. The protein package refers to what is in the rest of the protein source. For example, beef contains a lot of protein but also has saturated fats, which are correlated with cardiovascular disease and shorter lifespans. A less "bad fat"-filled protein option is salmon and other fish. You also can get protein from plant sources, which have even fewer fats associated with them.

If you don't get enough protein from your food, then a supplement is a good idea. How do you know if you're getting enough? Since protein is responsible for so many of your bodily functions, there are many possible signs, such as fatigue, mood changes, getting sick a lot, healing slowly, or hair, nail or skin problems.

A good way to calculate how much protein you get in a day is to keep a food diary for a few days or a week in an app and use that to determine your average weekly protein intake. It might be good to get used to knowing how much protein there is in the foods you normally eat. If you have Greek yogurt (18 g per cup) for breakfast, chicken breast (one-half breast, 28 g) on a salad for lunch, and salmon (fillet, 30 g) for dinner, you've had about 66 g for the day. This is plenty for most people, and that's not even including other protein that might be in other foods you eat.

Most people get sufficient protein from their foods, but there are times when protein or amino acid supplements may be useful. The best food sources for protein is animal protein because they contain all the essential amino acids or "complete" proteins. Fish, chicken, pork, beef, and bison have a lot of protein — about 20 to 40 grams depending on the portion size. Eggs and low-fat dairy are also great sources. An egg has about 6 g protein, and low-fat Greek yogurt can have as much as 20 g in a cup.

TIP

Vegetarian sources of protein don't contain complete proteins — they don't have all the essential amino acids — so it's always good to have a variety of foods each day. Eating a colorful diet helps to achieve this! The best vegetarian protein sources include nuts and nut butters, whey protein powder (if you include dairy in your diet), beans, tempeh, tofu, chickpeas, oats, lentils, pumpkin seeds, hemp hearts, chia seeds, and many raw vegetables.

Building muscles

There have been many studies on protein supplements and exercise. Protein is necessary for building, maintaining, and repairing muscle tissue. Exercise affects the muscle tissue and protein metabolism. Specifically, regular resistant exercise results in gradual accumulation of myofibrillar protein and increase in muscle size. When you do an aerobic workout, you also get an accumulation of protein in your muscle and improved mitochondrial metabolism that increases your cells' ability to use oxygen, which is helpful in converting stored energy into a usable form of energy. This powers up your muscles with adenosine triphosphate (ATP)!

When you get enough protein every day, you get the essential amino acids necessary for muscle protein synthesis. The protein feeds into the amino acid pool in your body (refer to Figure 8-1), which is then used for protein synthesis in the muscle.

How much you need depends on how much you exercise. If you mostly sit at your desk and work all day aside from a one-hour workout each day, you probably don't need extra protein. If you're a weightlifter or marathoner, you need more. If you're doing resistance training or other exercise to build muscle, you want to be sure to eat some protein within two hours post-workout. Muscle continues to be synthesized and also broken down for the next 24 hours, so you want to get enough protein to support this process.

REMEMBER

The recommended daily allowance (RDA) for protein intake is 0.8 grams per kilogram of body weight per day (g/kg/day) for healthy adults and 0.85 g/kg/day for adolescents. This translates to 0.36 grams per pound of body weight for an adult. For example, the recommended amount of protein for a 180-pound man is 64 g/day. For a 130-pound adult, the amount is 54 g/day. The average man in the United States gets 100 g/day, and the average woman gets 69 g/day. Most people get more than the RDA. Up to 2 g/kg/day is considered safe. A high protein intake for too long can overwork the kidneys, which are responsible for filtering waste products from your blood.

Athletes need 1.2 to 1.7 g/kg/day. It is recommended that athletes consume about 20 g of protein within two hours of working out and then having more protein every three to five hours throughout the day. There is some evidence that about 10 g of protein before sleeping can build muscle overnight. Two to three times the RDA is considered safe for an athlete to consume.

TIP

Recreational athletes (runners, gym rats, weekend warriors) doing moderate training of one or two hours a day, three to five days a week should eat between 1.2 to 1.4 grams of protein per kilogram of weight per day (g/kg/day). Elite athletes will need more — between 1.6 g/kg/day and 2.2 g/kg/day — depending on the number of hours of activity and the type of sport. Elite athletes include endurance athletes like runners and cyclists, strength and power athletes including sprinters and weightlifters, and team sports athletes such as basketball or soccer players.

TIP

Many elderly people eat less food as they get older, so a supplement may be the best way for them to get enough protein to prevent the breakdown of muscle. A protein shake using a scoop of protein powder, low-fat milk, kefir or soy milk makes a good high-protein drink as a meal, snack, or post-workout recovery drink.

Controlling appetite and aiding weight loss

It's important to get enough protein from your diet or supplements to control your appetite and manage your weight. Of the macronutrients (carbohydrate, protein, fat, alcohol), protein is the most satiating, meaning that it helps keep you feeling full because it increases the satiety hormones PYY (peptide YY) and GLP-1 (glucagon-like peptide-1). It also stimulates ghrelin (the hunger hormone) more effectively than fat and carbohydrates. Protein takes more time and energy to digest than fat and carbohydrates, so it sticks around longer, keeping you feeling full. Many clinical trials have shown that high-protein diets are good for weight loss, although weight loss and body composition is complicated. Also, a recent meta-analysis concluded that the amount of protein needed for weight loss is not clear.

Family history, your personal weight history, eating behavior, activity level, and genetics are important in weight-loss or weight-management success. This is why a personalized approach to weight loss can help you get started. Changing the foods you eat, controlling the portion sizes, creating a healthy food environment, and cutting back on restaurants and takeout are all things that can help. Specific genes have been isolated as "fat genes" that may be correlated with overweight or obesity, although having the gene or multiple genes doesn't necessarily mean that you will be overweight or obese. Although weight control is complicated, consuming more protein as part of a healthy diet and lifestyle may help with weight management.

Whether you are overweight, obese, or normal weight, it's recommended that you get between 10 percent and 25 percent of your calories as protein. The more protein in your diet, the more you might reduce carbohydrates and fats, which can help with weight loss. Because protein is more satiating, it's generally agreed that a higher-protein, lower-carbohydrate intake will help you lose weight.

Improving bone and skin

Collagen is the most abundant protein in your body and is the major structural protein in bones. Collagen creates the scaffolding for calcium and phosphorous in the formation of bone in your body. Collagen is synthesized in cells from the amino acid pool in your cells. Adequate protein is needed for bone remodeling and repair. Any protein, whether from food or a supplement will contribute to your amino acid pool and protein synthesis. With aging, bone breakdown can happen faster than repairs are made, leading to bone loss. Recent studies show that older adults should take more than the RDA for protein to prevent bone loss.

Collagen is also found in skin, hair, nails, tendons, and cartilage and helps to maintain skin elasticity, volume, and moisture. It helps make up proteins such as keratin that form skin, hair, and nails. Adequate protein will help keep your skin healthy.

Collagen supplements are currently popular and are advertised as something to reduce wrinkles and improve hydration and elasticity, so you may be wondering if they can actually improve your skin. Studies on collagen supplements do show some improvements among the people who take the supplements. However, the problem is that most of the products contain other vitamins and minerals and sometimes include additional substances such as hyaluronic acid. However, a randomized controlled trial (RCT) and a 2019 meta-analysis of 11 studies found that daily ingestion of a specific collagen hydrolysate, which contains prolylhydroxyproline (Pro-Hyp) and hydroxyprolylglycine (Hyp-Gly), improved skin hydration, elasticity, and roughness. This may be particularly beneficial as you age.

TIP

The bottom line is that adequate protein in your diet will help your bones and skin. Collagen hydrolysates or peptides (collagen broken down to smaller parts) may help your skin stay hydrated and healthier especially as you age.

Producing hormones, enzymes, and more

Proteins have many other functions in the body including the following:

>> Growth and maintenance of tissues

>> Catalyzing thousands of biochemical reactions

>> Acting as chemical messengers between cells, tissues, and organs

>> Acting as a buffer to keep the pH of your body regulated

>> Maintaining the body's fluid balance

>> Protecting against viruses and bacteria

>> Storing or transporting nutrients throughout body

>> Being broken down and used for energy, if necessary

Shopping for protein supplements

Here are things to look for when researching protein supplements:

TIP

>> Read the product labels to evaluate the quality and purity.

>> Check the kind of protein used in the product. It may include whey, soy, pea, or casein.

>> The first product on the ingredient list should be the protein.

>> The fewer the ingredients, the better.

>> Avoid added sugars and other fillers, especially if you can't pronounce it. An example of a filler is maltodextrin, which can spike insulin.

Some products may include added vitamins, minerals, and amino acids. Depending on your needs, this can be a good thing, but if you're simply looking for a protein supplement, added ingredients may just increase cost. Make sure to check the serving size. Generally, one scoop may provide 20 to 25 grams of protein, which is approximately 30 percent of what many people need in a day.

WARNING

Beware of claims. For example, if label says "low-carb," read the ingredient list to make sure it falls in line with that claim.

Essential Amino Acids

Amino acids are the building blocks of proteins and are part of other biological processes such as neurotransmitter synthesis and other biochemical reactions. There are 20 amino acids that get incorporated into proteins. This process is called translation, and the order in which they are added comes from ribonucleic acid (RNA), which is transcribed from deoxyribonucleic acid (DNA). Nine of these amino acids are *essential*, which means you must get them from foods.

TECHNICAL STUFF

The essential amino acids and their RDA is based on body weight. Table 8-1 lists the essential amino acids and the amounts needed for every 2.2 pounds of weight. To calculate how much you need, adjust for your weight.

TABLE 8-1   **Essential Amino Acids and Their RDA**

Amino Acid	Milligrams per 2.2 Pounds Body Weight
Histidine	14 mg
Isoleucine	19 mg
Leucine	42 mg
Lysine	38 mg
Methionine	19 mg
Phenylalanine	33 mg
Threonine	20 mg
Tryptophan	5 mg
Valine	24 mg

The nonessential amino acids (meaning your body can make them, and you don't need to get them from food or supplements) are alanine, arginine, asparagine, aspartic acid, cysteine, glutamic acid, glutamine, glycine, proline, serine, and tyrosine.

Conditionally essential amino acids are not essential except in times of illness and stress. Conditionally essential amino acids include arginine, cysteine, glutamine, tyrosine, glycine, proline, and serine. Some amino acids are both nonessential and conditionally essential.

Another function of amino acids in addition to protein formation is that they're precursors to (used to synthesize) other biological compounds. For example, tryptophan is a precursor for the neurotransmitter serotonin.

Signaling in your brain: neurotransmitters

Neurotransmitters send signals from neuron to neuron or neuron to tissue and are important to the nervous system. According to the Cleveland Clinic, there may be more than 100 known neurotransmitters, and there may possibly be many others that haven't been discovered yet.

The brain has a layer called the blood-brain barrier (BBB) that protects it from anything potentially harmful in the blood. Because of this, only certain substances can get into the brain. Glucose is one thing that can get through, and it's what the brain uses for energy (rather than fats or proteins). Certain amino acids have special transport mechanisms to get through the BBB. Table 8-2 lists the amino acid, the neurotransmitters that are synthesized from the amino acid, and their functions.

TABLE 8-2   **Amino Acids, Neurotransmitters, and Their Functions**

Amino Acid	Product	Functions
Tryptophan	Serotonin,	Mood, pain, food intake, arousal
	Melatonin*	Sleep
Tyrosine phenylalanine	Dopamine	Motor function, mood, arousal
	Norepinephrine	Arousal, anxiety, memory
	Epinephrine	Fight or flight response
Histidine	Histamine	Food intake, arousal, thermoregulation
Arginine	Nitric oxide	Arousal, anxiety, memory
Threonine	Glycine	Motor function
Glutamate	GABA (Gamma-aminobutyric acid) (inhibits)	Stress, anxiety, sleep
Glutamate	Glutamate (excitatory)	Stress, anxiety, sleep

Adapted from National Library of Medicine

Note that melatonin isn't considered a neurotransmitter technically, but it acts as one and is a commonly used supplement.

The BBB transport system works to regulate how much amino acids can get into the brain. It's important to have adequate blood levels of these amino acids for proper functioning of your brain and cognition. As with other nutrients, if you're deficient, then you may feel side effects. Animal and human research shows that sometimes deficiencies or excess can affect these functions.

Many foods contain these amino acids, but there isn't much evidence about their bioavailability and effects in people. A 2020 RCT in healthy middle-aged and older adults showed that intake of seven essential amino acids improved cognitive function and psychological and social function. This is encouraging, but. the significance of dietary neurotransmitters and their precursor intake needs to be further investigated to gather more data about their bioavailability and clinical implications.

Growing and repairing tissue

Leucine, isoleucine, and valine are called branched-chain amino acids (BCAA) and are particularly important for muscle protein synthesis and repair. Leucine acts to stimulate muscle protein synthesis by activating the mTOR pathway. BCAAs reduce muscle protein breakdown by serving as an energy source in the muscle. BCAAs can also reduce the severity and duration of muscle soreness after intense exercise.

A 2021 meta-analysis of more than 40 studies demonstrated that supplementation with either arginine and glutamine can positively influence wound healing or parameters related to healing. Arginine supplementation was significant in relation to hydroxyproline content, and glutamine supplementation had significant effect on nitrogen balance, patient mortality, and other measures related to the biochemical processes of wound healing.

Boosting your immunity

Amino acids contribute to the production of antibodies in your cells that recognize and destroy harmful foreign substances in your body. Amino acids support functions involved in the immune response, cellular repair and inflammation, and protein synthesis.

Cells of the immune system require energy in the form of ATP just as other cells in the body do. Amino acid metabolism contributes to this and also the synthesis of nucleotides, the building blocks of RNA and DNA, and other important biochemicals to support growth, proliferation, and function of immune cells.

Immune cells need glutamine — a conditionally essential amino acid that serves as a fuel for lymphocytes, macrophages, and neutrophils (cells involved in rapid immune response). Glutamine is also vital for gut health and preventing bacterial movement across the gut lining.

Arginine is important for immune function by boosting nitric oxide, which is involved in antiviral, antibacterial, and antifungal defense. Arginine also enhances T-cell function, which can help fight infections.

Leucine activates the mTOR pathway, which is important in activating and proliferation of the immunity boosting T- and B-cells. It also aids in protein synthesis to boost immune cell proliferation and response to pathogens.

Lastly, histidine is involved in the production of histamine, which helps to dilate blood vessels and get immune cells to an injury or infection site. Histamine also helps to improve immune cell response to pathogens and regulate an inflammatory response.

Breaking down your food

Digestion is a complicated process from beginning to end and involves proteins along the GI track. Your stomach, small intestine and pancreas — particularly the pancreas — produce digestive enzymes.

REMEMBER

Enzymes are proteins, and proteins are synthesized in the cells using amino acids as building blocks.

There are three main types of digestive enzymes:

>> Amylases break down complex carbohydrates into simple sugars that can be absorbed into the blood.

>> Lipases break down triglycerides (fatty acids connected to glycerol).

>> Proteases break down proteins into amino acids and peptides.

Two other enzymes important for digestion are the following:

>> Lactase breaks down lactose or milk sugar.

>> Sucrase breaks down sucrose (or table sugar) into glucose and fructose.

Providing energy

Amino acids can feed into the Krebs cycle or tricarboxylic acid cycle, a biochemical pathway involved in cellular energy production in the form of ATP. Some amino acids can also feed into the biochemical pathway that synthesizes glucose, an energy source in your body. When you need energy, you first use your blood glucose for cellular energy production. Then the storage form of glucose, called glycogen, is used by breaking down to glucose that feeds into the energy-producing pathways.

Once your liver stores are used up, you break down fat for energy. Protein and amino acids can be available to energy production once you've run out of glucose and fats. Ideally, you want to spare your body protein for energy production and instead use it to build muscle. If you're trying to lose weight, it's important you eat enough protein so you don't lose muscle as you lose fat and weight.

Helping you sleep

There is some evidence that 5-hydroxy-tryptophan (5-HTP), L-tryptophan, gamma-aminobutyric acid (GABA), and theanine alone or in combination help with temporary stress relief and improving sleep quality. Studies show that supplementing the diet with 5-HTP and tryptophan can help maintain healthy brain levels of serotonin. Serotonin is a brain neurotransmitter that's important for mood, emotions, and sleep.

GABA is a nonprotein amino acid that's important for central nervous system function and is a factor in human behavior. Specifically, it's involved in stress regulation, memory, mood, pain, and sleep regulation.

Theanine is found in green tea and is associated with a relaxed state. Sometimes theanine is added to melatonin supplements for sleep. It has also been found to enhance alpha brain wave activity, which is associated with a relaxed but alert state. Theanine helps with the release of GABA, which aids other neurotransmitters, dopamine and serotonin.

Amino Acids Supplements for Specific Claims

Most people get enough amino acids from their diets. However, there are some situations where amino acids supplements may be helpful.

Branched-chain amino acids for athletes

Valine, leucine, and isoleucine are the three essential BCAAs that are available as supplements. They are metabolized by skeletal muscle to provide energy to muscles during exercise. Athletes and exercise enthusiasts often take them to alleviate fatigue, improve athletic performance, and stimulate muscle recovery after exercise.

There have been a number of short-term clinical studies that show some improved performance and muscle recovery and decreased muscle soreness compared with those who took a placebo. Little evidence has been reported for improved performance in endurance-related aerobic activities or increased muscle mass from training.

Perking up your mood

There is much interest in the effects on amino acids, brain function and mood. Specifically, 5-HTP is a precursor for the synthesis of serotonin, and L-tyrosine is a precursor for the synthesis of dopamine. The availability and balance of these precursors can help optimize their transport into the brain and thus the synthesis of serotonin and dopamine, which are involved in mood. A few studies have shown that tryptophan or tyrosine supplementation can improve mood or reduce anxiety in people who have mood disorders.

WARNING

Much more research needs to be done to show that amino acid supplementation will help mood, including anxiety and depression.

Giving you energy

Getting all the essential amino acids and maintaining a balance of them are critical for metabolism. This can usually be accomplished by eating a balanced diet. It's difficult to know if you're getting a balance without analyzing your diet closely. However, by eating enough fruits, vegetables, and proteins, you will most likely be consuming enough and getting a good balance.

Amino acids are part of the biochemical pathways that produce cellular energy. The pool of amino acids is continuously turning over when proteins you eat are broken down to amino acids. This pool is used by your cells to build proteins and feed into biochemical pathways. If you're eating well and feeling fatigue, the cause is most likely not low levels of amino acids in your body, and supplements will not be helpful.

Beautifying your hair, nails and skin

Amino acids are the building blocks of the most abundant proteins in the skin: keratin, collagen, and elastin. L-cysteine and methionine help to build keratin, which is also an important protein in hair and nails. One study found that an L-cysteine supplement containing B vitamins helped to repair damaged hair and improve hair quality.

Another recent and very small open label study found that a product containing glycine, L-alanine, L-proline, L-valine, L-leucine, and L-lysine improved skin appearance, reduced hair loss, and improved nail conditions in some subjects. It makes sense that increasing the building blocks for proteins important in skin, nails, and hair might cause improvement, and there are some small studies that show great promise that specific amino acid supplements will work!

3

Using Supplements for Health Concerns

Support metabolism and energy needs for optimal health and to prevent chronic disease.

Understand brain and nerve function to determine supplement needs for mood, muscle function, cognition, and neurodegenerative diseases.

Get granular with cardiovascular health and disease and support your heart and brain.

Coordinate and balance your nutrition and lifestyle for a healthy, productive, and long life.

Chapter **9**

Supporting General Health and Wellness

A big question for many people is, "How do I determine what I need to stay healthy?" Understanding your health, your lifestyle, and the role of the foods you enjoy is part of the equation. Another factor is knowing what to choose from the tens of thousands of supplements available on the store shelves and online — and that can be overwhelming. These days, nutritionists focus on a personalized approach to optimize your metabolism to improve energy and mood, reduce oxidative stress, and promote overall health.

In this chapter, information is presented on maintaining body systems optimally to give you better immunity to fight disease, protect you against natural and environmental oxidative damage to cells, support your mood and muscle function through neuronal health, and keep your bones and teeth up to par. I present information using as much evidence as possible for use of supplements to keep you healthy and prevent disease. However, there are some ingredients (herbs, for example) that may be sold in supplements that have been used for thousands of years in their original plant form. There may not be enough clinical data to prove efficacy, but historically they have been advantageous and not harmful. Other supplements may have only a limited number of studies, or the studies may be conflicting, and you need to decide whether it is worth a try. In the next section, I explain a little about the various types of studies and research that form the basis of the information in this book.

Understanding the Research Options

Sifting through the information available in books and online, in advertisements, on talk shows, and at your local supermarket can be daunting. Sometimes there's a significant disconnect between the benefits of a supplement and the marketing around it. In this book, I've researched the scientific literature so I can be as accurate and succinct as possible.

There is a hierarchy of studies that can be done to prove that a nutrient or supplement is safe and effective. The first level of studies is done in either cells (called *in vitro*) or animal models (*in vivo*, meaning in a live organism). When vitamins were first discovered, their metabolism was often elucidated in animal studies first. *In vitro* and animal *in vivo* studies are called pre-clinical studies.

Clinical studies are done in people, and there are several kinds. The first is an *observational study*. In nutrition, an observational study is when information is collected about an individual's dietary patterns or nutrient intake and then correlated with health outcomes. The focus is relationships; there's no proof of cause and effect. An *epidemiological study* is when the information is collected from large groups of people who may be in different countries.

Another type of clinical study, which is truly the gold standard, is the *randomized controlled trial* (RCT). This kind of study involves recruiting subjects, using a control group, randomizing the subjects into different groups, and then testing a nutrient or diet as the intervention. This kind of study is planned for a certain amount of time that is relevant to looking at the outcomes and analysis to compare a treatment to a control group. The control group is made up of those who get no treatment or perhaps another product.

A *meta-analysis* is when scientists analyze several studies about the same subject, compare the results, and present an overview. This can be the most impactful type of analysis, especially if the results across the studies within the meta-analysis are consistent.

Another type of study you often see with supplements is done by the company that makes them; it's called a *marketing study*. These studies may or may not be done well (if at all) because they're expensive to conduct and aren't required by law.

WARNING

Note that to sell a supplement, companies do not have to confirm its effectiveness or safety. In addition, the FDA does not regulate these products.

Calming Inflammation and Reducing Oxidative Stress

Free radicals are a normal byproduct of your body converting food to energy. They're an important and useful part of your metabolism, but too many of them can cause oxidative stress. You have natural antioxidants in your body to offset the free radical damage to your cells. Sometimes, there's is an imbalance in this natural process. In this section, I explain the process and what you may be able to control with nutrition and supplements.

Explaining antioxidants and anti-inflammation

Free radicals — reactive oxygen species (ROS) and reactive nitrogen species (RNS) — are important for proper cellular metabolism. Both contain a free electron that can react with other things in your cells. Some of these things are essential for life. When there is an imbalance with too many free radicals and not enough other compounds to neutralize them in your cells, the result is a condition called oxidative stress.

Oxidative stress causes cellular damage and metabolic dysfunction and can lead to inflammation, disease, and other cellular changes. Some of the cellular processes from oxidative stress include oxidation of cell membranes, DNA damage and genetic mutations, and changes in functioning of proteins. Oxidative stress can also contribute to aging.

There are two types of inflammation. *Acute inflammation* is when your body responds to an injury. You may notice redness and swelling at the site of the injury. This inflammation is your body's immune response that it sends to heal a wound or combat a virus. If there is no injury or viral invader, and immune system inflammatory cells continue to travel through your body, they can cause damage. This is called *chronic inflammation*, which can cause damage that scientists link to a range of inflammatory diseases.

Chronic inflammation can be caused by several environmental and lifestyle factors. These include exposures to toxins, a low level of activity, overexercising, chronic stress, being overweight or obese, dysbiosis (imbalance in gut microbes), eating trans fats and sugar, poor sleep habits, smoking, and drinking alcohol.

Inflammatory diseases may account for more than half of deaths globally. Some of these include autoimmune diseases, cardiovascular diseases, some cancers,

Crohn's and inflammatory bowel disease, asthma, depression, anxiety, type 2 diabetes, and Alzheimer's.

There are good reasons to reduce oxidation and inflammation, and fortunately there are ways to prevent and reduce these processes.

Protecting your cells

Your cells have natural antioxidant systems that protect them against their naturally produced ROS. These systems protect cells by preventing the formation of free radicals, capturing and neutralizing ROS, and repairing molecules damaged by the ROS using repairing enzymes. There are two sources of antioxidants:

>> Endogenous antioxidants, which your body can synthesize

>> Exogenous antioxidants, which are supplied by foods and supplements

These can be further divided into enzymatic or nonenzymatic antioxidants. The enzymes are in your cells naturally, so the focus here is on the exogenous and nonenzymatic antioxidants.

Two vitamins that act as antioxidants are water soluble vitamin C and fat-soluble vitamin E. Vitamin C is one of the strongest natural antioxidants; it scavenges free radicals in the skin that are produced by ultraviolet (UV) radiation. This is helpful because it prevents aging of your skin by this method as well as by regulating collagen synthesis in the skin. Vitamin E or alpha-tocopherol protects your cell membranes against damaging effects of free radicals. It also protects the degradation of low-density lipoprotein (LDL) particles, which is the carrier form of cholesterol in your blood.

Carotenoids — in particular beta-carotene — are strong antioxidants. Polyphenols, which are found in a variety of plants, are also very good antioxidants.

One of the endogenous antioxidants found in every cell in your body is coenzyme Q10 (CoQ10). As you age, the levels go down. If you take statins, the levels go down more, and you may need a supplement. CoQ10 has low bioavailability, so it's probably best to take a low dose of 100 mg two times a day.

TIP

Bioavailability is the ability of a substance, like a supplement or drug, to be absorbed and used by your body. Some substances are readily absorbed through the GI tract after being swallowed. They go into the bloodstream and circulate throughout your body to exert their effect on various organs. Other substances, for example CoQ10, which is a fat-soluble compound, isn't readily absorbed, and the supplement formulation should be taken with food. Claims that the form ubiquinol is better absorbed than ubiquinone are not accurate. Bioavailability depends on many things, and in general, bioavailability of nutrients is better from foods than from supplements.

Glutathione is another antioxidant that is found naturally in your cells. It is made up of three amino acids — cysteine, glycine, and glutamic acid — and it plays a role in reducing oxidative stress, enhancing detoxification, and regulating your immune system. Your natural glutathione levels may decrease as you age or if you have certain conditions like cancer, type 2 diabetes, HIV, and Parkinson's. There are glutathione supplements as well as something called N-acetyl-cysteine (NAC), which makes and replenishes glutathione. However, some research suggests that your body doesn't really absorb oral glutathione very well. Fortunately, some foods may boost levels of glutathione in your cells, including spinach, avocados, asparagus, broccoli, garlic, and unprocessed meats.

Anti-inflammatory foods and supplements

Anti-inflammatory foods are also the foods that generally keep you healthy. Unhealthy foods like sugary drinks, deli meats, and processed foods can cause inflammation. An anti-inflammatory diet is essentially the Mediterranean diet, the Dietary Approach to Stop Hypertension (DASH) diet, the HUSS (Healthy U.S.-Style) diet, or the Healthy Vegetarian dietary pattern. All are plant-based and stress eating lots of fruits and vegetables, whole grains, good lean proteins, healthy fats, nonsugary drinks, and low-fat dairy.

According to the Centers for Disease Control (CDC), in 2019 only about 10 percent of Americans ate the recommended intake of fruits and vegetables per day! The recommendation according to the 2020-2025 Dietary Guidelines for Americans (DGA) is 2 cups of fruit and 2 to 3 cups of vegetables per day. Fruits and vegetables provide many antioxidants that help reduce inflammation, support healthy immune function, and help prevent obesity, type 2 diabetes, cardiovascular diseases, and some cancers.

Some anti-inflammatory dietary supplements include curcumin, fish oil, ginger, resveratrol, spirulina, vitamin D, bromelain, green tea extract, garlic, and other items mentioned in the following section.

Antioxidants prevent damage from ROS

ROS cause cellular and tissue damage because they are "free radicals" containing a free electron, which are unstable and react with other cellular components. Although the body has natural antioxidants or endogenous antioxidants, maintaining balance is important. If things are out of balance, you may need exogenous (from the diet or supplements) antioxidants to help reduce ROS and cellular damage.

Vitamins A, C, and E

Carotenoids (provitamin A) and retinol (vitamin A) are both good antioxidants. Vitamins C and E increase collagen synthesis and react with ROS. These three antioxidants are involved in many biochemical reactions in your body. Vitamins A and E are fat soluble and work to reduce ROS in cell lipid membranes. Vitamin A and beta carotene are water soluble and work by a different mechanism, but they also soak up ROS.

Dietary intake of these three antioxidants have been shown to reduce oxidation of fats in your cell membranes, decrease production of ROS, and DNA damage from oxidation. In the very large prospective Nurses' Health Study, vitamin A did not correlate to a reduction in some diseases, including cancer. In fact, in smokers, vitamin A may actually increase risk.

THE NURSES' HEALTH STUDY

The Nurses' Health Study is a large, prospective cohort study that is investigating risks associated with chronic diseases in women. The study began in 1976 with 121,700 nurses, continued in 1989 with 116,430 new participants (NHSII), and in 2010 enrolled more male and female nurses and nursing students (NHS3). It continues today. Overall, there have been more than 275,000 subjects in these studies.

The studies have provided key contributions to scientific knowledge about risks of chronic disease. For example, they have shown that cigarette smoking increases risk for coronary heart disease (CHD) and stroke, colon cancer, hip fracture, cataracts, and wet age-related macular degeneration (AMD). Data has also showed that obesity increased the risk of breast cancer in menopausal women, risk of CHD and stroke, colon cancer, cataracts, and AMD. There have been many observations about diet, including red meat increases risk of premenopausal breast cancer, Mediterranean diet reduces risk of CHD and stroke, and refined carbohydrates and trans fats increase risk of CHD. In addition, calcium supplementation and vitamin D reduces risk of bone fractures in women (with low-calcium diets) and vitamin A increases risk. Also, folate, vitamin B6, and vitamin D reduce risk of colon cancer. There are more interesting results that you may want to read about!

Many vitamin C and E supplement trials have not shown beneficial effects in certain medical disorders. This may be a problem with the design of the trials, but it can also mean that many of the study participants had adequate levels to begin with.

One study looking at several antioxidants and cognitive performance or decline show that a diet rich in vitamin E and carotenoids might reduce the likelihood of cognitive issues. The NHS study found that higher vegetable intake, especially of green leafy vegetables, reduces the risk of cognitive impairment. Otherwise, most studies have found little evidence of the beneficial effects of supplemental antioxidants in brain performance.

Selenium and zinc

Selenium is an important mineral in many biochemical processes. Selenium deficiency is associated with a higher level of inflammatory cytokines in your tissues. Cytokines are small proteins that promote inflammation by activating your immune cells. There are many kinds of cytokines and they play a role in fighting infections, wound healing, and tissue regeneration. Selenium is also involved in the regulation of mechanisms that defend you against viral diseases. Studies have shown that increasing selenium intake may help alleviate symptoms associated with HIV and hepatitis and perhaps other viruses such as Coxsackie or flu. Selenium is a component of selenoproteins, a group of proteins that are important in many functions, including antioxidant defense of cells from ROS, DNA synthesis and repair, sperm function, and thyroid hormone metabolism. A deficiency in selenium can result in oxidative stress and an impaired immune system.

Zinc is also very important in the structure and function of more than 300 proteins and enzymes that regulate cellular processes and signaling pathways. It's important in immune responses and also antioxidant anti-inflammatory activity in your cells. In particular, zinc increases the activation of glutathione, an antioxidant. Zinc protects proteins against oxidation and works with other metals, such as copper and iron, in preventing cellular oxidative injury.

Supplementation of both selenium and zinc may prove useful to reach the goal of 8 to 12 milligrams (mg) daily, depending on your stage of life. Some good food sources for selenium are Brazil nuts (just two will do it!), fish, meat, whole grains (whole wheat or fortified products), cottage cheese, and eggs. Good food sources for zinc include meat, shellfish, legumes, seeds, nuts and peanuts, dairy, eggs, and whole grains.

Phytochemicals

Some phytochemicals (also called phytonutrients) are the chemicals found in plants and are antioxidants that protect the body from ROS. Scientists estimate that there may be up to 4,000 phytonutrients. There are many common names for these including flavonoids, phytochemicals, flavones, isoflavones, catechins, anthocyanidins, isothiocyanates, carotenoids, allyl sulfides, polyphenols.

Phytochemicals are plentiful in fruits, vegetables, whole grains, seeds, and nuts. The phytochemicals are the sources of the color in fruits and vegetables. (This is why you sometimes hear that you should "eat the colors of the rainbow." The variety assures that you get all the phytochemicals you need.) Here are common phytochemicals and examples of food sources:

>> Beta-carotene: Orange foods (carrots, cantaloupe) and dark leafy greens (spinach, broccoli)

>> Lycopene: Red foods, such as tomatoes (cooked are absorbed better than raw), watermelon, red peppers

>> Lutein: Green foods, such as kale, spinach, broccoli, sprouts, lettuces

>> Resveratrol: Red wine, peanuts, grapes

>> Anthocyanidins: Red and purple berries

>> Isoflavones: Soybeans

It's always best to get phytonutrients from foods, but if you find that there are categories of fruits or vegetables you avoid, perhaps a supplement may be helpful.

Turmeric, curcumin, and botanical compounds

Turmeric is from the plant *Curcuma longa*. This plant is part of the ginger family and has long been used to enhance flavor in foods and for its potential health benefits. You can find it as a bright yellow powder and or ground from the fresh root. The active ingredient in this plant is curcumin, which has been used in Ayurvedic and Chinese medicine for thousands of years.

There have been many clinical studies to examine the efficacy, safety, and phar-macokinetics of curcumin. It has been shown to be involved in many cellular processes, including anti-inflammatory mechanisms. Clinical studies looking at effects on a variety of inflammatory diseases and cognitive functions have also been studied. It has been shown to be safe up to a high dose of 12 grams (g) per day for three months. The protective effect as an anti-inflammatory and in cognition look promising. However, more research is needed to better understand dosages, forms, bioavailability, and efficacy.

A good way to get curcumin is to use it as a spice in food. Another way is to use curcumin or turmeric supplements. These are generally recognized as safe (GRAS) by the Food and Drug Administration (FDA). Note that this doesn't mean that the FDA regulates the contents of specific products, however. Supplements are considered safe up to 3 tablespoons per day, but there can be side effects. They can interact with some medications such as blood thinners and chemotherapy. As with any supplement, make sure to consult with your doctor before trying it.

There are other antioxidant-rich herbs in addition to turmeric, including cloves, oregano, rosemary, cinnamon, ginger, and peppermint.

The National Institutes of Health (NIH) have a method to measure the antioxidant capacity of foods called the oxygen radical absorbance capacity (ORAC).For optimal health, the FDA recommends 3,000 to 5,000 ORAC units per day from high-ORAC-value foods. These foods include blueberries, tart cherry juice concentrate, prunes, blackberries, raspberries, strawberries, walnuts, artichokes, and dark chocolate. Check for ORAC levels on supplement labels.

Enhancing Immune Function

The immune system is complicated. An entire *Dummies* book could be devoted to it. Here, I'll give you a summary.

In short, your immune system includes several organs in your body and many different cell types. Nutrition plays an essential role by providing nutrients in correct amount to all these cells. As with other cells mentioned in this book, vitamins, minerals, and other biomolecules are an integral part of biochemical processes of the immune system's cells.

Understanding your immune system

Figure 9-1 shows the organs involved in the immune system, including the liver, spleen, appendix, lymph nodes, tonsils, and thymus. Figure 9-2 shows the cells involved in the immune system. Note that there are two main categories of immune cells according to their properties and defense mechanisms: cells of the innate immune systems and cells of the adaptive immune system. There are more and more studies about the effects of nutrition and supplements on immunity, and the list of nutritional-immuno-modulators is growing.

IMMUNE SYSTEM

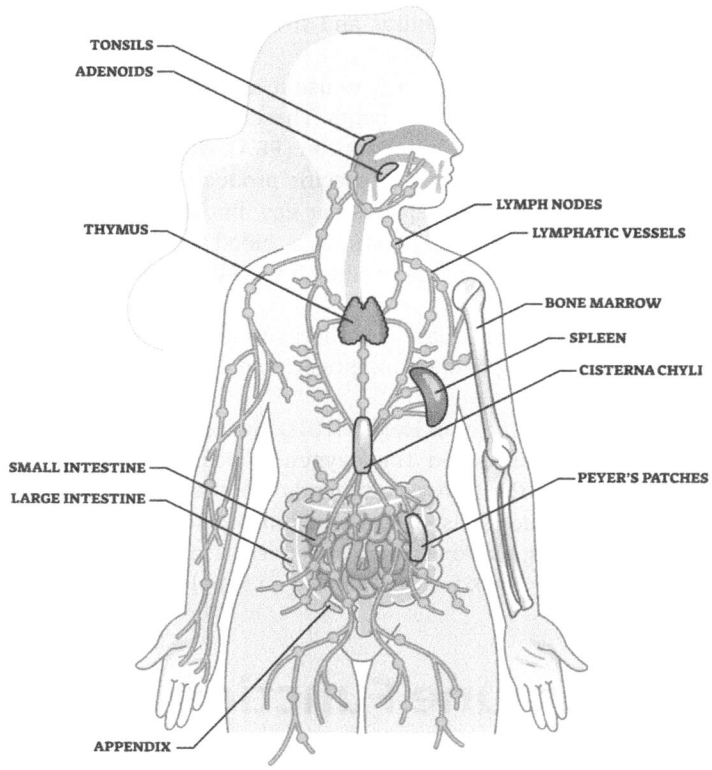

TONSILS

ADENOIDS

THYMUS

LYMPH NODES

LYMPHATIC VESSELS

BONE MARROW

SPLEEN

CISTERNA CHYLI

SMALL INTESTINE

LARGE INTESTINE

PEYER'S PATCHES

APPENDIX

FIGURE 9-1:
The organs involved in the immune system.

VectorMine/Adobe Stock Photos

Healthy cell turnover

About 330 billion cells in your body turn over every day. About 86 percent are blood cells, and 12 percent are gut cells. The cells that are replaced each day amount to about 1 percent of the total number of cells in your body. In 80 to 100 days, 30 trillion cells in your body will have been replaced!

This turnover process in your body requires nutrients and energy for myriad biochemical reactions. Overall health and good levels of essential nutrients are key to a healthy metabolism and immune system.

For example, zinc and vitamin A promote cell division and proliferations. Studies show that a deficiency in vitamin A results in impairment of many immune cell functions, decreases integrity of the gut lining, and increases risk of infection. Vitamin A supplementation decreases illness and death from infections and diarrheal diseases in children globally. Vitamins B1, B2, B3, and B12 act as coenzymes in many important cellular metabolic pathways that include enzyme reactions. These are therefore also important for cell turnover.

CELLS OF THE IMMUNE SYSTEM

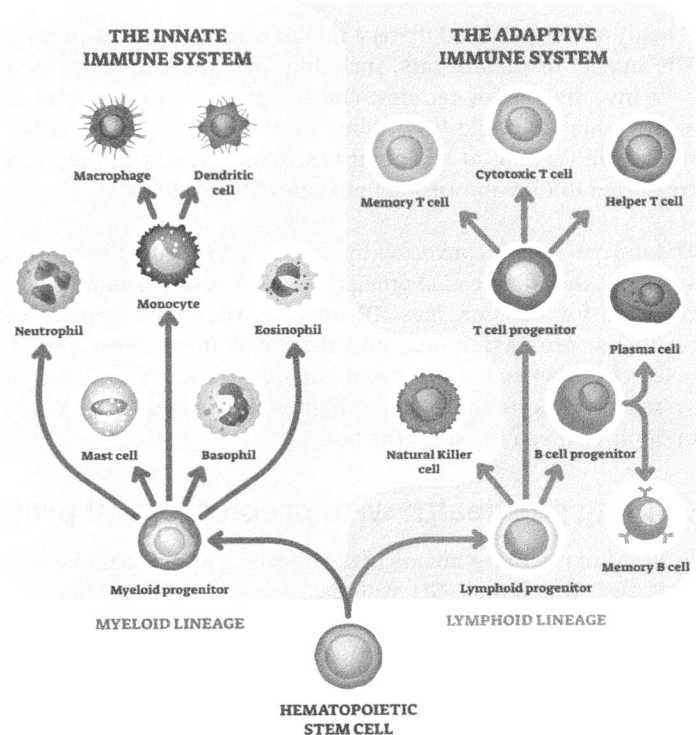

FIGURE 9-2:
The cells of the
immune system.

VectorMine/Adobe Stock Photos

Boosting immunity with antioxidants

Vitamins B1, B2, B3, and B12 play a significant role in anti-inflammatory functions. Vitamin B3, or niacin, is a precursor for nicotinamide adenine dinucleotide (NAD), and nicotinamide adenine dinucleotide phosphate (NADP) is critical for metabolic pathways, offers defense against ROS, has antitumor effects in animals, and promotes a variety of immune reactions. It's considered anti-inflammatory and antiaging. All the B vitamins are important for cell turnover and as antioxidants.

Vitamin A plays a key role in regulating immunity and antibody production. Research shows that vitamin A deficiency is associated with cytokine release and decreased production of natural killer cells, monocytes or macrophages, and impaired T and beta lymphocytes. Vitamins C and D are also antioxidants and reduce damage from ROS.

Combating with omega-3s

A healthy and balanced dietary intake is important for immune system function. The impact of dietary fats, including polyunsaturated fatty acids (PUFAs) have been investigated for decades. The omega-3 PUFAs are alpha-linolenic acid (ALA), eicosapentaenoic acid (EPA), and docosahexaenoic acid (DHA). EPA and DHA are the fats in fish oil. ALA is plant based and present in nuts and seeds. ALA can be converted to EPA and DHA by enzymes in your body.

The omega-3s are converted by enzymes to metabolites that affect the immune system. Other fats, called omega-6 PUFAs, use the same enzyme system and can compete for the enzymes. Ultimately, these compounds called leukotrienes, resolvins, prostaglandins, and thromboxanes, affect your immune cells. The research on omega-3 fatty acids demonstrates that all the cells in the immune system respond to these fats. A higher omega-3 to omega-6 ratio may be helpful in upping omega-3 use by the body.

Gaining gut health with prebiotics and probiotics

Trillions of microorganisms make up your gut microbiome — the environment in your gastrointestinal (GI) system. Your gut naturally has thousands of bacteria species, and intestinal bacteria cells outnumber human cells by ten to one!

The gut microbiome has many functions. One of those functions is immunity. About 80 percent of your body's immune cells live in your gut. The GI system is separate from the rest of your body and is exposed to the external world. When you eat or are exposed to pathogens, the microorganisms in your gut function to help digest your food and also to protect you. They clear out pathogens, compete with bacterial infections that can affect your gut, and maintain your gut walls to prevent leakage into your bloodstream. They are also anti-inflammatory.

You can maintain a healthy microbiome through a healthy diet that contains prebiotics and probiotics. Prebiotics are essentially the food for the probiotics. Plant foods such as fruits, vegetables, seeds, nuts, and whole grains are the best source of prebiotics. Some good sources include bananas, barley, garlic, kiwifruit, Jerusalem artichokes, legumes, oats, and potatoes. Prebiotic supplements should include fiber.

Probiotics, or good bacteria, are found in fermented foods. These good bacteria grow during the fermentation process. The best food sources for one of the most common probiotics — *L. acidophilius* — are kimchi, sauerkraut, yogurt, miso, tempe, kefir, and kombucha. Not all yogurts contain probiotics, so read the label to be sure!

There are many probiotic supplements on the market, and some studies show that most of them are dead and ineffective. The most commonly studied and recommended probiotics are *Lactobacillus* genus, including *L. acidophilus, L. rhamnosus, L. casei,* and *L. plantarum,* and the *Bifidobacterium* genus, including *Bifidobacterium longum* and *Bifidobacterium breve.* When looking for supplements, pay attention to colony-forming units (the number of bacteria per dose), types of bacterial strains used, need for refrigeration, and whether the supplement has been studied for effectiveness.

Supporting Nerve Function and Brain Health

The nervous system is a complex system made of a network of neurons and cells that communicates through electrical signals. (Refer to Figure 9-1.) Neurons send signals in the brain via chemicals called neurotransmitters, including serotonin, dopamine, and gamma-aminobutyric acid (GABA), which affect mood, sleep, focus, and thoughts. They also send signals to tissues, such as to tell muscle cells to contract. The central nervous system (CNS) includes the brain and spinal cord. The nerves branching out to the rest of the body are called the peripheral nervous system (PNS).

Critical electrolytes: potassium, sodium, calcium, and magnesium

Potassium, sodium, calcium, and magnesium are electrolytes important for many bodily functions. An imbalance in the cellular content can impact health. Electrolyte balance is critical for nerve cell processes in addition to other biological processes, including bone function, muscular physiology, and oxygen transport.

Potassium is very important for the regulation of nerve impulses, protein synthesis, blood sugar metabolism, and cell membrane potential, which is the regulation of the electrolytes that go in and out of cells. Sodium is also especially important in cell membrane potential. This regulation of the electrolytes going in and out of the cells keeps the fluid inside and outside the cells in balance, helps send nerve signals, and participates in muscle contraction.

Calcium plays a particularly important role in the formation and repair of bones, muscle physiology, nerve impulse transmission, hormonal regulation, and blood pressure stabilization. Magnesium is also important for energy metabolism, muscle and nerve function, and building bones and teeth.

Deficiencies in any of the electrolytes (potassium, calcium, or magnesium) can cause symptoms and sometimes severe effects. How can you be sure that you're getting enough? Some of the common symptoms to watch for are muscle cramps, fatigue, and numbness.

People who eat the Standard American Diet (SAD) probably do not get enough fruits and vegetables and whole grains. Therefore, they may be low in potassium, calcium, and magnesium. Most likely they are also high in sodium. Most sodium comes from sodium chloride (salt), which is very prevalent in restaurant foods, processed foods, and many packaged foods.

If you eat a healthier diet, you will probably still get enough sodium. If you're deficient, adding a bit of table salt to your food will give you enough. Deficiencies in potassium, calcium, and magnesium are more common and may result in some mild to severe symptoms. Some of the mild symptoms are listed here:

>> **Potassium:** Irregular heartbeat, high blood pressure, fatigue, muscle weakness, constipation and bloating, numbness or tingling in hands, arms, legs, and feet.

>> **Magnesium:** Fatigue, muscle cramps or weakness, numbness, decreased bone density

>> **Calcium:** Muscle cramps, fatigue, memory problems, fragile nails, dry skin

It's always best to try to get these minerals from foods, but sometimes you may need supplementation. If you are on certain medications, including diuretics, hydrocortisone, chemotherapy or antibiotics, you may be particularly in need of a supplement, and you should discuss this with your doctor. Another example is if you use an over-the-counter proton pump inhibitor for reflux for a long time, you may need a magnesium or calcium supplement.

TIP

Research supports that magnesium may help symptoms of migraines, help you sleep better, may aid cognitive function, boost energy and mood, reduce anxiety, regulate blood pressure, and alleviate muscle cramps. There are many forms of magnesium supplements, including magnesium citrate, magnesium oxide, magnesium glycinate, magnesium malae, and magnesium chloride. Some recommend a blend of glycinate, malate, citrate, and oxide because a high dose of certain types of magnesium can cause diarrhea, abdominal cramps, and nausea. Also, different types of magnesium are more effective for different ailments. For example, magnesium glycinate is better for sleep and anxiety, magnesium citrate helps with constipation, and magnesium malate may improve energy and muscle pain. The addition of B6 to a magnesium supplement will increase the body's use of magnesium.

See Table 9-1 for information about supplementation and food sources for potassium, calcium, and magnesium.

TABLE 9-1   ## RDA of Potassium, Calcium, and Magnesium

Mineral	RDA (depending on age and sex)	Food sources
Potassium	3,500 – 4,700 mg/day	Bananas, beet greens, salmon, white beans, avocado, potatoes, milk, mushrooms
Calcium	1,000 – 1,300 mg/day	Milk, cheese, spinach, tofu, yogurt, okra, trout, acorn squash
Magnesium	310 – 420 mg/day	Spinach, pumpkin seeds, lima beans, tuna, brown rice, almonds

Transmitting signals and aiding in muscle contraction

Neurons can transmit signals to other neurons, or a neuron can transmit a signal to tissue, such as muscle, via a chemical neurotransmitter such as acetylcholine. Acetylcholine is released from the motor nerve endings to receptors in your muscles. Sodium channels open, and sodium flows into the muscle cells to create depolarization, triggering a wave of events resulting in movement of actin and myosin filaments and ultimately muscle contraction.

Taming your brain

Your brain is a complex system of neurons and biochemical pathways that need a variety of nutrients to function and support your normal brain function to help your focus and control sleep and mood. Be sure to eat a variety of foods that include minerals for nerve signaling, amino acids for enzyme production and neurotransmitter synthesis, glucose for energy production, B vitamins for metabolism and neurotransmitter synthesis, and antioxidants for protecting against inflammation.

There have been numerous clinical studies on the effects of nutrients and herbs on anxiety. These interventions include using B vitamins, omega-3s, lavender, melatonin, passionflower, GABA, tryptophan, 5-hydroxy-tryptophan (5-HTP), S-adenosyl methionine (SAM-e), and kava. A 2010 meta-analysis showed inconstant results, and more recent studies are inconclusive. For mild anxiety or just to keep calm, be sure to get all your nutrients from foods and supplements if needed.

Fueling cognition with CoQ10

CoQ10 is a nutrient in all your cells that's involved in cellular energy production of ATP in the mitochondria. It also functions as an antioxidant and neuroprotective. As you age, cellular CoQ10 decreases and supplements may be beneficial. Statins, which work by lowering cholesterol synthesis in cells, also decrease CoQ10 production and can cause a deficiency in it. Many doctors recommend taking CoQ10 supplements while on statins to prevent muscle cramps and other side effects of low CoQ10.

CoQ10 deficiency is implicated in the pathogenesis of neurological disorders including epilepsy, stroke, multiple sclerosis (MS), depression, Alzheimer's disease, and others. There are several clinical studies suggesting the role of CoQ10 as part of the treatment of these diseases, but much more needs to be done.

Keeping Strong Bones and Healthy Teeth and Gums

Building bones and teeth are a part of normal childhood development. Children and adolescents create more bone than they lose and reach peak bone mass in their 20s. As you age, bone density can change, with bone loss becoming greater than repair and maintenance. In women especially, age-related bone loss significantly speeds up after menopause because of the decrease in estrogen. Teeth and gum maintenance is required throughout your life and includes a balanced diet, oral hygiene, and dental checkups. Staying as healthy and active as possible is an important goal, and there are lifelong nutrition and lifestyle things you can do to keep your bones and teeth healthy.

Oral health (the health of your mouth) encompasses your teeth, bones, and the gingival tissue (gums). The most common diseases of the mouth are tooth decay and periodontal (gum) disease. What you eat and drink affects your mouth, and the health of your mouth can affect what you eat and drink. Specific nutrients are very important. For example, tooth enamel requires calcium, phosphorus, and vitamin A. Eating foods high in fiber like fruits and vegetables help balance sugars and help to clean your teeth and stimulate saliva. Vitamin C is important for your gums and healing. Calcium, phosphorous, and vitamins C and A are important in tooth development, and vitamin D is also important because it helps the body absorb calcium. Lastly, fluoride strengthens tooth enamel and helps prevent cavities and is in many fluoride toothpastes and in some water.

Maintaining bone health and density

It's critical to include plenty of foods rich in calcium and vitamin D for bone growth, repair, and maintenance. Foods rich in these nutrients include dairy products, almonds, broccoli, kale, sardines, and soy. The RDA for calcium is 1,000 mg/day up to age 51 for women or 70 for men. After age 51 for women and 70 for men, you will need 1,200 mg/day. Calcium supplements are useful to be sure that you are getting the RDA.

Your body needs vitamin D to absorb calcium. The RDA of vitamin D for adults ages 19 to 70 is 600 international units (IUs) a day. After age 70, and for pregnant and lactating women, the recommendation increases to 800 IUs a day. It's hard to get enough vitamin D only from sun exposure (depending on where you live and time of year) and food, so it's important to know your vitamin D status and take a supplement to get to normal levels, but more may not be better! It may be better to take lower doses — 400 to 600 IU/day — than higher amounts 4,000 to 10,000 IU/day — according to a 2020 meta-analysis.

Preventing conditions like osteopenia and osteoporosis

About 54 million Americans have osteoporosis, which is a gradual thinning out of the bones — or low bone density. Osteopenia is the start of bone loss that can sometimes proceed to osteoporosis. Bone loss and low bone density can mean it's easier for bone fractures to occur, especially in older people. Women typically start out with lower bone density than men, and loss of estrogen over time can increase the risk for osteoporosis.

The best way to prevent osteopenia and osteoporosis is through nutrition and lifestyle throughout your life. This means getting enough calcium and vitamin D, protein, and other nutrients through food, as well as exercising regularly. Weight-bearing exercise (for example, walking, running, tennis) and resistance exercise (weights) help to stimulate the cells responsible for building bones.

Calcium, phosphorus, magnesium

Most of the calcium in your body is in your bones — about 99 percent. Adequate calcium is essential, and getting the RDA is important for good bone health and maintaining good bone density as you age. Surprisingly, many randomized clinical studies and meta-analyses have not shown that calcium supplements alone improved bone density or prevent bone fractures in older adults. Calcium with 400 IU of vitamin D showed improvement in bone density. A good source of this combination is from fortified dairy. Getting the RDA of calcium is important, but calcium supplements may not help reduce bone loss and fractures as you age.

Sixty percent of the magnesium in your body is found in bones. Research regarding magnesium supplements on osteoporosis and bone fractures is mixed. Since more research is required for definitive understanding of the benefits of magnesium supplements, it's best to be sure that you are getting the RDA for your stage of life from your foods, including legumes, nuts, seeds, and whole grain.

Phosphorous and calcium form hydroxyapatite to create bone and both are essential to good health. It's important to get adequate amounts of both from foods. Most people get enough phosphorous from foods and supplements aren't necessary.

Supporting your gums with vitamin C

Centuries ago, sailors learned that the lack of certain foods caused a disease called scurvy, which resulted in swollen and bleeding gums, loose teeth, hemorrhaging under the skin, and slowed healing of wounds, and sometimes death. These symptoms were cured by intake of citrus fruits containing ascorbic acid or vitamin C.

If you eat a diet rich in fruits and vegetables, you most likely get enough vitamin C. Unfortunately, many Americans do not eat five servings of fruits and vegetables as recommended. Some vitamin C–rich foods include

>> Citrus fruit, such as oranges, lemons, and orange juice

>> Peppers (red, orange, yellow, green)

>> Potatoes, both white and sweet

>> Strawberries

>> Blackcurrants

>> Broccoli

>> Brussels sprouts

Vitamins and oral health

The American Dental Association recommends reducing the consumption of added sugar and sugar-sweetened drinks and limiting ultra-processed foods as two ways you can maintain good oral health. They support fluoridation of water because fluoride helps strengthen teeth and prevent cavities.

A recent review of the literature showed that certain supplements improved dental health. Specifically, vitamin A helps preserve mucosal membranes, salivary glands, and teeth. Vitamin D is essential for absorption of calcium, magnesium, and phosphorus, which are used to form enamel and dentin. Vitamin C acts as an anti-inflammatory, promotes collagen formation, and prevents periodontitis. The B vitamins, folate, and B12 contribute to mucosal and bone health. Zinc helps with gingival inflammation. Vitamins and minerals in general contribute to immune response, which also improves oral health.

Herbs and oral health

Some herbs have been used historically for oral health, most of which have anti-oxidant and anti-inflammatory properties. Some of these are found in toothpaste, such as mint. So, it not only freshens breath but also is an anti-inflammatory agent. Here are some other herbs that may help maintain a healthy mouth:

> » Green tea naturally contains fluorine and may help prevent dental decay.

> » Licorice root has antimicrobial properties.

> » Neem sticks or leaves destroy cavity-causing bacteria.

> » Turmeric helps heal gums because of its anti-inflammatory action.

> » Chewing on a clove of garlic can reduce tooth pain.

> » Thyme leaves are antiseptics and antifungal.

> » Tulsi leaves from holy basil are well-known as an antibacterial.

> » Clove oil is antimicrobial and effective topically to numb and relieve tooth pain.

Maintaining Your Vision

Vitamin A is an essential part of the complex biochemical pathways involved in the retina in your eye. Very simply, a form of vitamin A (called all-trans-retinol), combines with a molecule called opsin to form rhodopsin. Rhodopsin reacts with light, forms photorhodopsin, undergoes changes in shape and structure, and sends a signal to the brain via the optic nerve to form an image.

Vitamin A is essential for maintaining healthy vision. Vitamin A deficiency is generally not an issue in the United States and western countries where people get sufficient amounts from their foods. If you aren't getting enough for some reason, the following foods high in vitamin A or beta-carotene can help you get the RDA: beef, chicken, fish, cheese, eggs, carrots, kale, spinach, mango, and guava. If your diet is limited for any reason, a supplement is always an option. Since vitamin A is fat soluble you do not want to take more than the tolerable UL of 3,000 micrograms (mcg) per day for adults. This means that you don't want to consume more than 3,000 mcg of vitamin A per day from both food and supplements because it could be unsafe.

Preventing blindness and protecting against eye damage

A deficiency in vitamin A affects over 2 billion people globally, and there is a great need for supplementation and food fortification, especially in pregnant women and children younger than five. Vitamin A deficiency is more prevalent in Sub-Sahara Africa and parts of Asia, where diets are low in vitamin A, and childhood infections like measles and diarrhea are common. Lack of vitamin A in the fetus or child can cause vision loss, impaired immune system leading to increase in risk of infectious disease, and death in infants and toddlers. There are public health efforts to address this problem, including food fortification and supplementation. These efforts are supported by UNICEF and WHO. Other organizations, including the Bill and Melinda Gates Foundation, also work to reduce mother and infant malnutrition, risk of infectious disease through vaccination, and help supply supplements to people in affected countries. There are government efforts worldwide to require fortification of food to address malnutrition. In the United States, breakfast cereals and milk are fortified with vitamin A.

Blindness isn't the only issue to be concerned about, though. When you stare at devices or are exposed to sunlight, you're exposed to something called blue light. Blue light can affect your ability to go to sleep, but according to the American Academy of Ophthalmology, blue light doesn't appear to affect your eyes. So, in terms of blue light's effects on you, the types of supplements you may want to use are those to help you sleep.

Age-related macular degeneration (AMD) is a devastating eye disease that can develop into vision loss. In some patients, vitamins have been shown to delay progression of advanced AMD. In a landmark study called the Age-Related Eye Disease Study or AREDS, researchers found a vitamin formulation that helped delay progression of advanced AMD. This vitamin formulation included vitamin C, 500 mg; vitamin E, 400 IU; zinc, 80 mg; copper, 2 mg; lutein, 10 mg; and zeaxanthin, 2 mg. They also found that eating a good diet, especially one that included fresh fish, fruits, nuts, and vegetables, was helpful to prevent certain eye diseases, such as cataract glaucoma and diabetic retinopathy.

Considering helpful carotenoids

Lutein and zeaxanthin are two helpful carotenoids that are useful in preventing some eye disease. These accumulate in parts of your eye and act as antioxidants protecting your eyes from free radicals. Your body can't make these two carotenoids, so getting them from foods or supplementation is important. Good food sources include kale, spinach, broccoli, peppers, corn, egg yolks, pumpkin, Brussels sprouts, and avocados. If you don't like any of these foods and you want to supplement for good eye health, then taking 10 mg of lutein and 2 mg of the zeaxanthin would give you enough.

Capturing Beauty Inside and Out

Some nutrients work from the inside, and others work from the outside, as in skin care. A number of beauty companies like the idea of promoting supplements as well as products that work together to help you look and feel better.

Nutrients to help from the inside include healthy fats, like the omega-3 fatty acids, and other mono- and polyunsaturated fats. Proteins and amino acids make collagen and keratin and protect against UV rays. Vitamin A protects as an antioxidant. Vitamin C helps form collagen and is also a good antioxidant. Vitamin E is an antioxidant and anti-inflammatory. Zinc is concentrated in the outer layer of skin and helps in healing and cell biochemistry, and it's also an antioxidant. Selenium protects against UV radiation. *Polypodium leucotomos*, a species of fern, may also protect from sunlight.

Protecting your skin from the outside

Skin is the largest organ in your body and covers and protects your body from the outside elements. It has a complex structure (see Figure 9-3) made up of the epidermis, dermis, and subcutaneous fat. The middle layer, dermis, is held together by collagen, which provides strength and flexibility. Kertinocytes are a large part of the epidermis; they also contribute to the skin's structure and ability to protect.

Aside from protection, other functions of the skin include sensation, heat regulation, control of evaporation, synthesizing vitamin D, aesthetics, storage, and synthesis of lipids, excretion of sweat, and absorption of medications and hormones. It's also water resistant. The different types of cells and variety of functions means that skin relies on most nutrients to stay healthy.

SKIN ANATOMY

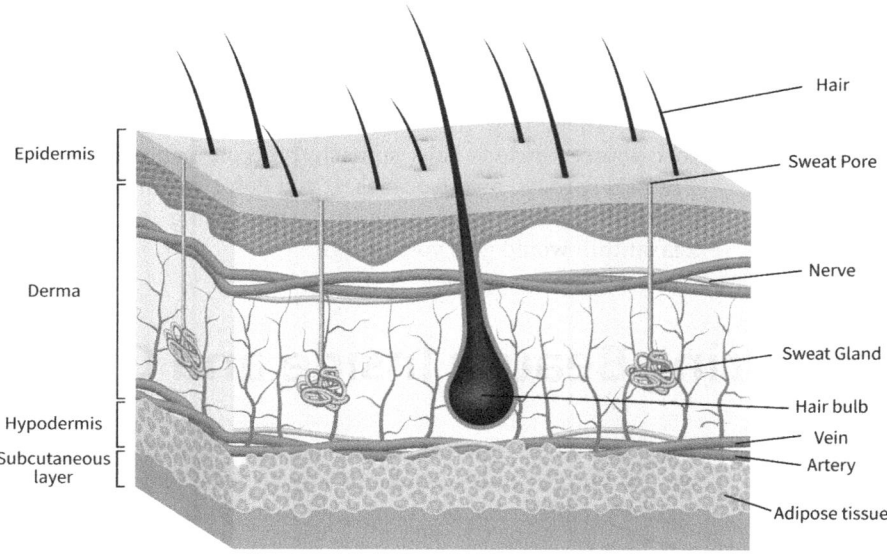

Epidermis

Derma

Hypodermis

Subcutaneous layer

Hair

Sweat Pore

Nerve

Sweat Gland

Hair bulb

Vein

Artery

Adipose tissue

FIGURE 9-3:
The layers of skin.

MicroOne/Adobe Stock Photos

Care of your skin will keep it looking good as well as maintain its ability to perform its functions listed above. Many supplements are advertised to improve your skin. Research on many of the important nutrients shows that deficiency can cause skin issues, so it's good to eat a healthy diet for glowing skin. If your diet is poor, then it may be wise to supplement.

Analyzing antiaging products

One recent report estimated the cosmetic industry at $108 billion and growing. Skin care is responsible for about one-third of this! Chronological skin aging is the natural aging of your skin according to your age and genetics. You can't prevent it. Photoaging is damage to your skin from UVA (linked to wrinkles and some cancers) and UVB light (sunburn and most skin cancers). You can prevent sun damage by staying out of the sun, covering your skin, or using sunblock. You also can treat sun damage to improve signs of photoaging such as wrinkles, sunspots, decreased elasticity, and increased roughness and redness.

Excellent scientific evidence exists that retinol or the synthetic version — tretinoin — that's found in prescription or over-the-counter antiaging products exert biological effects such as collagen synthesis, fibroblast activity, and inhibition of zinc-dependent enzymes involved in aging and skin health in cells or animals. Some small clinical trials have shown some improvement in photoaging with retinol products, vitamin C, and other antioxidants. However, most current clinical studies using a variety of retinol formulations have shown negligible effect on facial aging except for some improvement of fine-line wrinkles. Also, not everyone tolerates retinol; some find their skin becomes dry and red from these products.

Hyaluronic acid is another naturally found molecule in your skin that attracts water and keeps your skin hydrated and flexible. A 2021 study in 40 women demonstrated that hyaluronic acid improved skin hyaluronic acid content, smoothness, plumping, and hydration, with some improvement in fine lines and wrinkles. Most people tolerate it very well.

Glycolic acid and lactic acid belong to the alpha hydroxy acid (AHA) family. They're water-soluble organic compounds that, in cosmetic formulations, may help prevent or treat fine lines and wrinkles. They're exfoliants and also can hydrate. Because they are exfoliants, they aren't for daily use and may cause redness.

To prevent or treat the results of photoaging with over-the-counter creams and other products, here are things to consider:

>> Retinoids seem to be best for treating early signs of aging and moderately treating fine lines and wrinkles.

>> Vitamin C and other antioxidants added to creams or serums may reduce ROS damage.

>> Hyaluronic acid is a great hydrator. The improvement may be seen as soon as 8 to 12 weeks.

>> In general, just using a moisturizer, as demonstrated in controls in some of these studies, offer some improvement in fine lines as well.

TIP Many skin products with supplements are expensive, so I recommend trying and comparing different products for visible improvement.

Sculpting with collagen

Collagen accounts for 30 percent of your body's protein and is important for structure and support of your skin. As you age, your body produces less collagen (especially after menopause), and collagen in your skin may break down faster. Too much sun, smoking, and too much refined carbohydrates and sugars make collagen breakdown worse.

To improve skin collagen, sunscreen is important to protect from UV radiation. Eating a well-balanced diet such as the Mediterranean diet will give you the nutrients you need to produce collagen naturally. Dermatologists can use collagen cosmetically as a filler to decease lines and wrinkles.

Supplements of collagen (a protein) are broken down to amino acids in your gut and are absorbed into your body. These amino acids are used to create all proteins in your body including collagen. Ingesting collagen supplements doesn't mean more collagen in your body. Some research on collagen peptide supplements show small improvement of skin hydration and elasticity, but more studies need to be done to prove this effect.

Supporting Athletic Activities

Whether you're a weekend warrior or a serious athlete, you need a balanced diet rich in carbohydrates, protein, fat, vitamins, and minerals to support your muscles, joints, and energy level. The amount of exercise you get in a day affects your needs for these macro- and micronutrients. You need carbohydrates for energy, protein for your muscles, and healthy fats for overall health. You need vitamins and minerals from a well-balanced dietary intake for peak metabolism. If you exercise for 30-60 minutes a day and do not have a physically strenuous job, then you probably do not need to change your diet or take any supplements.

If you're very athletic, work out in the gym more than an hour a day, or do strenuous sports, then you may want to include supplements in your routine. Common supplements that athletes use include the following:

>> **Protein:** Endurance athletes need between 1.2 g/kg/day and 1.4 g/kg/day, and strength training athletes need between 1.4 g/kg/day and 2.0 g/kg/ day.

>> **Creatine:** Creatine from food and supplements can give you a boost of energy and help build muscle. Studies show that it's generally safe and increases muscle in 18 to 30 year olds when used along with regular exercise and weightlifting.

>> **Caffeine:** Taking caffeine before a workout or event can increase alertness, reduce fatigue, improve endurance and power output.

>> **Beta alanine:** Taken before exercise, beta alanine can balance lactic acid buildup in muscles, improve endurance, and delay fatigue.

>> **BCAAs:** When taken during or after exercise, BCAAs support muscle recovery, increase muscle protein synthesis, and reduce muscle soreness.

Other supplements for general health that also support muscle, joint, bone, and immune system health include

>> Vitamin D

>> Iron

>> Omega-3's

>> Iron

>> Glutamine

Chapter **10**

Targeting Preventable Chronic Diseases

Metabolism is your body's process of breaking down the food you eat. Myriad biochemical reactions digest and break down proteins, fats, and carbohydrates for energy that fuels your body and keeps your tissues and organs functioning. A metabolic disorder is when your body experiences a disruption in these processes that can lead to chronic diseases such as obesity, heart disease, and diabetes.

Chronic diseases as defined by the Centers for Disease Control (CDC) are conditions that last one year or more and require ongoing medical attention, limit to activities of daily living, or both. Six out of ten Americans have one chronic disease, and four out of ten have two. With age, those numbers increase, and 94 percent of people older than 60 have one chronic disease, and 78 percent have two or more. Chronic diseases that are related to nutrition or lifestyle include cardiovascular disease, diabetes, hypertension, cancer, and neurodegenerative disease (such as Alzheimer's). In addition to nutrition, lifestyle factors can include smoking, alcohol, environmental factors, and lack of exercise.

Genetics also plays a part in chronic diseases. Some research suggests that environmental, genetic, and lifestyle factors each contribute equally to the development of chronic disease.

Metabolic syndrome is when you have three of the following contributors: high blood pressure, low levels of high-density lipoprotein (HDL), high triglycerides, high blood sugar, and large waist size. Metabolic syndrome puts you at a higher risk for heart disease, stroke, and diabetes.

In this chapter, I present information on how some specifics of metabolism are related to disease states and how you can reduce your risks of getting chronic diseases. Lifestyle, including nutrition and exercise, play a role in the underlying metabolic processes involved in development of some chronic diseases.

Turning Food into Energy Pathways

Your body utilizes the food you eat for cellular energy that fuels many metabolic processes. Food, made up of proteins, fat, and carbohydrates, undergoes catabolism to digest and convert to cellular energy called adenosine triphosphate (ATP). Amino acids, glucose, and fats (as fatty acids) can also be used to make proteins, store glucose as glycogen, or make and store fats.

Figure 10-1 shows how food gets metabolized to energy. All these pathways require vitamin and minerals to aid in the enzyme-catalyzed biochemical reactions. The need for essential vitamins and minerals in these processes has been well known, and their roles are understood on a cellular level.

Contributing to the energy-producing pathways in cells

The need for essential vitamins and minerals in the metabolic process has been well known for some time, and experts understand their roles on a biochemical level. The pathways are involved in producing energy as well as reducing fatigue and improving cognition and mood.

All the B vitamins are involved in energy metabolism from food. Thiamine (B1), riboflavin (B2), and niacin (B3) are essential for breaking down glucose, and pyridoxine (B6) and biotin (B7) are important for amino acid and lipid metabolism. Recommended daily allowances (RDA) for these have been established to optimize energy metabolism. A deficiency in any of the B vitamins upsets the dynamics of these metabolic pathways.

METABOLISM

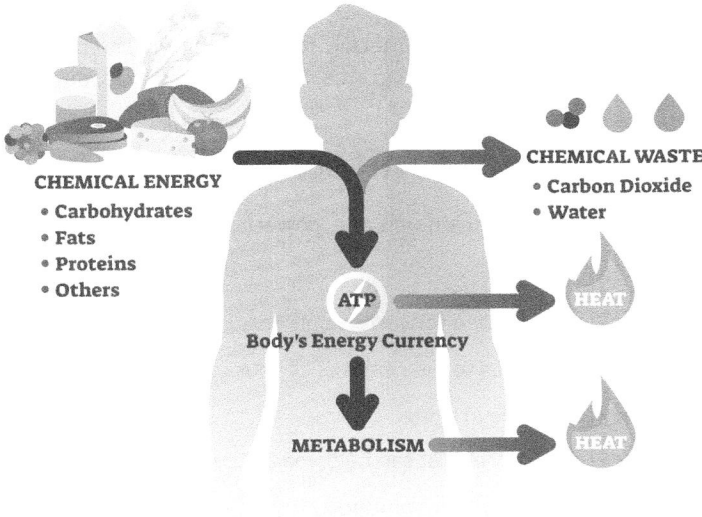

FIGURE 10-1: Componants of the food you eat are metabolized to produce energy.

Vitamin C, iron, and magnesium are also very important in cellular energy production of ATP. Sending oxygen to your organs via hemoglobin is important for energy production in organs' cells and tissues. Iron-deficiency anemia reduces blood transport and supply of oxygen to muscle, which impairs endurance capacity and energetic efficiency. Other types of anemias can occur if B12, B6, or B9 are low because that can decrease oxygen transport in the blood. Neurotransmission and brain health are also important for mental energy and mood. Vitamins B3, B5, iron, magnesium, and zinc are all important for brain function.

Clinical studies have shown that suboptimal levels or deficiencies of vitamins and minerals important in cellular energy production can lead to physical and mental fatigue. True deficiencies of vitamins and minerals can lead to clear symptoms of physical or mental fatigue, and supplementation works to alleviate these. In subjects with low (or suboptimal) but not deficient levels, the symptoms might be vague, but a review of many clinical studies showed that taking supplements improved symptoms in people with suboptimal levels.

If you often feel physically or mentally tired or moody, or you have trouble thinking clearly, the first step is to see your doctor to determine if anything is medically concerning. If you're otherwise healthy, eating foods high in the B vitamins, iron, and magnesium might help you, especially if you have lower-than-normal blood levels.

TIP

Foods high in B vitamins include whole grains (not processed grains), eggs, legumes, citrus fruits, avocados, meat, poultry, fish, liver, and fortified cereals. Foods high in iron are red meat, seafood, beans, dark leafy greens, and iron-fortified cereals. Magnesium-rich foods include dark chocolate, avocados, nuts, legumes, tofu, seeds, whole grains, fatty fish, bananas, and leafy greens.

Minding your mitochondrial health

Mitochondria are considered the powerhouse of the cell. Here are some ways they're important:

>> They're essential to converting nutrients into cellular energy.

>> They're essential to the health of all your cells, tissues, and organs.

>> They play a role in aging.

>> They contain DNA that can be damaged by mutations and aging.

>> They're important for immune function.

There are several serious mitochondrial diseases — mostly genetic. For some of those diseases, there are few, if any, randomized controlled trials (RCTs). The studies that have been done have not shown much success treating the diseases with supplements. If you have a primary mitochondrial disease, you're probably already consulting your doctor and looking for the best treatments. Some small studies or case reports (some with only one subject!) show some beneficial effects in specific conditions for alpha-linolenic acid (ALA), arginine, carnitine, citrulline, coenzyme Q10 (CoQ10), creatinine, folinic acid, riboflavin, and thiamin when used alone and in some combination.

FORMS OF B9

The natural form of vitamin B9 is folate. That form is found in foods. Folic acid is the synthetic form that is used in fortified foods and supplements. They're both converted to the active form — 5-methyltetrahydrofolate or 5- MTHF — in the body. Synthetic folinic acid is easily absorbed and mostly used in a medical setting.

The evidence for supplements supporting general mitochondrial processes and health are not always easily interpreted. For example, nicotinamide adenine dinucleotide (NAD in either its NAD+ or NADH forms) is an important cofactor in ATP (energy) production in the mitochondria and crucial for cellular processes. The body converts niacin (B3) into NAD+, which transports electrons within mitochondria for energy production. NADH is the form of NAD that holds these electrons plus a hydrogen ion. In one study, scientists found that people with primary mitochondrial disease had low blood levels of niacin, and supplementing with niacin increased blood levels and relieved some symptoms. Animal studies have also shown that niacin can increase blood levels of NAD as well. However, increased blood levels does not necessarily translate to increased mitochondrial levels. If you're deficient in niacin, your mitochondrial health may be affected. Foods rich in in niacin, tryptophan, and other B vitamins help to increase NAD levels naturally. If you're getting enough niacin from foods, there isn't much evidence that supplementing with niacin is beneficial. In fact, too much niacin can cause side effects, such as skin flushing, dizziness, and upset stomach.

There are several animal studies and recent small clinical studies that show the benefit of NAD metabolites: nicotinamide mononucleotide (NMN) or nicotinamide riboside (NR). Oral supplements of these is well tolerated, stimulate NAD+, and are promising in reducing risk factors of cardiovascular disease as people age.

The best thing that you can do for your mitochondrial health is to eat good foods and get your nutrients. In absence of a diet with a variety of good foods, it can be worthwhile to take a multivitamin and CoQ10 supplement. This combination provides niacin for NAD production, all the other B vitamins for mitochondrial metabolism, plus antioxidants (vitamins C and E) to protect against reactive oxygen species (ROS) damage. CoQ10 is not in most multivitamins, so it's a good addition for mitochondrial health.

Exercise is also important for metabolic health because it can increase the number of mitochondria in muscle cells. It also increases the efficiency of the mitochondria to produce more energy. These enhancements of mitochondrial function improve strength and endurance and reduce oxidative stress and resulting damage to cells.

Keeping Up with Prediabetes and Diabetes

About one-third of people in the United States have prediabetes, a condition in which a person's blood glucose (sugar) levels are higher than normal. A normal fasting level of blood glucose is less than 100 milligrams per deciliter (mg/dl). If the levels are higher than that, it can eventually lead to type 2 diabetes.

Another measurement is hemoglobin A1c (HbA1c), which measures a person's average glucose attached to hemoglobin in the past two to three months. It is best if this number is less than 5.7 percent.

If you develop diabetes, your body will not be able to effectively use the hormone (insulin) that helps glucose get into your cells, a condition called insulin resistance. The good news is that prediabetes can be prevented or reversed! But if you don't address it, it leads to diabetes, which is the eighth leading cause of death in the United States and can cause cardiovascular disease, kidney failure, loss of toes or feet, nerve damage, and blindness.

The exact cause of prediabetes isn't known, but genetics and family history may play a role in its development. Some other risk factors include being overweight or obese or having a waist size larger than 35 or 40 inches for women and men, respectively. Other risk factors are diet, a sedentary lifestyle, age, race, polycystic ovary syndrome (PCOS), high blood pressure, high triglycerides, and low HDL. Many of these factors are controllable by making some behavioral or lifestyle changes.

Regulating blood sugar

When you eat food, it is digested in your stomach and intestines and nutrients are released into your blood. (Refer to Figure 10-1.) Carbohydrates are generally broken down to a smaller digestible sugar called glucose, which circulates in your blood and then gets into your cells where it is further metabolized to form energy in the form of ATP. Insulin is the hormone that helps glucose get into your cells.

Blood levels of glucose go up and down throughout the day. When you eat food, blood glucose goes up. Insulin is then released by your pancreas to help the cells take glucose up, and the blood levels go down. When your glucose gets low, you can experience fatigue, hunger, and sometimes moodiness (you know, being hangry!). In prediabetes, your pancreas may be making or secreting less insulin and/or your cells may not be responding to it normally.

Eating food regularly — perhaps every three to four hours — helps to keep your blood sugar relatively even throughout the day. Regular food intake prevents very high blood levels and very low levels of glucose, and maintaining stable levels is less demanding on your pancreas.

Eliminating fatigue

If you feel tired, it's important to try to understand why. Did you sleep well the night before? Are you stressed? Have you eaten lately? If you're prediabetic, the most important thing to do is eat well and treat the predicating reasons for developing the disease. Losing weight and exercising may be what the doctor has prescribed. Both of these can help relieve fatigue.

Dealing with hunger, thirst, headaches

Symptoms of prediabetes include hunger, thirst, and headaches. The best thing to do is treat the condition to reduce symptoms. Dehydration is common, and drinking more water is recommended. Some supplements mentioned in this section may help with insulin control in general, which may help alleviate hunger, thirst, and headaches.

Using berberine, cinnamon, mushrooms, and chromium

Using berberine to help treat diabetes is well researched. Berberine is from the herb rhizoma coptidis and has been used in many formulas for treatment of diabetes for thousands of years. In a 2021 systematic review and meta-analysis, the efficacy of using berberine for diabetes care was studied. This large analysis showed that berberine could lower blood glucose as effectively as metformin, a prescription medication. It also showed that along with other treatments, it helped to lower HbA1C. These results further suggest that berberine may be most effective in people under 60 and who have had the disease for less than five years. The effective dose is 1 to 2 grams per day.

These results also demonstrated lowered fasting blood insulin, decreased body mass index (BMI), and improved insulin resistance. Berberine alone or combined with other therapies also reduced triglycerides, cholesterol, and low-density lipoprotein (LDL) and moderately increased HDL.

Cinnamon is spice containing many bioactive phytochemicals, including cinnamaldehyde, a polyphenol. These compounds in cinnamon have demonstrated antidiabetic properties, including lowering blood sugar and lowering blood lipid levels. It has been used for years to treat or complement diabetes treatment. Clinical trials have clarified these effects and also that cinnamon is an anti-inflammatory, which may act beneficially in diabetes. It seems to work by mimicking insulin and also improving enzyme activity.

A recent review of the literature confirmed these benefits of cinnamon, and a good dose to use for diabetes is 3 to 6 grams in your diet per day. Cinnamon may also include iron and aluminum. At 3 to 6 grams of cinnamon per day, most products will be safe.

Knowing what to look for in combination supplements

Other supplements that may help with diabetes include the following:

>> Magnesium, which may help with insulin resistance

>> Fiber, which can slow the release of glucose in the bloodstream

>> Vitamin D may slow the transition from prediabetes to diabetes

>> B12 if you take taking metformin, which can cause B12 deficiency

>> Apple cider vinegar (1 to 2 tablespoons in a glass of water) to possibly lower blood sugar levels (more studies need to be done)

>> Ginger to possibly lower blood glucose and regulate insulin production

TIP

More research on ginger is needed, but adding ginger to your diet is a good way to get some if you want to try it. Don't exceed more than 4 grams per day.

WARNING

Whenever you see a supplement that says it's for diabetes control, read the label carefully to see what nutrients are included and the suggested dose. Also look at the product's claims and marketing strategy. For example, a statement that it's "clinically tested" can be misleading.

There are many kinds of clinical studies (discussed in detail in Chapter 7). They could include a small marketing study conducted by a company on its own product or a large, well-designed scientific study, such as a randomized controlled clinical study (RTC). Just because a product claims "clinical study" on its label doesn't mean it underwent reliable testing in humans. Also, make sure to read the ingredients to look for fillers and additives and other things you can't identify.

Addressing Heart Disease and Hypertension

Heart disease includes several conditions that affect the heart and blood vessels. According to the CDC, about one in five people in the United States died from heart disease in 2022. The most common heart condition is coronary artery disease, which is when arteries are diseased and cause a decrease blood flow to the heart. Other conditions include arrhythmias or irregular heartbeats, congenital heart defects, and disease of the heart muscle or valve.

Hypertension is high blood pressure, which is when the pressure of the blood against your artery walls is too high. Your arteries bring blood to your heart, and if the pressure is abnormally high, it can lead to bigger problems like a heart attack or stroke. Your healthcare provider will tell you if you have high blood pressure because it, along with high cholesterol and smoking, are risk factors for heart disease.

Substituting fish oil for fish

Studies show that eating fish at least twice a week reduces your risk of dying from heart disease. Fish contains omega-3 fatty acids — docosahexaenoic acid (DHA) and eicosapentaenoic acid (EPA) — which must come from foods because your body doesn't produce them. Good sources of omega-3s are salmon, mackerel, trout, and shellfish, including mussels, oysters and crabs. Flaxseeds, chia seeds, and walnuts are good vegetarian sources of ALA, which gets converted to omega-3s. Several systematic reviews and meta-analyses have shown that higher consumption of fish and higher dietary or plasma levels of omega-3s are associated with a lower risk of heart failure, coronary disease, and fatal coronary heart disease

Many excellent and large studies have been done to examine the relationship between fish consumption and fish oil supplementation and heart disease and hypertension. The scientific research supports that consuming fish as part of a balanced diet promotes heart health by reducing heart failure, coronary disease, and fatal coronary heart disease. This is especially true if the fish replaces unhealthy foods and is baked or broiled.

Fish oil and other omega-3 supplements lower triglyceride levels and might reduce the risk of some cardiovascular disease, especially in people who are otherwise deficient in omega-3s. However, supplementation does not have the same health benefits as eating fish. This may be because it's not only the omega-3s in fish that may be heart healthy. If you already have heart disease, then your doctor may prescribe omega-3 supplements because they've been shown to be more effective in people who already have heart disease than for healthy people. Several studies have demonstrated a slight decrease in blood pressure with fish oil supplement use, so there may be a stronger effect in people with higher blood pressure.

You may see an FDA-qualified claim on supplement bottles that says, "Supportive but not conclusive research shows that consumption of EPA and DHA omega-3 fatty acids may reduce the risk of coronary heart disease and hypertension." The FDA allows supplement companies to add this claim on omega-3 products because there it meets the "credible scientific evidence" of being supportive enough (but not conclusive) to support the claim. It does not mean that the FDA has tested or specifically approved the product buying. The FDA also specifies that the labels of dietary supplements should not recommend a daily intake of EPA and DHA higher than 2 grams.

Multiple studies report modest reductions in blood pressure in people who take fish oil supplements. There's some evidence that the beneficial effects of fish oil might be greater for people with moderate to severe high blood pressure than for those with mild blood pressure elevation.

The bottom line is that it is best to eat fish, but if you don't eat fish, then a supplement may be helpful if you're not getting enough omega-3s from other dietary sources. If you've already been diagnosed with heart disease, then it is a good idea to take a fish oil supplement according to your doctor's instructions.

Filling up on fiber

There are two types of fiber in food: soluble and insoluble. Soluble fiber dissolves in water and forms a gel-like material as it goes through your gastrointestinal (GI) system. Soluble fiber helps slow down digestion, which can help regulate blood sugar. It also lowers cholesterol and is food for your microbiome and can increase the healthy gut bacteria leading to lower inflammation. Insoluble fiber doesn't dissolve in bodily fluids as it travels through your gut and adds bulk to stool. Insoluble fiber improves bowel health, prevents constipation, and reduces risk of hemorrhoids and diverticulitis.

Studies show that both kinds of fiber are good for your health. Fiber can help lower cholesterol and may help prevent and control high blood pressure. Soluble fiber can reduce LDL cholesterol (the bad cholesterol) and overall cholesterol. It may do this by physically binding to cholesterol as it goes through your GI tract, and then it helps to eliminate the cholesterol from your body. Other studies show that fiber may lower the risk of stroke and type 2 diabetes, both of which are linked to higher risk of heart disease. Another clinical study showed that a high-fiber diet lowered blood pressure after just 12 weeks. In a large study of 300,000 participants, eating lots of fiber led to a longer life.

The best sources for insoluble fiber include beans, nuts, whole grains, vegetables, and berries. Good sources of soluble fiber include citrus fruit, oats, peas, apples, barley, beans, carrots, and psyllium, which can be used as a laxative. A balanced diet of whole foods will give you plenty of fiber. Women should aim for about 22 to 28 grams per day, and men need about 28 to 34 grams per day.

Most Americans do not get enough fiber from their diets because they don't eat enough fruits and vegetables. Supplements can help you reach a daily goal. There are many types of fiber supplements on the market to choose from. If you have high blood sugar or cholesterol, you may choose a soluble fiber supplement that has psyllium husk, inulin, or wheat dextrin. Inulin is considered a prebiotic fiber because it is food for gut bacteria. If you have constipation or IBS, you may choose a supplement with insoluble fibers of calcium polycarbophil, flaxseed, or methylcellulose. These fiber supplements may come as gummies, powders, pills, or bars.

Magnesium and potassium

Magnesium is important in more than 300 enzymatic reactions in your body, so it's not surprising that it's important for heart health. Numerous studies support this idea. Both adequate dietary intake and circulating levels of magnesium in your blood are correlated with a lower risk of heart disease and high blood pressure. In addition, adequate magnesium also protects against metabolic syndrome and type 2 diabetes, which are both risk factors for heart disease. In most clinical nutrition studies, it's hard to separate the effect of magnesium from other components of food, so it's always best to get it from your diet. Following the DASH (Dietary Approach to Stop Hypertension) diet has been shown to reduce blood pressure. This diet increases intake of magnesium but also potassium and calcium that are associated with reductions in blood pressure. Some magnesium-rich foods include avocados, nuts, legumes, tofu, seeds, fatty fish, bananas, leafy greens, and whole grains.

There are many forms of magnesium supplements on the market, which makes it hard to choose. Some have better absorption, so they will more easily address magnesium deficiency. Here is a list of the different forms and their uses:

» **Magnesium citrate:** Common form that's absorbed by the body well and used to increase magnesium levels and to treat constipation

» **Magnesium oxide:** Not absorbed well, but may help with digestive symptoms

» **Magnesium chloride:** Absorbed well and used to raise magnesium levels and treat constipation or heartburn or topically for sore muscles

» **Magnesium lactate:** Food additive or supplement that may be gentler on the digestive system and better tolerated than other forms

» **Magnesium malate:** Well absorbed and good for raising magnesium levels but with less laxative effect

» **Magnesium taurate:** May be the best form to control blood sugar levels and blood pressure

» **Magnesium L-threonate:** Easily absorbed and may support brain health

» **Magnesium sulfate:** Can treat constipation or be used in bathwater (as a component in Epsom salt) to sooth sore muscles

>> **Magnesium glycinate:** Easily absorbed and may have calming effects and improve sleep

>> **Magnesium orotate:** Easily absorbed, lacks laxative effects, and may promote heart health

Potassium is important for regulating blood pressure, lowering cholesterol, and regulating your heartbeat. It doesn't treat or prevent heart disease, but it is good to make sure you're getting the RDA of 4,700 milligram per day (mg/day) from foods. Fruits and vegetables, dairy, whole grains, meat, and fish are all good dietary sources for potassium.

WARNING

Do not take a potassium supplement without talking to your doctor first. Too much can lead to kidney issues or interact with medications.

Lowering your blood pressure

According to the World Health Organization (WHO), an estimated 1.28 billion adults worldwide have hypertension. Because it is a major cause of premature death worldwide, it is important to diagnose and treat it. About 20 percent of people with hypertension have it under control. Your doctor may prescribe medication for treatment and recommend some lifestyle changes to reduce your risk, such as losing weight, being more physically active, no longer smoking, or cutting down on alcohol. You can help yourself lose weight and get important nutrients that help bring down blood pressure by eating a healthy, low-salt diet that is also low in saturated fats and sugar.

There are supplements that may help bring your blood pressure down, especially if you don't have optimal levels in your system because you don't eat a variety of foods. High blood pressure is nothing to fool around with, so always check with your doctor about using supplements!

Studies indicate that, in addition to fish oil, magnesium, and potassium, the following supplements may lower blood pressure:

>> Vitamin D: If your blood D3 levels are low, be sure to take a supplement to bring it up.

>> Riboflavin: May lower blood pressure, especially if you have the methylenetetrahydrofolate reductase (MTHFR) gene mutation

>> Folate: A supplement may lower levels in people with heart disease and may prevent younger people from developing heart disease later in life.

>> Here are some other supplements that may help, but more research is needed:

- CoQ10
- L-arginine
- Vitamin C
- Beetroot
- Garlic
- Probiotics
- Green tea
- Melatonin

Sprinkling in some helpful spices and herbs

Cinnamon, celery seeds, and cardamom are spices that may help lower blood pressure. The studies in support of using these spices for this purpose are small and suggestive but not conclusive. If nothing else, adding these spices will help make food taste good, and they may possibly help your health as well.

Garlic contains allicin, which may help your heart. Raw garlic, cut and allowed to sit out for ten minutes allows peak allicin activity. However, when you cook garlic, the allicin activity is greatly reduced, and more of the allicin is most likely destroyed in your GI tract. Garlic supplements that are made of aged garlic extract (AGE) have been shown to retain activity, and research shows that garlic supplements reduce blood pressure significantly. AGE may also improve cardiovascular health by reducing arterial stiffness, elevated cholesterol levels and blood "stickiness."

Thyme, parsley, and basil have shown some blood pressure–lowering activity in animal studies. It's unclear if this benefit translates to humans because no clinical studies have been done. However, adding these herbs, especially if fresh, to your diet is tasty, and they contain a number of healthy nutrients. For example, they all contain carotinoids that have health benefits, and parsley has a lot of iron and vitamin C in it.

Limited studies show that ginger may also lower blood pressure. It is easy to add ginger to your cooking, and supplements are available.

Two other herbs you may be less familiar with — Chinese cat claw and Bacopa monnieri — have been used to lower blood pressure, but there is little or no human trial information supporting their use.

Protecting Your Heart Health

Keeping your heart healthy has become easier than it once was because we know a lot more than our grandparents did! There are modifiable and nonmodifiable risk factors. The Framingham Heart Study started in 1948 and is now studying its third generation of participants. This very large study identified risk of cardiovascular disease, and other studies have followed.

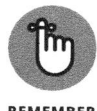

REMEMBER

The nonmodifiable risk factors (things you cannot change) for heart disease are age, gender, ethnicity, and family history. The modifiable risks — those you can change — include hypertension, hyperlipidemia, diabetes, obesity and overweight, smoking, poor diet, sedentary lifestyle, and stress.

Lowering your cholesterol

High cholesterol, high triglycerides and other lipids, and low HDL (good cholesterol) contribute to the risk of heart disease. It's important to keep your cholesterol in the normal range which is less than 200 mg/dl. You make cholesterol in your cells because you need it to form cell membranes and hormones and perform other important functions. You also get cholesterol from your foods.

Your annual blood test will include a lipid panel that typically measures the following:

>> Total cholesterol, where normal is less than 200 mg/dl

>> LDL ("bad") cholesterol, which should be less than 100 mg/dl

>> Very low-density lipoprotein (VLDL), which is usually a low level and comes from foods you eat

>> HDL ("good") cholesterol, which should be greater than 60 mg/dl

>> Triglycerides, a type of fat that comes from food you eat and should be less than 150 mg/dl

The best way to keep your blood cholesterol down is to reduce your intake of saturated fats and sugars from food. Both contribute to increasing blood cholesterol. Sugar and saturated fat intake are more important than the cholesterol concentration in foods. Exercise also is known to lower LDL cholesterol and increase HDL cholesterol.

Supplements that may help control cholesterol include these:

>> Red yeast rice extract contains trace amounts of monacolin K (the same chemical as in the medication lovastatin). Doses aren't regulated, and it may cause some side effects.

>> Niacin may lower LDL and triglycerides and increase HDL. High doses can cause side effects such as flushing.

>> Berberine may reduce LDL and triglycerides. You should not take it during pregnancy and while lactating.

>> Fish oil may reduce triglycerides, but it may interact with blood thinner medications.

>> Ground flaxseed may reduce triglycerides, but it may interact with blood thinner medications.

>> Green tea extract may decrease LDL.

>> Plant stanols and sterols may reduce LDL in familial hypercholesterolemia.

All of the above may have side effects, including GI issues such as diarrhea and gas.

Keeping the heart rhythm with potassium, magnesium, and calcium

Your heart works to pump blood through your body, and you don't even have to think about it. It uses an electrical system that coordinates your heartbeat very rhythmically. There are times when you may feel your heart at work, especially when you increase your exercise or physical activity. These rhythmic changes are normal during physical activity but may also be triggered by other things like mild dehydration or a change in medication. Be sure to drink water and also be aware of medication side effects.

The electrical system that works to keep your heart pumping is fairly understood at a cellular level. Potassium, magnesium, and calcium (and sodium) are electrolytes important for maintaining cellular function, fluid balance, signal conduction, intracellular signaling, and contraction of muscle fibers in your heart. An imbalance of these electrolytes can cause issues; therefore, it's critical to get what you need from your diet or supplements. Good sources of magnesium and potassium are covered in the "Magnesium and potassium" section earlier in this chapter. Good sources of calcium include diary, including hard cheeses, such as cheddar, Parmesan, and Emmental; fortified soy milk and tofu; sardines with bones; yogurt; and milk.

There are several forms of calcium in supplements. The two main forms are calcium carbonate and calcium citrate. Calcium carbonate is absorbed best when taken with food. Tums and Rolaids use this form of calcium. Calcium citrate can be taken with or without food, and this form is absorbed better if you're taking medications that lower your stomach acid or as you age. Other forms include calcium sulfate, calcium ascorbate, calcium microcrystalline hydroxyapatite, calcium gluconate, calcium lactate, and calcium phosphate.

Supplementing your meds: statins and CoQ10

If your lipid panel comes back with numbers out of normal range, resulting in an increase in risk for heart attack or stroke, your doctor may prescribe statins. These are medications known to lower cholesterol and inflammation.

Statins work by blocking the cholesterol synthetic pathway in your cells. This pathway also leads to the creation of CoQ10. Therefore, taking a statin reduces the amount of CoQ10 created in your cells, and a deficiency in CoQ10 can cause muscle aches and possibly neurological damage. It's hard to get CoQ10 from your food, so a supplement can help avoid or treat muscle aches caused by statins.

Reducing atherosclerosis with vitamin K

Atherosclerosis is when you have a gradual buildup of plaque in the walls of your arteries, which are the vessels that carry blood to your organs and tissues throughout your body. Plaque is made up of fat, cholesterol, and calcium. As it gets thicker, the opening of your artery narrows, and the blood has a harder time getting through. This gradual buildup of plaque can begin when you're young and may be worsened by high LDL cholesterol and triglyceride levels, smoking, high blood pressure, and diabetes. If plaque gets bad, it can rupture, causing a blood clot that can lead to a heart attack or stroke.

The Danish Diet, Cancer, and Health Study observed that people with adequate vitamin K1 and K2 levels (from food intake) had a lower risk of being admitted to the hospital for atherosclerotic cardiovascular disease (ASCVD). Vitamin K may work by reducing plaque formation and reducing clot formation.

WARNING

It is important to have a diet rich in vitamin K as part of a healthy diet. However, there is not enough evidence to warrant taking vitamin K supplements to prevent or treat plaque formation.

Keeping the heart muscle pumping

Your heart is a muscle that pumps about 2,000 gallons through it each day. Blood comes into the heart lacking oxygen, is reoxygenated in the heart, and pumped back out to your tissues and organs. As the blood flows through your body, tissues and organs take up the oxygen from the blood, which then circulates back to the heart for more oxygen. This complex process involves heart muscle tissue for structure and pumping, heart valves opening and closing between the heart's four chambers, energy metabolism, other metabolic processes, and nerve function. You need nutrients for all of this.

The best thing you can do is eat healthily, exercise, not smoke, and limit alcohol intake. And be sure that you are getting all your vitamins and minerals.

Managing Your Weight to Deter Obesity

According to the WHO, one out of eight people in the world are living with obesity, and the number has more than doubled since 1990. Adolescent obesity has quadrupled since 1990. In the United States, two-thirds of people are either overweight or obese. If you're overweight, you have an excessive amount of fat deposits in your body. Obesity is a little more complicated because fat deposits can impair your health. Being obese is a risk factor for type 2 diabetes, heart disease, and some cancers. Obesity is measured using BMI. Sometimes your doctor may also measure your waist and arm circumferences.

Generally speaking, adults are considered to be overweight when their BMI is greater than or equal to 25; obesity is the descriptor when the BMI is greater or equal to 30. These numbers are slightly lower for people of Asian background. BMI may be high in an athlete who is not overweight or obese because their increased muscle mass contributes to their weight. Children and adolescents have separate growth charts to measure their rate of growth and the percentile they are in for height and weight to determine if they are in the normal range.

It is important to be normal weight to avoid risk factors due to excessive fat. The best way to do this is to eat a healthy diet, such as the Mediterranean diet or Dietary Approach to Stop Hypertension (DASH) diet, the Healthy U.S.-Style (HUSS) diet, or an otherwise balanced way of eating. The key is not to eat too much and to keep your weight within normal range.

In the following sections, I will discuss some supplements that may help with efforts to lose weight.

Reducing appetite

There are several supplements on the market that claim to reduce appetite. They claim to work by a number of mechanisms including increasing your feeling of fullness, suppressing appetite, slowing stomach emptying, blocking nutrient absorption, breaking down fat, and boosting energy burning.

WARNING

These products include fenugreek seeds, glucomannan (a viscous fiber), *Gymnema sylvestre*, *Griffonia simplicifolia* (5-HTP), *Caralluma fimbriata*, conjugated linoleic acid, garcinia cambogia, and yerba matte. There is not enough evidence to say that any of these work to suppress appetite in people. It does seem reasonable that fiber in a supplement such as glucomannan could help to make you feel fuller and less hungry, but so could eating an apple!

TIP

In my opinion, the only thing that may help is caffeine and green tea or green tea extract that has epigallocatechin gallate (EGCG). EGCG and caffeine may boost metabolism for a short time after you've consumed them. Caffeine may also be a metabolism booster and may decrease your appetite.

Supplementing after weight-loss surgery

According to doctors at Johns Hopkins University, some daily supplements are necessary after bariatric surgery. Note that there are three different types of surgery, and the recommendations may vary depending on which you have. In any of these cases, you will be eating less, so there is a danger of not getting enough nutrients from food. Absorption of nutrients may also be affected.

The recommendation is to take vitamin D, B12, calcium, and an over-the-counter multivitamin. Total vitamin D should be 3,000 international units per day (IU/day), B12 should be 350 to 500 micrograms per day (mcg/day), and calcium citrate should be 1,200 to 1,500 mg/day over two or three doses for better absorption. The multivitamin may contain enough B12 and D if it is a bariatric multivitamin. There should also be some iron (13 to 30 mg) in the multivitamin.

Supporting weight loss on GLP-1 medications

Glucagon-like peptide-1 (GLP-1) medications work by enhancing insulin secretion from the pancreas to help sugar get into your cells, cut your appetite by telling your brain that you're full, and also slow down the rate at which your stomach empties. Some of the side effects include GI issues, nausea, vomiting, stomach pain, and indigestion. Also, Since you're eating less food, you may not be getting enough of the essential vitamins and other nutrients.

If you take a GLP-1 medication, it's important to eat enough protein and a variety of vegetables. In addition, whole grains, nuts, omega-3s, and fruit are also important as part of a nutritious diet. The GLP-1s work in ways that are not yet completely understood and may affect absorption of some vitamins, such as B12. These deficiencies are not necessarily treated with a simple multivitamin. If metabolism is changed, it may then be possible to get too much of the fat-soluble vitamins (A,D,E,K), which can be toxic.

TIP

There's supporting evidence for taking a few supplements while taking a GLP-1. You may want to consider taking multivitamin, vitamin B12, magnesium, omega-3 fatty acids, and probiotics to support gut health and manage GI side effects. Electrolyte balance is important, and magnesium levels may drop. Be sure to drink plenty of water because dehydration is also common. There are also several vitamin and mineral supplements specifically for people taking GLP-1s that include combinations of these nutrients.

When taking GLP-1 medications, it's important to eat well to support the action of the medications, the release of your natural GLP-1 hormones, and other hormones that help you feel full. Some of the best foods to eat while on GLP-1 medications include eggs, healthy fats, whole grains, berries, legumes, and vegetables. A growing field of companies — including BistroMD, CookUnity, Hungry Root, MealPro, and Territory Foods — are now providing packaged foods and food delivery services for people on weight-loss medications, and these may be quite helpful if they provide adequate protein and nutrients.

Looking for a magic supplement

GLP-1 medications are effective for weight loss and treating diabetes, but if you don't qualify for these prescription medications and are hoping that there is a supplement that works for weight loss, then you may be disappointed.

Weight-loss supplements advertise that they help you lose weight by curbing your appetite, speeding up your metabolism, or reducing the absorption of fats or carbohydrates. There's little scientific evidence for these claims, and supplements can be expensive and dangerous. Here are some of the ingredients in products on the market for weight loss:

>> **African mango:** May help a little and seems to be safe

>> **Beta-glucans:** Soluble fiber that may slow down digestion and is safe but doesn't seem to reduce weight

>> **Bitter orange:** May slightly increase the number of calories you burn and reduce appetite a little but may not be safe

>> **Caffeine:** Might burn calories and increase fat breakdown to contribute to a little weight loss; safe up to four or five cups of coffee a day but may have side effects

>> **Calcium:** Claims to burn fat and decrease its absorption but probably doesn't work for weight loss

>> **Capsaicin:** Claims to help burn fat and calories and make you eat less but hasn't been studied enough for weight loss

>> **Carnitine:** In meat and dairy and helps break down fats, safe for use, and may promote weight loss

>> **Chromium:** Regulates blood sugar and may help you lose a little weight

>> **Conjugated linoleic acid (CLA):** Found in meat and dairy and purported to lower body fat so may help you lose a very small amount of weight

>> **Garcinia cambogia:** Claimed to limit weight gain because of hydroxycitric acid in the fruit but has no effect on weight loss and may have side effects

>> **Green tea and green tea extract:** May increase metabolism and decrease fat absorption and the amount of new fat your body makes but taking the extract may not be safe so stick to the tea

>> **Probiotics:** Good for gut health but have no known effect on weight or body fat

>> **Pyruvate:** Claimed to reduce body weight and body fat and may help you lose a little weight

>> **Raspberry ketone:** Purported to be a fat burner but effects on body weight are unknown; more studies need to determine effectiveness

>> **White kidney bean/bean pod (*Phaseolus vulgaris*):** Extract from a legume that may block carbohydrate absorption, suppress appetite, and help you lose a small amount of weight

>> **Yohimbe:** Claimed to increase weight loss but no evidence that it works and may not be safe due to known side effects

Neurodegenerative Diseases

Neurons need nutrients to function, and an adequate dietary intake is essential for neuronal health. Neurodegenerative diseases are disorders characterized by a progressive loss of neurons, neuronal structure, and/or neuronal function. The most common are Alzheimer's disease, Parkinson's disease, amyotrophic lateral sclerosis (ALS), motor neuron disease, Huntington's disease, and spinal muscular atrophy.

These diseases are progressive, and many studies have been done to examine lifestyle and diet influence in the progression of these diseases. There are many things you can do to help prevent the onset or progression of declined neuronal function, which I talk about in the following sections.

The MIND diet takeaways

The MIND diet is the Mediterranean–DASH Intervention for Neurodegenerative Delay, which combines scientifically backed ways of eating to support the health of your aging brain. Both the Mediterranean and the DASH diets are known to prevent and improve cardiovascular disease and diabetes and promote healthy weight loss. Newer studies show that the MIND diet may prevent and slow neurodegenerative diseases, but more clinical research is needed to determine long-term clinical outcomes.

The MIND diet guidelines stress eating more "brain foods," such as fruits, vegetables, nuts, beans, berries, whole grains, some chicken and fish, and olive oil. You should limit or avoid unhealthy foods like saturated and trans fats, sugar, and alcohol.

Vitamin supplementation appears to be more effective in people with early disease rather than in people with more advance neurodegeneration. Some supplements may be helpful because they are antioxidants and anti-inflammatory. Others may be involved in the complex pathology of the proteins amyloid beta and tau.

Researchers at Mass General Brigham have led a large study called the COcoa Supplement and Multivitamin Outcomes Study (COSMOS). There have been three published papers from this nationwide, randomized trial that rigorously tests cocoa extract and multivitamin supplements. The results confirm consistent and statistically significant benefits of a daily multivitamin versus placebo for both memory and global cognition.

The only other supplement with scientific evidence for preventing cognitive decline is omega-3 fatty acids. There is very limited and inconsistent evidence for others including ginkgo biloba and curcumin.

Gene regulation

Epigenetics is when DNA can be modified but not changed. This can then modify gene expression, which may affect physiological processes including aging and carcinogenesis. This is also inheritable and can be passed down to offspring. Nutrients and food components can influence this by inhibiting enzymes or altering the availability of things needed for enzymatic reactions of DNA methylation and other modifications.

Nutrients that affect DNA methylation include folate, methionine, choline, betaine, and B12. Research on other bioactive food components, including tea polyphenols, genistein from soybeans, and isothiocyanates from plants, show that these might inhibit cancers by inhibiting methylation of DNA. Several studies show that alcohol and total diet can affect DNA methylation and then gene expression.

Another epigenetic effect is on something called histone modification, which modifies DNA but doesn't change its actual structure. Some things that may affect this include resveratrol, choline, calorie restriction, curcumin, and choline. Note that much of the work determining these biological effects has been done in animal studies.

Nerve function

There are some supplements that support your nervous system as well as to help improve neuropathy (nerve dysfunction that results in weakness, numbness, and pain). Some of these are also antioxidants.

WARNING

Consult with your healthcare professional before taking any of the supplements listed here so they can help decide what's appropriate based on your situation and the cause of any dysfunction.

B vitamins — especially B1, B6, and B12 — are essential for proper neurological function. B12 deficiency can actually cause neuropathy when it's severe. Acetyl-L- carnitine is derived from an amino acid and is a conditionally essential nutrient because your need sometimes exceeds your ability to synthesize this nutrient. It has been studied in Alzheimer's disease and dementia, and results are unclear as to whether there is any benefit.

Fish oil is an anti-inflammatory and may repair nerve damage and slow or reverse the progression of neuropathy. There have been several systematic reviews and meta-analyses assessing the effects of omega-3 supplementation on cognitive function and dementia in healthy older adults and those with Alzheimer's disease or cognitive impairment. Overall, these studies indicate that omega-3 supplementation does not affect cognitive function in healthy older adults or in people with Alzheimer's disease. They may improve certain aspects of cognitive function in people with mild disease, although more clinical research is needed to confirm.

Antioxidants

N-acetyl cysteine (NAC) is sold as a supplement but is actually classified by the FDA as a drug. It's used for a variety of things and is involved in synthesis of glutathione, an important antioxidant. In this way, it may help with nerve damage and pain and improve motor coordination.

ALA is an antioxidant that may be beneficial for the brain and skeletal muscle energy metabolism. There are no good clinical trials to support clinical efficacy. However, there are no safety concerns or adverse effects known.

Curcumin is an antioxidant that may help with nerve function. In particular, one animal study showed some improvement in diabetic neuropathy; however, clinical studies are needed to confirm this in people.

Ongoing research is being done on other antioxidants that may have neuroprotective benefits. Some of these are vitamins E and C, coenzyme Q10, resveratrol, ginkgo biloba, astaxanthin, and beta-carotene. Because many of these protect the body from ROS, there's promise that these supplements may have some benefit. Following the MIND diet will provide plenty of good antioxidants to keep your nervous system healthy.

Confounding Cancer

Cancer is caused by DNA mutations that can be inherited. They can also be caused by environmental and lifestyle factors. If you have an inherited DNA mutation, you may or may not develop cancer. Sometimes you need a second trigger (or carcinogen exposure) to develop the cancer. According to the WHO, about a third of cancers may be caused by modifiable risk factors such as tobacco use, high alcohol consumption, unhealthy diet, lack of physical activity, air pollution, radiation, and too much sun. Viral or bacterial infections can also cause certain types of cancers.

There are things you can do to control these risk factors, including eating well and getting all your nutrients, including those antioxidants that help prevent damage to your cells from ROS. The theory is that antioxidants may prevent cellular damage and inflammation that may lead to cancers.

To support you while going through cancer treatment, some supplements may be helpful, and others may cause harm.

Possible benefits

Some large population studies (epidemiological studies) correlate high fruit and vegetable consumption with lower risk of most cancers. The belief is that this could be due to high levels of vitamin C or carotenoids. However, all kinds of clinical studies — case controlled, prospective, and RCTs — over many years in many people have not demonstrated this as cause and effect. In other words, there is no proof that vitamin C or A supplementation or any other dietary supplement helps prevent or cure cancers. Some supplements are still being investigated — including vitamin C, oral glutamine, and melatonin — for helpfulness with side effects of cancer treatment. For example, one study found that intravenous vitamin C with chemotherapy may help patients with pancreatic cancer. A good source of information is the list of Dietary Supplement Fact Sheets from the National Institutes of Health Office of Dietary Supplements.

Proven harm

While undergoing treatment for cancer, it's important to consult with your doctor about any supplements you're taking. Some types of treatments have antimetabolic effects, which helps to kill off cancer cells. For example, some cancer drugs decrease folate metabolism, which will inhibit mitosis or replication of cancer cells. You can imagine that this affects normal cells also, so a patient is walking a fine line between killing off cancer cells and maintaining healthy cells. In most cases a multivitamin to keep your cells healthy is fine and recommended. Larger doses of some nutrients — especially folate and B12 — are not recommended because they may counteract the chemotherapy action.

REMEMBER

There are many kinds of cancer and treatments. You must be careful about anything you take, especially while going through chemo, radiation, or other treatments. It's always recommended that you eat well and get your nutrients from food. However, getting those nutrients from supplements may not be a good idea.

Chapter **11**

Taking Supplements for Other Conditions

From time to time, you may experience nutrient deficiencies in your life due to illness, a particular treatment, or a condition. The deficiency may be temporary or chronic. Sometimes it may be because you aren't getting enough food; other times, you may be eating too much of the wrong foods.

In this chapter, I address a variety of conditions or disorders that may be improved or supported with supplements. Sometimes these arise from nutrient deficiencies and other times from the condition or treatment.

Understanding Nutrient Deficiencies

Nutritional deficiencies can develop for several reasons, but it's frequently because of a reduced intake of foods that provide essential nutrients. This can happen for several reasons, including digestive issues, anorexia and other eating disorders, eating the wrong foods, and unavailability of enough food or of good foods. Chronic malnutrition effects over 934 million people worldwide. In 2023, there were 47.4 million people in the United States living in food-insecure homes, which includes 14 million children. Some health issues — such as type 2 diabetes, obesity, and heart disease — are related to poor nutrition.

Aside from food insecurity, some people overeat non-nutritious foods, and although they may carry extra weight, they're undernourished. In the United States, fast foods are readily available and inexpensive, but fast food isn't as nutritionally dense as whole food prepared at home.

In addition to the availability of fast foods and cheap processed foods, some of the foods we eat are less nutritious than they were in the past. The nutritional quality of fruits, vegetables, and food crops including rice, potatoes, wheat, and corn has declined because of changes in farming practices and nutrient reduction in soil.

TIP

Some common nutritional deficiencies include the following:

>> **Protein:** This macronutrient should be at least 10 percent of your caloric intake. You can figure out your recommended amount of protein by multiplying your weight in pounds by .36. Signs of protein deficiency are edema (swelling); hair, nail, and skin problems; slow-healing injuries; mood changes; hunger; and fatigue. Good sources of protein include meat, fish, dairy, eggs, and nuts. Protein supplements mostly come in the form of powders, shakes, or bars.

Note that many healthcare professionals believe that the popular view that Americans need more protein is not warranted. Most people in the United States get the Recommended Dietary Allowance (RDA) of protein, and many get much more that. According to the Mayo Clinic, high-protein diets for a long period of time may limit carb intake so much that nutrients from fiber are reduced, a high-protein diet may increase your intake of saturated fats, and can lead to increased risk of heart disease and put stress on your kidneys.

>> **Fats, especially omega-3 and omega-6 polyunsaturated fatty acids (PUFAs):** Lower omega-3 intake is correlated with a higher risk of mortality by heart disease. During pregnancy, omega-3 supplementation decreases the risk of premature births. Omega-3s are also recommended for people with hypertriglyceridemia (too many triglycerides in the blood). Omega-6s are important for energy production, cell membrane structure, and lowering LDL. Too much omega-6 can promote inflammation. A balance of both of these PUFAs is crucial for optimal health.

TIP

Good food sources of omega-3 fats include fish, seeds, canola oil, and olive oil. Good sources of omega-6 fats are vegetable oils and fish. According to Harvard Health, to maintain a good ratio of the two important fats, eat more omega-3, not less omega-6!

- **Fiber:** Most Americans need about 25 to 30 grams of fiber a day. You get fiber from fruits, vegetables, and whole grains. Fiber is good for healthy and regular bowel movements, reducing cholesterol by increasing excretion, and increasing your sense of fullness after meals. It also may help you eat less and control weight blood sugar.

- **Vitamin D:** Ninety-four percent of people in the United States do not meet the recommended daily allowance (RDA) for vitamin D. Lack of vitamin D can cause fatigue, mood change (depression), muscle cramps or weakness, and bone pain. A deficiency can happen because of a lack of sunlight or vitamin D–rich foods such as fish, dairy, and fortified milks and orange juice.

- **Magnesium:** A deficiency, which affects 52 percent of U.S. residents, may start with fatigue, weakness, numbness, and/or muscle contractions. Severe deficiency results in low calcium or potassium and a disruption in mineral metabolism. Some good sources for magnesium include fatty fish (salmon, halibut, and mackerel), spinach and other leafy greens, tofu, nuts, seeds, legumes, quinoa, and avocado.

- **Calcium:** Getting enough calcium is important for bone and tooth health throughout life. A deficiency can lead to osteoporosis (especially in women as they age), cataracts, dental changes, and rickets in children. Vegetarians may be especially at risk for deficiency. Good sources are dairy products, fortified milks and juice, kale, broccoli, and oranges.

- **Iodine:** Deficiency in iodine can lead to changes in thyroid function that can impact metabolism and development. Goiter is a disease that results from insufficient iodine, although it's no longer common in the United States. The best source of iodine is iodized salt and seaweed.

- **Folate (folic acid B9):** This nutrient is vital for women of childbearing age and early in pregnancy to prevent neural tube birth defects. If you're thinking of becoming pregnant, B9 is essential for three months before conceiving. A prenatal vitamin is the best source for this and all the other essential vitamins and minerals needed for pregnancy. Food sources include beef, spinach and other greens, beans, and fortified cereals and other grains.

- **Vitamin C:** A lack of vitamin C can lead to bleeding gums, bruising, poor wound healing, and, ultimately, scurvy (which is uncommon in the United States, but rates are rising). The mild deficiency we see in the United States is because many people do not eat enough fruits and vegetables due to lack of availability or high cost. Good sources include citrus fruits, kiwifruit, strawberries, peppers, broccoli, cantaloupe, and tomatoes.

- **Vitamin E:** Most people in the United States (88 percent) do not meet the RDA for vitamin E. Good food sources of vitamin E are wheat germ oil, nuts, seeds, vegetable oils, tomatoes, avocados, spinach, and mangos.

>> **Vitamin A:** Forty-three percent of people in the United States do not get the RDA for vitamin A. Good sources of vitamin A are leafy greens, tomatoes, red peppers, cantaloupe, mango, beef liver, fish oils, milk, eggs, and fortified foods.

>> **Zinc:** Zinc deficiency isn't as common, but about 12 percent of people (and up to 40 in the elderly) are deficient in this nutrient. Good sources of zinc include oysters, beef, breakfast cereals, pumpkin seeds, pork, turkey, cheese, lentils, peanuts, and sardines.

>> **Potassium:** According to the 2020–2025 Dietary Guidelines for Americans, underconsumption of potassium is a concern for people in the United States. Good sources of potassium include dried apricots, lentils, acorn squash, prunes, raisins, potatoes, kidney beans, orange juice, soybeans, bananas, milk, spinach, dairy, tomatoes, chicken, salmon, and beef.

Using Supplements for Specific Medical Conditions

When you're diagnosed with a medical condition, you work with your healthcare providers to come up with the best plan of action. Often this will involve medications and possibly lifestyle changes. In addition, there may be some benefits to supplement use.

Supplements are often used to complement conventional medical treatments. Sometimes they provide support for overall health — especially when a person is deficient in certain nutrients or prescribed medications contribute to deficiencies. Complementary supplements offer additional support in managing symptoms, improving quality of life, and enhancing overall health in various medical conditions. Your doctor should always help you determine what supplements are appropriate for your situation.

WARNING

Supplements are meant to *complement* your treatment but *never* intended to replace your treatment. Work with your healthcare providers to complement your medical treatment before adding them to your plan.

Alcoholism

Drinking excessive amounts of alcohol can result in the reduced intake of nutritious foods because alcohol (which lacks nutrients) replaces calories from nutrient-dense foods. In addition, alcohol can reduce the absorption of nutrients in the intestines. It can cause changes in the storage and metabolism of some nutrients. The result can be more health problems, such as gastrointestinal (GI), neurological, and liver damage.

Treatment for deficiencies related to alcoholism include healthier food intake and supplements. But the underlying disease of alcoholism needs to be addressed in consultation with health professionals.

Possible deficiencies include the following:

>> **Protein and amino acids:** A person can be deficient in protein and amino acids because of both decreased intake of foods and altered metabolism. Deficiency can cause muscle wasting, weight loss, impaired immunity, loss of hair, and skin issues.

>> **Sodium and potassium:** Drinking alcohol increases excretion and alters electrolyte balance. This causes dehydration, which can lead to irregular heartbeat and muscle weakness.

>> **Vitamin B1 (thiamine):** In this case, alcohol interferes with the absorption and functioning of vitamin B1. Some symptoms may include fatigue, confusion, memory loss, and muscle weakness. A deficiency can lead to Wernicke-Korsakoff syndrome, which includes severe neurological damage.

>> **Vitamin B9 (folate):** Alcohol interferes with absorption from the intestines and storage in the liver. Low folate can cause fatigue, mood changes, and weakness.

>> **Vitamin B12 (cobalamin):** Alcohol causes a reduced intrinsic factor (a protein in the stomach) secretion that can lead to decreased B12 absorption. Low B12 can cause pernicious anemia, numbness, tingling in hands and feet, memory loss, and other neurological damage.

>> **Vitamin A:** Alcohol can impair liver function, which affects vitamin A metabolism. Low levels can cause dry skin, increased infections, and night blindness.

>> **Vitamin D:** Impaired liver function reduces conversion of vitamin D to its active form. Symptoms include osteopenia or osteoporosis and bone pain.

>> **Vitamin C:** If alcohol consumption interferes with food intake, a person can be deficient in vitamin C due to not getting enough fruits and vegetables. Deficiency can lead to scurvy, which causes bleeding gums, bruising, fatigue, and joint pain.

>> **Calcium:** Alcoholism interferes with absorption and metabolism of calcium. Deficiency causes bone weakness and higher risk of fractures and muscle cramps.

>> **Magnesium:** The diuretic nature of alcohol results in increased excretion, which affects magnesium levels. Absorption of this mineral is also decreased because of alcohol. Symptoms include muscle cramps, tremors, and heart abnormalities.

>> **Zinc:** Zinc can become depleted because of decreased absorption and increased urinary excretion. Symptoms include loss of taste and smell, immune dysfunction, and poor wound healing.

>> **Iron:** A person with alcohol addiction can experience impaired absorption and storage of iron, leading to iron-deficiency anemia. Symptoms include fatigue and weakness.

Weight-loss surgery and GLP-1s medications

If you've undergone weight-loss surgery (bariatric surgery) to address obesity and related health issues, then you will need supplements. The different types of surgeries, including bypass and sleeve, lead to reduced food intake, altered digestion, and altered absorption of nutrients. As a result, you won't get enough of many nutrients from foods. Specifically, you may not get enough of the fat-soluble vitamins A, D, E, K, folate, B12, iron, calcium, zinc, and copper.

Your healthcare provider will monitor your post-surgery and will give you a list personalized to your specific needs. Supplements recommended by your healthcare provider after bariatric surgery may include these:

>> A multivitamin that will cover most of these deficiencies

>> Extra fat-soluble vitamins A, D, E, and K

>> Iron supplements if you're anemic

>> B12 sublingual or intravenous (IV) infusion

>> Folic acid

>> Calcium

>> Zinc and copper

Another approach for managing type 2 diabetes and its complications and obesity is the use of glucagon-like peptide-1 agonists (GLP-1s). They're recommended for use along with diet and lifestyle changes. These drugs include liraglutide, dulaglutide, semaglutide, and tirzepatide (brand names include Ozempic, Wegovy, Monjourno, and Zepbound). They work by enhancing insulin secretion in response to meals, slowing gastric emptying, and reducing appetite. These drugs can help reduce "food noise" so that you're no longer as interested in eating food. When you eat less, it will be hard to get all the nutrients you need in the necessary amounts.

GLP-1s are being studied for a number of other medical conditions, including addiction, dementia, neurodegenerative diseases, kidney disease, and psychiatric disorders.

If you take a GLP-1, it's a good idea to meet with a nutritionist or dietitian to get a personalized assessment and recommendations about food and supplement intake. Here are some things to consider if you're taking a GLP-1:

>> Concentrate on staying hydrated and be sure to get all your electrolytes.

>> Focus on protein by having protein at each meal to prevent muscle wasting. Protein shakes and supplements can be helpful.

>> Supplement with essential vitamins and minerals to avoid developing deficiencies. Recommended supplements include

- A daily balanced multivitamin.

- Vitamin B12 (sublingual or IV).

- Vitamin D and calcium citrate.

- Iron with vitamin C (to enhance iron absorption). Ferrous salts (ferrous fumarate, ferrous sulfate, and ferrous gluconate) are the most bioavailable.

- Magnesium (citrate or glycinate).

- Folic acid or use methylfolate, especially if you have the MTFHR gene mutation.

Hormonal issues

Hormones are chemical messengers that are synthesized in the body and can then be transported through the body to cells where they control specific cellular functions. Here are some:

>> **Insulin:** A hormone synthesized in the pancreas. Its main function is to control sugar metabolism. When you can't make insulin or your body doesn't process it correctly, the result is insulin resistance, prediabetes, or diabetes.

>> **Estrogen:** One of the female sex hormones. It's responsible for ovulation, menstruation, breast development, and bone density. Having too much estrogen can cause weight gain, sleep difficulties, menstrual issues, and

anxiety. Too little estrogen, which happens naturally with aging, can cause menstrual issues, mood disorders, fertility issues, and loss of bone density (osteoporosis).

>> **Progesterone:** Another female sex hormone. It's important for menstruation, uterine health, and pregnancy. Low progesterone can cause menstrual and fertility issues.

>> **Testosterone:** An androgen, which is a hormone associated with male reproduction. Women can produce testosterone and other androgens as well. In both men and women, testosterone can contribute to sex drive, fat distribution, muscle strength, bone mass, and red blood cell production.

>> **Cortisol:** Often referred to as the stress hormone because your body increases production as a reaction to stress. Cortisol, which is produced in the adrenal glands, helps regulate metabolism and blood pressure. It's also anti-inflammatory. Too little may cause low blood pressure, weakness, and fatigue. Too much cortisol for long periods can cause hypertension, anxiety, sleep loss, and autoimmune problems.

>> **Adrenaline:** Also a stress hormone produced in the adrenal glands as well as within some cells of the central nervous system. This is the fight-or-flight hormone that prepares your body in dangerous or stressful situations. Too much may lead to high blood pressure, anxiety, heart palpitations, irritability, or dizziness.

>> **Thyroid hormones:** Regulate metabolism. An imbalance of thyroid hormones can cause problems with energy levels and weight and can be linked to serious conditions like Grave's disease or Hashimoto's disease.

The following hormonal conditions occur when the hormones from the preceding list are too high or too low:

>> **Diabetes:** Blood sugar levels are too high

>> **Hypothyroidism:** Thyroid doesn't produce enough thyroid hormones

>> **Hyperthyroidism:** Thyroid gland produces too much hormone

>> **Graves' disease:** Thyroid gland produces too much hormone

>> **Hashimoto's disease:** An autoimmune disease where the body attacks the thyroid gland

>> **Cushing's syndrome:** High levels of cortisol

>> **Polycystic ovary syndrome (PCOS):** Enlarged ovaries, cyst-like follicles, and irregular periods

>> **Menopause:** Age-related decline in hormones

>> **Addison's disease:** A rare disease where not enough cortisol and adrenaline is produced

Nutritional deficiencies can sometimes impact hormonal balance and cause thyroid dysfunction, insulin resistance, adrenal fatigue, and irregular menstruation. Be sure to get enough of the following key nutrients to help keep hormonal balance:

>> **Vitamin D:** Deficiency is linked to low sex hormone levels, PCOS, infertility, insulin sensitivity, and thyroid dysfunction.

>> **Magnesium:** Deficiency can disrupt estrogen and progesterone balance, increase cortisol, and contribute to insulin resistance.

>> **Omega-3s:** Deficiency can lead to increased inflammation, disrupt reproductive and thyroid hormones, and increase anxiety and depression.

>> **Zinc:** Deficiency impairs sex hormone metabolism, fertility, and libido; contributes to hypothyroidism, and decreases insulin sensitivity,

>> **B12 and folate:** Deficiency may reduce cellular energy production, decrease metabolism, promote adrenal fatigue, enhance estrogen levels, contribute to an imbalance of sex hormones, and affect mood by increasing anxiety and depression.

>> **Iron:** Deficiency is linked to heavy menstruation, low energy, thyroid dysfunction, mood disorders related to dopamine and serotonin production, and impaired oxygen transport (fatigue).

>> **Iodine:** Deficiency leads to reduction in thyroid hormones, hypothyroidism, weight gain, risk of goiter, and cognitive issues.

>> **Selenium:** Deficiency reduces conversion of T4 and T3 (thyroid hormones), increased estrogen levels, and increased oxidative stress.

>> **Vitamin C:** Deficiency weakens the adrenal glands and increases production of stress-related hormones, affects progesterone levels, and impairs immune function.

>> **Protein:** Without enough protein or amino acids, you can experience a decrease in all hormone synthesis, an impairment of neurotransmitter synthesis that affects mood and sleep, muscle loss, fatigue, and poor blood sugar control.

>> **Myo-inositol:** This supplement may improve insulin sensitivity and ovarian function in polycystic ovary syndrome (PCOS).

Some botanicals that may help include

>> **Ashwagandha:** May help balance cortisol levels and reduce stress (adrenal fatigue, stress-related hormone imbalances)

>> **Chaste tree berry (vitex):** Supports hormonal balance (PMS, menopause)

>> **Black cohosh:** May relieve some symptoms of menopause

Taking the supplements when you're deficient in these nutrients can help contribute to hormonal balance. In addition, other lifestyle adjustments will contribute to hormone balance, including eating a nutrient-dense diet; reducing processed foods, sugar, and inflammatory foods; getting enough sleep; exercising regularly; and managing stress.

Type 2 diabetes or prediabetes

To really dive into details about prediabetes and type 2 diabetes, check out Chapter 10. Here, I've provided a list of supplements that may help with blood sugar control, energy production, and preventing complications from the disease.

REMEMBER

The recommended doses for supplements below may differ for you depending on your nutrition and lifestyle, medications, and severity of disease. Always discuss supplement types and dose with your healthcare provider.

>> **Magnesium glycinate or citrate:** 200 to 400 mg

>> **Vitamin D3:** 1,000 to 5,000 IU/day

>> **Chromium picolinate:** 200 to 1,000 mcg/day

>> **Zinc citrate or picolinate:** 15 to 30 mg/day

>> **ALA (alpha-lipoic acid):** 300 to 600 mg/day

>> **Omega-3 (EPA, DHA):** 1,000 to 2,000 mg/day

>> **B vitamins (methylated B-complex):** One multivitamin or B supplement a day

>> **Coenzyme Q10 (CoQ10):** 100 to 300 mg/day

>> **Fiber via dietary intake or a supplement:** About 25 to 30 g/day

>> **Cinnamon:** Quantity undetermined but the amount of cinnamon in foods is safe, so use liberally

>> **Berberine:** Up to 1.5 g/day for six months and may slightly reduce blood sugar in people with diabetes

Hypertension and heart disease

Some supplements may be helpful if you have hypertension or heart disease.

WARNING

Supplements for any condition should complement your medications and be taken only after consulting your doctor. Supplements may be helpful, but primarily when your diet is lacking or you're clinically deficient in a nutrient; it's always best to get nutrients from foods if you can. Note that the clinical evidence for efficacy of these supplements is limited and mostly valuable if you have a deficiency.

Suggested doses vary based on your individual situation so always check with your healthcare provider. The doses I list here are general guidelines and may not be for everyone. The effectiveness may also vary depending on lifestyle and health factors. Lastly, these doses are not necessarily backed by a sufficient number of scientific studies.

>> **Magnesium:** 300 to 420 mg/day

>> **Potassium:** 3,500 to 5,000 mg/day through food

>> **Omega-3 fatty acids:** Up to 1,000 mg/day

>> **CoQ10:** 30 to 200 mg/day

>> **Garlic:** 600 to 2,400 mg of garlic powder or aged extract per day

>> **Vitamin C:** 500 mg/day for eight weeks

>> **Turmeric (curcumin):** 500 to 2,000 mg of turmeric powder/day

>> **L-arginine:** 3 to 9 g/day

>> **Green tea extract:** 380 mg/daily

WARNING

Before you start taking something, verify whether any supplements you're considering are contraindicated for certain conditions. For example, high blood pressure and heart disease are serious concerns, and it's important to know what supplements *not* to take. Avoid the following if you have heart disease: arnica, ephedra, ginseng, guarana, and licorice.

Osteopenia, osteoporosis, and joint health

If you have osteopenia or osteoporosis, medications, supplements, and lifestyle modifications help to enhance bone density and reduce risk of fracture. Osteopenia is when your bones have less minerals in them and they become less dense. Osteoporosis is when the loss of bone density gets worse and can lead to bone fractures. Some of the risk factors for losing bone density include being older than 50, being female, being postmenopausal, smoking, drinking alcohol, having diabetes, having calcium or vitamin D deficiency, experiencing hormonal imbalance, having rheumatoid arthritis, and having disordered eating. Some medications may increase your risk including hormonal cancer therapy, proton pump inhibitors, diuretics, and corticosteroids.

The recommendations for preventing and treating osteopenia are typical of preventing most diseases. First, be sure to see your healthcare provider. Stay physically active, get plenty of calcium and vitamin D from foods daily, limit alcohol, and don't smoke. If you're diagnosed with osteoporosis, the recommendations are similar. Always be cognizant of possible interactions between supplements and medications to ensure safety and efficacy. Supplements recommended for prevention and treatment of osteopenia and osteoporosis may include the following:

» **Calcium:** Women younger than 51 years need 1,000 mg, and women older than 51 need 1,200 mg daily from food and supplements combined but be aware that calcium interferes with the absorption of some medications for osteoporosis. If you take supplements, take them at a different time than your oral bone medications for the best results. Be sure to follow directions for your medication. For example, if you're taking bisphosphonates, take them on an empty stomach with water and wait 30 minutes before ingesting anything else, including supplements.

» **Vitamin D:** People older than 50 need 800 to 1,000 IU daily. Vitamin D helps calcium absorption.

» **Vitamin K2:** The recommended amount is 100 to 200 mcg/day. K2 regulates calcium deposition to promote bone formation and studies show that combining it with bisphosphonates may prevent vertebral fractures better than taking bisphosphonates alone. Be sure to take this and any supplement separately from the medication.

» **Magnesium:** Having 300 to 400 mg/day supports bone structure.

» **Omega-3:** These fatty acids may benefit bone health. The dose varies, so it is best to eat good food sources such as salmon, flaxseeds, and walnuts.

» **Collagen peptides:** Having 5 to 10 g/day of collagen peptides may help bone health, especially if your protein intake is low.

Some supplements may help to ease joint pain and arthritis. Some of these include:

» **Glucosamine:** Your body produces glucosamine to help grow and repair cartilage. There are no major food sources of glucosamine, so supplements may be helpful to lubricate joints and help maintain cartilage structure and function.

Cartilage naturally has both glucosamine and chondroitin, so a supplement with both may help relieve pain. The anti-inflammatory properties of glucosamine and chondroitin also may help relieve pain from arthritis and decrease joint pain.

>> **Curcumin:** This is a powerful anti-inflammatory and may help with symptoms of osteoarthritis and rheumatoid arthritis. Some studies say it might be better than anti-inflammatory drug treatment.

>> **Green tea:** The active ingredient in green tea (epigallocatechin gallate or EGCG) may help your joints and muscles. Animal studies show that it may protect cartilage and bone and lower the risk of rheumatoid and osteoarthritis.

>> **Vitamin D:** This vitamin fights inflammation and is necessary to help your body absorb calcium to support bone health. Studies show that people with rheumatoid arthritis are often deficient in vitamin D.

>> **Omega-3 fatty acids:** These help control inflammation and may decrease the autoimmune-related inflammatory symptoms in rheumatoid arthritis. Omega-3s may also reduce arthritis pain and joint stiffness.

Autoimmune diseases

Autoimmune diseases are conditions in which the immune system attacks the body's healthy cells, tissues, and organs. The immune system becomes overactive and targets normal body structures instead of fighting off foreign intruders like viruses and bacteria. This can then lead to inflammation, tissue damage, and dysfunction.

The exact causes of autoimmune diseases are unknown but may involve a combination of genetics, environmental triggers, and, in women, hormones. The root of many of these diseases is inflammation and enhanced immune response. The treatments include medications, lifestyle changes, and supplements. Supplements that may support immune function are vitamin D, omega-3, and probiotics. Lifestyle changes include dietary adjustments to reduce inflammation and ensuring adequate nutrient intake to support the immune system.

The following list includes some of the more common autoimmune diseases and supplements that may help. In some cases, these supplements address inflammation or support immune function. In other cases, such as with celiac disease, supplements may help manage deficiencies due to malabsorption because of the disease. Probiotics that support gut health may also contribute to supporting immune responses.

>> **Psoriasis:** Topical or oral vitamin D, omega-3 fatty acids, probiotics, and zinc

>> **Type 1 diabetes:** Vitamin D, ALA, and magnesium

>> **Rheumatoid arthritis (RA):** Omega-3 fatty acids, vitamin D, turmeric, and probiotics

>> **Lupus:** Omega-3 fatty acids, vitamin D, and probiotics

>> **Hashimoto's thyroiditis:** Selenium, vitamin D, and possibly iodine

>> **Celiac disease:** Vitamin D, folic acid, and iron

>> **Inflammatory bowel disease, Crohn's, and ulcerative colitis:** Vitamin D, omega-3 fatty acids, probiotics, and folic acid

>> **Multiple sclerosis:** Omega-3 fatty acids, vitamin D, B12

Mental health and cognitive disorders

Complementary use of the following supplements may be helpful if you have anxiety, depression, ADHD, dementia, or Alzheimer's, but take them only after consulting with a healthcare provider. Some of these work by supporting metabolism of neurotransmitters or gut health. This topic is covered in more detail in Chapter 10.

>> Omega-3 fatty acids

>> Vitamin B complex

>> Probiotics

>> Ginkgo biloba

>> Ashwagandha

Digestive disorders

Digestive disorders include everything from occasional indigestion to more chronic problems like IBS (irritable bowel syndrome). There are often things that you can do to relieve symptoms and also address the underlying causes. Addressing most GI disorders also involves making dietary changes as well. Some common digestive disorders include indigestion, GERD (gastroesophageal reflux disorder), irritable bowel syndrome, inflammatory bowel disease, celiac disease, lactose intolerance, constipation, gastritis, bloating, and nausea.

Some helpful supplements for general GI distress include the following:

» **Ginger:** Helps reduce nausea, vomiting, and indigestion. It may also improve gastric emptying and reduce bloating.

» **Probiotics:** Reduces symptoms of IBS, IBD, and generally promotes gut health.

» **Peppermint oil:** Relieves bloating and cramps in general or from IBS.

» **Digestive enzymes:** Assist the enzymes in your body to break down food and help nutrient absorption.

» **Glutamine:** Supports gut health and may help with leaky gut, IBS, and irritable bowel disease (IBD).

» **Fiber (psyllium, acacia):** Helps relieve constipation generally and from IBS.

» **Licorice root extract:** May help relieve symptoms from heartburn, acid reflux, and indigestion.

Here are some of specific common digestive disorders and diet recommendations and supplement recommendations to discuss with your doctor:

» **Gastroesophageal reflux disease (GERD):** Follow a lactose- and gluten-free diet low-fat diet and avoid chocolate, tomatoes, spicy food and caffeine but include a ginger tea or supplement.

» **IBS:** Eat a low-FODMAP diet (see www.monashfodmap.com for more information) and supplement with probiotics, fiber supplements, peppermint oil, and glutamine.

» **Celiac disease:** Follow a strict gluten-free diet and take a multivitamin with folate and vitamin B12.

» **Crohn's disease and ulcerative colitis:** Eat a low-residue diet during flare-ups and avoid high-fiber foods, raw fruits, vegetables, nuts, seeds, and dairy. When you've recovered from the flare-up, add whole grains, fruits, vegetables, and lean proteins and take vitamin D, omega-3 fatty acids, and probiotics.

» **Lactose Intolerance:** Follow a dairy-free diet and take lactase enzymes if you consume dairy.

» **Constipation:** Increase fiber intake from food and supplements and take magnesium citrate.

» **Diverticulitis:** Eat low-fiber foods during a flare-up and then increase fiber during recovery with food and supplements. Also, take probiotics for gut health and to prevent flare-ups.

Skin conditions

A wide range of skin conditions exist, and in most cases, the causes are multifactorial. Diet, hormones, autoimmune responses, allergies, or general health are all possibilities. The skin microbiome plays an important role in maintaining skin health. The gut-skin axis describes the skin and gut microbiome connection, which isn't completely understood. But if the gut microbiome and the immune system are impaired, effects may be triggered on the skin. Treatments are often holistic, perhaps involving diet, hormone products, topical treatments, medications, and supplements including probiotics. Some common skin conditions are acne, eczema, psoriasis, rosacea, and dry skin.

Acne is complicated and can be caused by stress and sex hormones, oily skin, salt from sweat, inflammation, diet, genetics, and environmental factors. Treatment may involve some trial and error, and the advice of a dermatologist is always recommended. That said, some supplements — both topical and oral — may be helpful:

>> Vitamin A and topical retinol help to maintain healthy skin. Topical retinol can help prevent dead skin cells from clogging pores, treat acne, and prevent signs of aging.

>> Topical alpha-hydroxy acids (AHA) or glycolic acid help promote cell turnover. Lactic acid is an AHA that can improve skin texture and tone, reduce dark spots, and smooth fine lines. It's a natural substance that's present in the skin and can be found in many skin care products. AHAs are exfoliants. They improve hydration, stimulate collagen production, and balance skin tone and hyperpigmentation. They're sometimes used in chemical peels.

>> Salicylic acid is also helpful for acne because it helps unclog pores.

>> Benzoyl peroxide kills bacteria on the skin.

>> Probiotics improve gut health, which impacts your skin.

>> Zinc may help reduce acne flare-ups.

>> Vitamin C may also help reduce inflammation and prevent scarring.

>> Niacinamide (B3) is an anti-inflammatory and may help both topically and orally.

>> Vitamin B5 may help reduce oil production.

>> Vitamin B6 may help with hormonal acne.

>> Tea tree oil may also be helpful as a topical for acne.

HERPES SIMPLEX VIRUS

Herpes simplex virus (herpes) is a common viral infection that can cause symptoms, including painful blisters. There are two types of herpes: HSV-1 and HSV-2. HSV-1 is the most common and spreads by oral contact; it causes blisters or cold sores around the mouth. It can also cause genital blisters. HSV-2 spreads by sexual contact and causes genital symptoms. Antiviral medications are used to treat herpes. There are some studies that show that taking a lysine supplement every day may reduce recurrences of herpes outbreak.

TIP

Staying hydrated and eating a balanced diet filled with fruits, vegetables, whole grains and staying away from sugar, dairy, and processed foods can support your skin and possibly reduce acne flare-ups.

Here are some supplements to include in your overall health plan if you have other skin issues:

>> **Zinc:** Supports skin health and may reduce flare-ups of eczema

>> **Vitamin A:** Helps maintain healthy skin and healing of skin tissue and may help with psoriasis

>> **Omega-3 fatty acids:** May decrease skin inflammation and help keep skin affected by eczema and psoriasis hydrated

>> **Probiotics:** Supports gut health, which can influence skin conditions including eczema

>> **Biotin:** Supports hair and nails and perhaps dry skin

Sleep disorders

Sleep disorders include insomnia, sleep apnea, and restless leg syndrome. Supplements that may help you regulate sleep include the items in the following list. The dose for all of these will vary depending on the product and your needs. The supplement label on the product provides information on best way to use these products:

>> **Melatonin:** This natural hormone helps control your sleep/wake cycle. Melatonin acts on receptors in your body to encourage sleep. As people age, natural melatonin declines. Taking melatonin supplements can add to your body's natural supply of the hormone. This is particularly helpful with jet lag and insomnia. The dose is usually between 1 and 5 mg.

>> **L-theanine:** This amino acid may help promote relaxation and improve sleep. It's often added to melatonin supplements or separate supplements are taken together.

>> **L-tryptophan:** This amino acid (found in turkey and possibly responsible for its well-known sedative effect) produces melatonin and calming neurotransmitters. A supplement may help quiet anxiety and improve the quality of your sleep.

Cannabis: Cannabinoids in the cannabis plant are known to have sleep-promoting properties. The natural or synthetic cannabinoids in sleep aids are cannabidiol (CBD) and delta-tetrahydrocannabinol (THC). Smoking marijuana or ingesting gummies, where legal, are other ways to get CBD or THC.

>> **Chamomile tea:** This herbal tea may promote calm and help with sleep. The dried flowers of chamomile contain many terpenoids and flavonoids, which contribute to its medicinal properties for sleep and other issues, including gastrointestinal disorders.

>> **Magnesium:** This mineral is important in many body processes, and magnesium levels have been shown to influence both sleep quality and quantity. Magnesium glycinate is the best magnesium supplement for sleep because it's absorbed well and has calming effects. Magnesium taurate and magnesium L-threonate are also beneficial for sleep because of good absorption. The recommended dose depends on which form you choose, so read the label carefully.

>> **Valerian root:** This supplement may help with relaxation and sleep. It is thought to work by increasing levels of gamma-aminobutyric acid (GABA) — a neurotransmitter that has calming and sedative effects. The body's natural production of GABA typically declines after age 60.

>> **Glycine:** Glycine is an amino acid and neurotransmitter that's important in sleep. A small dose (3 g) may improve sleep quality and reduce daytime sleepiness. It works by causing a slight drop in body temperature that helps you fall asleep and stay asleep.

>> **Passionflower:** This supplement may work by increasing the body's natural production of GABA.

Magnolia bark: This traditional Chinese medicine is known for its natural sedative properties. The magnolol and honokiol found in the bark activates GABA receptors in the brain to be calming and promote sleep.

Lemon balm: The compounds in this plant that is often used as a tea helps slow the breakdown of GABA, thus maintaining higher levels of GABA longer and promoting sleep.

>> **Lavender oil:** The essential oil of the lavender plant may also calm and improve sleep quality. This oil can be applied topically to skin, used with a diffuser, or inhaled after a few drops are put on a cloth.

Macular degeneration and other eye issues

Age–related macular degeneration (AMD) is a common eye disease that causes blurring of your central vision. The most common type is when the light sensitive cells in the macula (located in the center of the retina) break down. This is called dry AMD. Risk factors include a high-fat diet, being overweight, having high blood pressure, being White, and having a family history.

There is no cure for AMD, but according to the National Eye Institute Age-Related Eye Disease Studies (AREDS), you can slow down the progression by eating a good diet, taking medication, and using some supplements. The AREDS and AREDS2 found that a combination of vitamins and minerals might slow the progression of dry AMD.

TIP

The current AREDS supplements contain vitamins C, E, zinc, lutein, zeaxanthin, and copper. There are many brands of AREDS supplements available, and you can choose the best one for you by reading the labels, looking for third-party certifications, and determining whether there are additional ingredients included that you may not want to take.

Eating a healthy diet is important to protect your eyes from other diseases, including glaucoma and cataracts. An eye-healthy diet is consistent with other well-balanced healthy eating such as the Healthy U.S.-Style (HUSS) diet, Mediterranean diet, or vegetarian diet that will also protect you from heart disease, diabetes, and obesity.

Diets high in fruits and vegetables provide carotenoids, which your body can convert to vitamins, such as vitamin A. These are naturally found in your eye's retina, and their concentration may go down with age. These also act as antioxidants to protect your eyes from damaging free radicals.

Lutein and zeaxanthin are carotenoids that are highly concentrated in the macula and filter out damaging radiation from sunlight. They also act as antioxidants. Lutein and zeaxanthin are found at high levels in dark green leafy vegetables and herbs, as well as in orange bell peppers and egg yolks.

Your retina contains high concentrations of omega-3 fatty acids. Eating fatty fish, such as salmon, tuna, halibut, and herring may help prevent eye disease. Omega-3 fatty acids are also in in flaxseed, chia seeds, walnuts, and canola oil.

Women's sexual health

There is some evidence that some supplements may help women's libido and lubrication, including these:

>> **DHEA (dehydroepiandrosterone):** The body converts this hormone to estrogen and testosterone. There is mixed scientific evidence that it helps women's libido; it may be most effective in women who are premenopausal and have low sexual function to begin with. Because DHEA has side effects, such as increased facial hair and acne, it may not be the best option.

>> **Vitamin E plus ginseng:** This combination was shown to boost libido in a study of 62 women. More fine-tuned studies showed that this combination seemed to enhance sexual desire in menopausal but not premeno-pausal women.

>> **Zinc:** A small study showed that zinc supplements increased testosterone and sexual desire in women. Taking excess zinc is not recommended, so for general well-being, including sexual health, be sure that you are getting enough zinc from your food sources.

>> **L-arginine:** L-arginine is an amino acid involved in many body functions. There are several small, randomized studies that show that L-arginine improves libido and vaginal dryness in pre- and postmenopausal women. This supplement is well tolerated and may be worth a try. To increase L-arginine in your diet, include meat, poultry, fish, dairy, legumes, and pineapple.

>> **Tribulus terrestris:** This is an herb from a Mediterranean fruit that people have taken to improve sexual issues, including infertility. Some research supports its use, but more research is needed to prove the benefits. Short-term use is safe; however, it can interact with some medications. With limited data and some side effects, do your research and talk to your healthcare provider before deciding to use Tribulus.

There are some supplements that are marketed for increasing libido and improving women's sexual health but lack enough scientific studies to recommend taking. They include maca root, kanna, red clover, fenugreek, saffron, and ashwagandha.

WARNING

Beware of online betel nut supplements. Although they may work by triggering dopamine release and may boost libido, they can be very dangerous. There are adverse side effects (insomnia and anxiety), and it can be addictive. Eating high doses of 8 to 30 g can cause death.

Menopause

Supplements to ease the symptoms of menopause include black cohosh, a member of the buttercup plant family. It's found in many supplements for relief of menopausal symptoms. Black cohosh contains many botanical compounds that may be responsible for its effects, but the exact mechanism isn't clear. The latest research suggests that it may increase serotonin, which may help reduce hot flashes and affect mood. Black cohosh has a long history of being used by American Indians for menstrual problems, childbirth, and other women's issues. It's been widely used in Germany since the 1940s and is approved by the German health authorities at a dose of 40 mg/day of black cohosh (as Remifemin) for six months for relief of menopausal symptoms, premenstrual syndrome, and dysmenorrhea.

More recently, randomized controlled trials, the 2012 Cochrane Review, a 2016 systematic review, and meta-analysis of randomized clinical trials have been done, and the conclusions are mixed. As a result of years of studying black cohosh, the American College of Obstetricians and Gynecologists in 2015 concluded that data doesn't support herbal dietary supplements like black cohosh as beneficial for treating symptoms like hot flashes and night sweats. The North American Menopause Society also advises clinicians against recommending herbal therapies such as black cohosh because they are not effective for relieving symptoms.

Health risks of taking black cohosh are low. However there have been reports of liver damage. Always consult with a healthcare professional before taking this supplement.

Other supplements that may help with menopausal symptoms have been studied less, but they may reduce symptoms. Here are some examples:

>> **Red clover:** Contains phytoestrogens (plant estrogens) that may help reduce hot flashes.

>> **Soy isoflavones:** Contains estrogenlike compounds that may relieve hot flashes.

>> **Omege-3 fatty acids:** Support heart health, decrease inflammation, and may improve mood.

>> **Vitamin D and calcium:** Helpful throughout menopause for reducing risk of osteoporosis and bone fracture.

>> **Evening primrose oil:** An omega-6 fatty acid and anti-inflammatory that may help with hot flashes, mood swings, and skin dryness.

>> **Rhodiola rosea or golden root:** May reduce stress, fatigue, and cognitive issues.

>> **Purified cytoplasm of pollen (PCP):** A nonhormonal herbal remedy used to manage vasomotor symptoms and sleep and mood disorders in menopausal women.

TIP

The Bonafide brand has a product that contains curcumin, green tea extract, and spirulina extract that may be a helpful combination. Another product called Estroven is plant based and has rhapontic rhubarb root extract. Other established brands include Fem EstroPlex, Femarin, Femguard + Balance, MedCaps Menopause, and Menovair.

Vaginal dryness

Menopausal women often experience general dryness (including skin, eyes, and oral) as well as vaginal dryness. Maintaining overall hydration is a good start to balancing your body as much as you can by drinking enough water, eating a balanced diet with plenty of fruits and vegetables (which provide phytoestrogens), getting enough omega-3 fatty acids that support hydration, reduce inflammation, and support elasticity in tissues.

Along with omega-3s and phytoestrogens, be sure to get enough vitamin E, protein, and vitamin C. Along with foods and oral supplements, there are nonprescription and nonhormonal supplements that can be inserted vaginally to address dryness. You can take vitamin E and DHEA (converted to estrogen and testosterone in your body) orally or insert it vaginally. Probiotics may also help to maintain health of the vaginal microbiome, which can maintain tissue elasticity and moisture.

Hyaluronic acid is a compound that attracts water and is used as a moisturizer in topical skin creams. It's s also a component of vaginal suppositories that are effective at moisturizing vaginal tissues and improving elasticity. There are a several suppositories available for vaginal dryness that contain hyaluronic acid, DHEA, or vitamin E or combinations of these. Some of these brands include Bonafide, Hydro Gyn Vaginal Moisturizer, Julva, ReNewed by Nature's Naturopathic, Replens, and Revaree. There also are drugstore brands and other online brands that may be good. Always check the ingredient labels to see what they contain.

Men's sexual health

Several supplements have been studied for their effects on men's sexual health, including libido, erectile function, testosterone levels, and overall well-being. The following list includes some of the most well-researched options:

>> **DHEA:** DHEA is a precursor to testosterone production. As you age, testosterone production declines, so it makes some intuitive sense that a supplement might increase testosterone levels and improve your age-related issues and sexual function. Some small studies support some limited improvement in erectile function in older men whose hormone levels are low. Studies have

mixed results as to whether DHEA improves overall sexual health in men, although it may help with cognitive function, bone density, and immunity. This is something to discuss with your doctor.

>> **L-citrulline and L-arginine:** These amino acids help increase nitric oxide production, blood flow, and erectile dysfunction.

>> **Maca root:** This supplement may enhance libido and sperm quality.

>> **Ashwagandha:** In infertile men, this supplement may increase testosterone levels and sperm quality.

>> **Tongkat ali:** This herb may boost testosterone, reduce cortisol, and improve libido and sexual function.

>> **Fenugreek:** This herb may support testosterone production and sexual function.

>> **Panax ginseng:** Traditional forms of medicine have used ginseng for improving erectile functions and sexual health, and some clinical trials also support its use.

>> **Zinc and other micronutrients:** Zinc deficiency is linked to low testosterone. Other deficiencies may also influence reproductive health, so it is important to get your RDA for these and all your nutrients.

COVID and long COVID

Persistent symptoms after having COVID-19 can impact your quality of life. The underlying mechanisms involved in long COVID may be chronic inflammation, compromised immune processes, changes in your gut metabolism, and malfunction in protective cells that line all your blood vessels. Eating a nutritionally balanced diet and maintaining a physically and emotionally active life can create a controllable foundation for addressing some of these physiological issues. Seeing a healthcare professional who is knowledgeable about long COVID or going to a long COVID clinic is a good first step to addressing this illness. Taking their advice and any medications they recommend is critical.

When you first get COVID, there may be some supplements that can help you by supporting your immune system and alleviating symptoms. Some supplements that might help are:

>> Vitamin D can enhance immunity.

>> Vitamin C may help to fight infections.

>> Zinc helps with immunity and fighting viral infections.

>> N-acetyl cysteine (NAC) produces glutathione, a powerful antioxidant.

>> Probiotics support gut health and immunity.

>> Fish oil is anti-inflammatory and may modulate your immune response.

Long COVID is when you have long-lasting symptoms such as cough, shortness of breath, fatigue, brain fog (difficulties with memory or concentration), and GI or musculoskeletal problems. These can continue months to years post–COVID infection and can negatively impact your life.

Specific treatments for long COVID have not been determined, but there are many research studies currently looking into the best medical treatment. There are also excellent long COVID clinics in many parts of the country.

In addition, there is a plethora of dietary supplements and natural bioactive substances to address long COVID. There are many scientific articles with continuously changing up-to-date information. You can work with a health professional to understand your symptoms and come up with a personalized supplement plan if you have long COVID.

The following list includes some of the supplements that are being tested that may help with long COVID. Remember that the field is new and changing as researchers gain more understanding of the condition and how to treat it. Supplements are only part of the treatment along with medications, diet, and lifestyle changes. Supplements that may help include these:

>> **Amino acids:** Glutamine, branched-chain amino acids (BCAAs), and arginine supplements help with increased metabolic demand.

>> **Hydroxy-beta-methyl butyrate:** This is the active metabolite of leucine. It stimulates something called mTOR-dependent pathways, which are important in several physiologic processes, including protein metabolism, insulin activity, skeletal muscle hypertrophy, cell apoptosis (cell death), and muscle stem cell proliferation and differentiation. This supplement could help reduce muscle loss and aid inflammatory and immune responses.

>> **Tricarboxylic acid metabolites:** These metabolites feed into cellular energy production. Along with amino acids and micronutrients, they address mitochondrial health and energy production, which may be key to helping long COVID sufferers.

>> **Micronutrients including selenium, iron, zinc, and magnesium:** Deficiencies in these micronutrients — especially in older people — can increase the risk of fatigue, cardiometabolic disease, musculoskeletal disorders, and cognitive impairment.

>> **Bromelain:** This proteolytic enzyme is anti-inflammatory.

- >> **Troxerutin (vitamin P4):** This is a flavonoid found in tea, coffee, cereals, fruits, and vegetables. It has many biological effects, including as an antioxidant, anti-inflammatory, neuroprotective, antidiabetic, and antithrombotic.

- >> **Lactoferrin:** This protein is found in milk that prevents microbial and viral adhesion to human cells.

- >> **Probiotics:** These may help with GI symptoms associated with long COVID. Specific combinations are being tested, and there is some evidence that they may prevent some secondary infections of COVID.

- >> **Vitamin D:** Low levels can worsen fatigue, muscle pain, and general health. Therefore, adequate intake from food and supplements is important for long COVID.

- >> **Beetroot juice:** Studies show beetroot juice may help preserve metabolic homeostasis, reduce inflammation, and support pulmonary function. It may modulate inflammation associated with long COVID.

- >> **Pollen-based herbal extracts:** These are a mixture of amino acids, carbohydrates, minerals, and bioactive substances that may help with numerous symptoms associated with long COVID, including mood alterations.

- >> **Vitamin C:** This vitamin helps with immunity and inflammation.

- >> **N-acetyl-cysteine (NAC):** It has antioxidant properties to help alleviate lung symptoms and inflammation.

- >> **L-carnitine:** This supplement helps with energy function and supports mitochondrial function to produce energy and reduce fatigue.

- >> **B vitamins:** They support energy production, mitochondrial health, and nerve function to help with several symptoms, including brain fog.

Cold and flu

To prevent and reduce symptoms of colds and flu starts by working on controllable factors to boost your immunity: eating healthily, getting all your essential nutrients, and staying active. Beyond doing those things, you can try using supplements to boost your immunity, reduce symptoms, and cut down on the duration of the illness.

REMEMBER

Vitamin C has been studied for years as an immunity booster for prevention and shortening the duration of colds. Numerous clinical studies have shown that vitamin C will not prevent infection with the cold virus but will shorten the duration of the illness. The Linus Pauling Institute recommends 400 mg/day, which is sufficient for most people. Megadoses of vitamin C don't make a difference.

The institute recommends that you ingest no more than 2,000 mg/day because there can be side effects. Once an illness begins, taking vitamin C will not make much of a difference, so you may want to be sure that you are getting 400 mg/day normally!

Other supplements may help fight infections or reduce symptoms, especially if you are deficient. Be sure that you get your daily amounts of all your essential vitamins and minerals to support your metabolism and immune system.

Along with getting enough vitamin C and the rest of your nutrients, here are additional supplements that may help prevent a cold or flu:

>> **Vitamin D:** This vitamin reduces risk of respiratory infections.

>> **Probiotics:** Gut health supports immune function and may reduce upper respiratory infections, and probiotics support gut health.

>> **Echinacea:** This herb (2,400 mg/day) helps prevent and reduces severity of the infection.

>> **Garlic:** Garlic contains allicin, which is a natural antiviral and antibacterial compound. You can eat it or take a garlic extract supplement (600 mg/day) to help prevent illness.

>> **Elderberry:** A dose of 600 to 900 mg reduces symptoms and the length of the illness.

Once you're sick, adding the following supplements may help you to reduce the severity of your illness:

>> **Zinc:** May shorten symptoms when taken as soon as you feel sick

>> **Elderberry extract:** Reduces symptoms and length of illness (600 to 900 mg)

>> **NAC:** Increases glutathione, an antioxidant, and reduces mucus in lungs and sinuses (600 to 1,200 mg/day)

>> **Quercetin:** A natural antihistamine and anti-inflammatory and may be good for reducing a cold's severity once you're sick (50 to 1,000 mg/day)

Support during Health and Illness

Supplements can be a great addition to your healthcare plan. The word *supplement* means "something added to" — in this case, added to your diet.

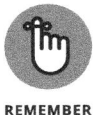

REMEMBER

Supplements are not intended to treat, cure, or prevent diseases. This book explains some uses of supplements to stay healthy and help prevent certain conditions. This covers some medical conditions where supplements may be helpful. It's always important to note that scientific evidence for these supplements isn't always clear and absolute. Sometimes the decision to take a supplement is based on a small amount of evidence combined with other considerations.

In this section, I help you determine whether you need supplements, what testing you may want, and how to go about choosing supplements to buy.

Identifying need

There are ways to identify your need for taking supplements including consulting with healthcare professionals, evaluating food intake and lifestyle, having blood tests, monitoring your symptoms, and considering your life stage.

The first thing to determine is whether you're getting the necessary nutrients from your diet. Understand and review the recommended consumption of foods to reach the Recommended Daily Allowance for essential micro- and macronutrients. You can find them on the websites for MyPlate and the Dietary Guidelines for Americans. You can also do this with a healthcare professional or by using online tools or apps to keep a food record and evaluate your food consumption for all the nutrients.

TIP

There is a simple online tool to get a list of all of the nutrients that you need at www.nal.usda.gov/human-nutrition-and-food-safety/dri-calculator.

Next, consider your lifestyle. Do you sit at a desk all day, smoke, drink alcohol, or exercise? Are you a vegetarian, or do you avoid eating certain foods? Are you stressed, or do you use food to comfort yourself during stress or emotional times? Are you a snacker? Do you get enough sleep? The answers to these questions could help you determine your needs.

When you meet with your doctor and get your annual blood tests, you hopefully find that everything is in the normal range. However, there are some things that can be checked, such as vitamin D, folate, B12, iron, and calcium. If these are low, then you may need a supplement.

If you have symptoms such as dizziness, fatigue, or mood swings, it could be related to a nutrient deficiency. Self-monitoring is always a good idea. If symptoms persist, see your healthcare provider.

Nutrient needs vary with age, sex, and life stage and are reflected in the Dietary Reference Intake tables that you can use as a resource. Pregnant and lactating people need more of certain nutrients to support their increased needs. Aging adults often need more vitamin B12.

Speaking to your doctor

One of my recurring themes throughout this book is consulting with your healthcare professional. Ultimately, and especially if you have health issues or a disease, you must discuss supplement use with your doctor and/or a dietician or nutritionist. This professional will help you evaluate all the information to help you come up with a personalized plan.

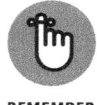

REMEMBER

In addition, if you're taking any medications, you want to be sure that there are no negative interactions with any supplements you are thinking of taking.

Testing

Your doctor orders tests to determine whether you're low in some vitamins or minerals and monitors other health indicators, such as your lipid panel or blood sugar.

Several companies now sell home testing kits without a doctor's prescription. This can be useful for self-monitoring a variety of things, but it should not be used for self-diagnosing. For example, if your vitamin B12 levels are low and you are taking a supplement for that with your doctor's approval, perhaps you want to monitor it between doctor visits. More on testing can be found in Chapter 12.

Monitoring quality, form, and dose

The Food and Drug Administration (FDA) does not regulate dietary supplement production. The efficacy of a supplement is supported by scientific research but does not have to be proven by the manufacturers. When you buy a supplement, there are certain things to look for while deciding which ones are the best for you.

TECHNICAL STUFF

There are three third party certifying companies that test supplements to assure that what you are getting in the bottle matches the label. They are USP, NSF, and ConsumerLab.com, and you can refer to Chapter 4 for more information.

There are also certifications for supplement manufacturing companies that you can look for if researching the company:

>> GMP (Good Manufacturing Practice)

>> QAI (Quality Assurance International)

>> USDA Organic

Additional certifications that you may find on labels include these:

>> Certified gluten-free

>> Non-GMO Project Verified

>> International Fish Oil Standards (IFOS)

>> Certified Vegan

The best form and dose of a vitamin or mineral or other supplement will depend on your specific health need. Usually, the best form is the most bioavailable or easily absorbed. Here are some examples of good forms of some supplements:

>> **Vitamin D:** D3, cholecalciferol (with food)

>> **Magnesium:** Magnesium citrate, glycinate, malate or taurate or L-threonate depending on the use

>> **Calcium:** Calcium citrate, calcium carbonate

>> **Iron:** Iron bisglycinate or ferrous sulfate (take with vitamin C for better absorption)

>> **Folate:** L-methylfolate

>> **B12:** Methylcobalamin, adenosylcobalamin, cyanocobalamin (take sublingually [under the tongue] for better absorption)

>> **B6:** Pyridoxal-5-phosphate (P5P)

>> **Zinc:** Zinc picolinate or zinc glycinate, zinc citrate (with food)

>> **Protein:** Whey protein isolate or pea, hemp, soy for vegetarian options

The best dose of any supplement will depend on you and your needs. You usually want a dose that will bring you up to the levels recommended by the U.S. Department of Agriculture (USDA). There may be some nutrients that you may need more of, but you should always discuss this with your healthcare professional.

Integrating with medications

Combining dietary supplements with prescription medications can have dangerous and sometimes life-threatening effects. Supplements can sometimes reduce the effectiveness of medications. They can do this by interfering with the absorption from the gut or by reacting with the drug to change it.

Here are some examples of drug-supplement interactions to avoid:

>> Vitamin K and blood thinners

>> Gingko and blood thinners

>> St. John's wort and birth control, antidepressants, drugs for HIV/AIDS, and heart disease

>> Vitamin C and antacids

>> Vitamin E and blood thinners

>> Supplements that affect the liver, such as kava and comfrey

>> Vitamin A and beta-carotene if you're a smoker

>> Licorice root and blood pressure medications or ACE inhibitors

>> Calcium, magnesium, iron, and soy with thyroid medications

>> Calcium, magnesium, iron, and zinc with antibiotics like fluoroquinolones and tetracycline medications

>> Calcium and bisphosphonates

4

Getting Practical with Your Vitamins and Supplements

Chapter **12**

Choosing the Right Vitamins and Supplements

Before you run to the store or visit an online supplier, you need to assess your dietary intake, your overall health, and your lifestyle. Until you've done that, you don't know what supplements you may need. In this chapter, I explain the various things you need to consider as you determine what vitamins and supplements to take.

Assessing Your Needs

Unfortunately, assessing your needs isn't easy — even for professionals. To make this assessment, you need to pay attention to nutritional recommendations and what you're eating to nourish yourself.

You can start with guidelines like the new 2025–2030 Dietary Guidelines for Americans. It can help you determine whether you're eating well. It discusses the

Healthy Eating Index (HEI), which was developed in 1995 to assess how well Americans were eating. It asks questions regarding intake and totals a score between 0 and 100, where 100 is the best. The information is mainly from data in the What We Eat in America (WWEIA) database, the dietary intake interview portion of the National Health and Nutrition Examination Survey (NHANES). To provide the data for WWEIA, participants report what they eat and drink over a 24-hour period. The information from the survey is then used to calculate national average HEI for toddlers through adults. Table 12-1 shows the most recent HEIs for various age groups.

TABLE 12-1

HEI by Age Group

Age Group	Score out of 100
Younger than 2	63
2–18	54
18–59	57
Older than 60	61

As you can see from the table, everyone has quite a way to go to improve their food intake!

You can find online ways to calculate your HEI, but it's complicated. An easier method is to use one of the online food diary apps, such as MyFitnessPal or Lose It! These are free to use and can give lots of info. For example, log your food intake for one week. It will then give you a weekly average nutrition intake including macros — protein, fat, carbs — *and* other nutrients such as vitamins and minerals. I highly recommend assessing your dietary intake this way, and taking a week's average of essential vitamins, minerals, and macronutrients.

Comparing Nutrients from Diet versus Supplements

TIP

Eating a good diet is the best way to get all your nutrients, including vitamins and minerals, because foods also provide other good things. For example, although you can get vitamin A from a supplement, getting it from a carrot is better because carrots also have some carbohydrate, plant protein, sugar, vitamins K and C, potassium, fiber, calcium, magnesium, phosphorous, and iron. Cooked carrots improve the availability of some of these nutrients, but raw carrots are an even better option for nutrition-packed excellence.

Another reason for getting nutrients from foods is because studies have shown health benefits from certain good diet intakes, but when assessing how individual nutrients affect health outcomes, the data has not been as good. For example, a big study with more than 280,000 subjects called the Nurses' Health Study showed that eating a diet rich in vitamin A had benefits in that it reduced some cancers. This effect was not observed in people who took vitamin A supplements.

Looking at the Dietary Guidelines for Americans

The Dietary Guidelines for Americans (DGA) is an informative document available to the public, although it's generally used by professionals to help guide policy or programs such as school lunches or SNAP (Supplemental Nutrition Assistance Program) that provides food benefits to low-income families.

The information in the DGA is based on science and addresses dietary needs at all life stages. There are details on different healthy diets, including the following three recommended ways of eating:

>> The Healthy U.S.-Style (HUSS)

>> Healthy Mediterranean Style

>> Healthy Vegetarian

The DGA includes tables for adapting these diets as needed for your age and sex, and it makes suggestions for how to fill your plate with the healthy foods needed to get the necessary nutrients. (See Figure 12-1.) If you are interested in more details, visit the site at www.dietaryguidelines.gov.

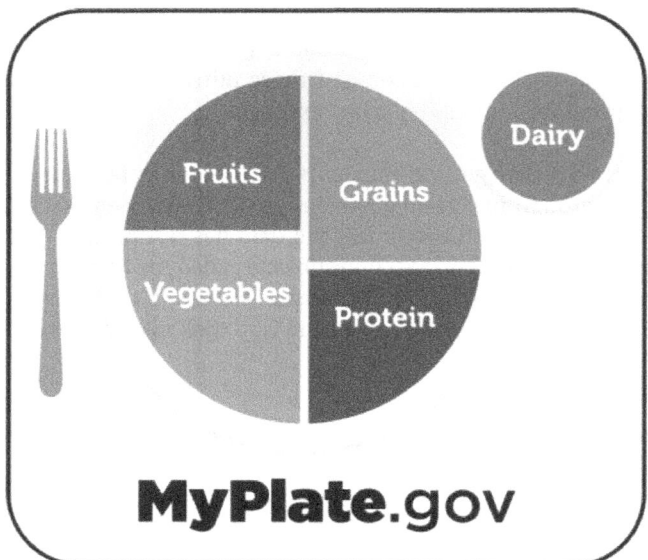

FIGURE 12-1:
The MyPlate
visual can help
you determine
how to distribute
components of
your meal across
the food groups.

Considering Special Diets

Although it's always best to get vitamins and other nutrients from your diet, it isn't always possible. If you have dietary restrictions or choose to eat a certain way, you may need to use supplements to be sure that you're covering your basic nutritional needs. Pay attention to macros to ensure you're getting enough protein, carbs, and good fats you need, but also consider micronutrients — vitamins and minerals. In this section, I suggest some things to watch for if you're following a particular type of diet.

Vegetarian

Being a vegetarian rather than a vegan makes it a little easier to easily get all your nutrients. According to the American Dietetic Association, "appropriately planned vegetarian diets, including total vegetarian or vegan diets, are healthful, nutritionally adequate, and may provide health benefits in the prevention and treatment of certain diseases."

There are multiple forms of vegetarianism:

>> Vegans are described in the next section.

>> Lacto-ovo vegetarians eat plant-based food plus dairy and eggs.

>> Lacto vegetarians eat plant-based food plus dairy only.

>> Ovo vegetarians eat plant-based food plus eggs.

Eating eggs and dairy helps you to get all the nutrients you need. If your daily intake is well balanced and has a variety of foods, you may not need any supplements. However, many vegetarians may not get enough protein, B12, iron, or omega-3 fatty acids. It is important to understand your food intake and activity level to be sure that you get what you need.

Good sources of plant-based protein include those listed in the following section, Eggs and dairy (such as plain Greek yogurt) are other good sources. Dairy and eggs also provide B12 and eicosapentaenoic acid (EPA) and docosahexaenoic acid (DHA), the good fats that you need.

TIP

Most vegetarians get enough iron from their food sources. However, note that absorption from plants is not as efficient as from animal products. Fortunately, this is something your doctor can measure to see if you are deficient and need a supplement.

TIP

I often find that vegetarians need B12, iron, and sometimes vitamin D. You can get these through fortified grains and cereals and milk (dairy and plant-based milks) or always by supplements. In addition, adequate vitamin C will help promote iron absorption from plant-based sources.

Vegan

Strict vegans don't eat any animal products like meat, fish, dairy, eggs, or honey. Reasons for being a vegan include eating a plant-based diet for better health and/or ethical reasons of not wanting to harm any animal life, conserve earth's resources, and protect the environment.

A vegan diet is comprised of all plant-based foods, both raw or cooked. There are many vegan options of cheese, yogurt, and meat substitutes available on the market. If you're a vegan for health reasons, it's always good to read labels to determine if vegan options meet your standards of good ingredients for optimal health. For example, vegan substitutes for meats are highly processed foods, but you may be willing to accept that compromise because they're good sources of protein. There are also vegan substitutes for cookies, cakes, and ice cream, but these foods may have fats or chemical ingredients that aren't as healthy as you want to opt for.

TIP

Vegans and vegetarians still need to get enough protein each day. A variety of foods helps to get all the amino acids necessary to make complete proteins — for example, when you mix beans and rice.

If you've chosen a vegan diet, the biggest challenges are getting enough protein, omega-3s, vitamins B12 and D, calcium, and iron. High-protein plant-based foods include

>> Nuts and seeds

>> Beans

>> Tofu or bean curd

>> Quinoa

>> Seitan (made from wheat gluten)

>> Tempeh (a fermented soy product)

>> Oats

>> Vegan meat

>> Protein powder from soy or peas

Vegans may need to work a bit more work to create a healthy diet, but eating a variety of the following foods is a great start:

>> **Fruits and vegetables:** Eat a variety of all colors of fruits and vegetables because the different colors represent different nutrients. They are a great source for vitamin C, vitamin E, folate, magnesium, potassium, fiber, and antioxidants. Green leafy vegetables (except spinach) and dried fruit are good sources of calcium and vitamin C.

>> **Legumes:** Peas, beans, and lentils can be pared with rice so that you meet your protein needs and get the full amino acid profile. These are also a good source for iron.

>> **Nuts, seeds, and olives:** These are good sources for omega-3 fatty acids, zinc, and folate.

>> **Breads, cereals, rice, and pasta:** Eat whole grain options when possible. Healthy items in this category include whole wheat bread, brown rice, whole grain pasta, and nonsugary whole grain cereals. In the United States, most store-bought breads and cereals are fortified with B vitamins and iron.

>> **Vegetable oils:** Olive oil is especially good for getting omega-3s.

>> **Plant-based milks:** Soy milk has the most protein amounts of the plant-based milks and about the same as cow's milk (6 to 8 g). Rice, coconut, cashew, and almond milk do not provide significant amounts of protein (<1 g). Certain oat and hemp milk products may provide some protein (2 to 9 g). All of these products are fortified with calcium, vitamin D, and sometimes other vitamins and minerals. Be sure to check the label for the nutrients, levels of fats, and calorie count to decide which is best for you. I mostly recommend soy milk because it's higher in protein and lower in calories.

>> **Nutritional yeast:** This is a good source of B12. Nutritional yeast can be a flavorful addition to some foods in place of Parmesan cheese. It tastes good on popcorn as well!

If you eat a variety of foods every day, you may be getting all your necessary nutrients from your diet. If you're concerned you're missing out on some things, then be sure to include the following foods for specific nutrients. If you don't eat all of these foods, or don't get enough of them, consider using supplements to fill in the gaps!

>> **Vitamin B12:** Foods supplemented with B vitamins, such as nutritional yeast, breakfast cereals, and breads

>> **Omega-3s:** Dark leafy greens, seaweed, soybeans, hemp and chia seeds, walnuts, flaxseed

>> **Calcium:** Orange juice (fortified with calcium), tofu, plant milk, soy yogurt, molasses

>> **Vitamin D:** Fortified orange juice, fortified cereals and breads, and plant-based milks

>> **Iron:** Fortified breads and cereals, dark leafy greens, rice, pasta, soybeans

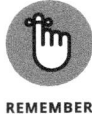

REMEMBER

If you're on a low-carb vegan diet, you may need B12. If you're on a low-fat vegan diet, you may need more omega-3s. Young women may need more iron. I recommend you be tested and discuss a supplement with your doctor.

Pescatarian

A pescatarian diet is sometimes categorized as a variation of vegetarianism. Pescatarians eat mostly vegetarian but add some fish and seafood. They may or may not eat eggs or dairy. Adding fish to the vegetarian diets has advantages because it's a very good source of protein, B12, and omega-3s.

If you eat fish two to three times per week as well as eating a variety of vegetables, fruits, grains, dairy, and eggs, you will potentially get all the nutrients you need. As with any way of eating, if you don't eat certain foods and these foods supply essential nutrients, then you will need supplements.

WARNING

No matter what diet you follow, it's difficult to get vitamin D from foods. Therefore, if you test low at your annual doctor appointment, you should supplement with vitamin D.

TIP

Too much mercury can cause damage to the nervous system and cause insomnia, memory loss, headaches, and cognitive and motor dysfunction. It may also cause oxidative stress and heart disease, but these effects are not understood yet. If you're concerned about eating fish because of mercury levels, the best low-mercury fish to eat to ensure you get your omega-3s are salmon, cod, sardines, scallops, shrimp, anchovies, Atlantic mackerel, catfish, clams, crab, crawfish, flounder, haddock, mullet, oysters, and pollock.

Keto

I first want to talk about what is meant by a *keto* diet. A true keto diet is a medical diet used to help children with epileptic seizures and sometimes people with type 1 diabetes. A true keto diet is when your body uses stored fat to produce energy in the form of ketone bodies. For your body to do this, you must deprive it of carbohydrates, eat some (but not too much protein), and eat a lot of fatty foods. It takes a few days to be in a true state of ketosis — something that can be determined by measuring ketone bodies in your urine.

This type of diet of burning fat may result in weight loss, which is what many people use the keto diet for. However, it's difficult to maintain the diet long term, and all that fat — including saturated fats — may increase your low-density lipoprotein (LDL) and increase your risk for cardiovascular disease. In addition, if you eat a low-carbohydrate diet, your intake of vegetables, fruits, and grains is low, and you may develop micronutrient deficiencies. Also, you'll get less fiber and possibly too much fat and protein, which will overload your liver and kidneys.

When following a true keto diet, you may need to supplement with the following:

>> Selenium

>> Magnesium

» Phosphorus

» B vitamins

» Vitamin C

In addition, if you are doing a true keto diet for weight loss, it's hard to sustain for a long period. Once you go off it — as with most "diets" — you may gain the weight back.

Some people try a modified keto diet for weight loss. You may be trying a higher-protein, lower-carb, and higher-fat diet. If you eat lower carb and higher fat and protein, it can reduce your appetite and help with weight loss. Choose good fats, lean proteins, and lots of vegetables. If you instead eat meats high in saturated fats like salami, beef, and bacon, and you're not eating fruits, vegetables, or whole grains, then your diet isn't good for you and can lead to risk for heart disease as well as being hard on your liver and kidneys. You may need the supplements listed above for the true keto diet.

Standard American Diet

By definition, the Standard American Diet (SAD) consists of ultraprocessed foods, added sugar, fat, and sodium. Generally, people do not consume enough fruits, vegetables, whole grains, legumes, and lean protein on this diet. This way of eating is very common in the United States — especially with the increasing number of fast-food restaurants, large portions sizes, the increase in take-out food options, and the higher cost of healthy foods.

About half of Americans suffer from chronic diseases that are related to poor diet. A contributing factor is that about 60 percent of Americans are overweight or obese. The SAD diet may put you at risk for some cancers, cardiovascular disease, diabetes, hypertension, and metabolic syndrome.

Eating a better diet will improve health. Unfortunately, for many people, the SAD diet is more affordable and convenient. In addition, supplements that you may need, such as vitamin D, calcium, potassium, and fiber, may also be expensive. More home cooking and bulk shopping makes eating healthier more affordable.

REMEMBER

If your diet fits the SAD definition, supplements may be necessary, particularly vitamin D, calcium, potassium, and fiber.

Testing Your Levels

One way to determine your need for supplements is through testing. At your yearly checkup your doctor will often order some blood tests, including comprehensive metabolic panel, lipid screening, and other tests based on your age. The tests most relevant to the discussion of vitamins and supplements include the following tests:

>> Vitamin B12

>> Vitamin D

>> Iron and ferritin

>> Homocysteine to diagnose vitamin B6, B9 or B12 deficiency

>> Fasting blood glucose (see Figure 12-2) and HbA1C

>> Lipid panel (total cholesterol, LDL, HDL, triglycerides, and so on as shown in Figure 12-3)

>> Magnesium

>> Thyroid panel

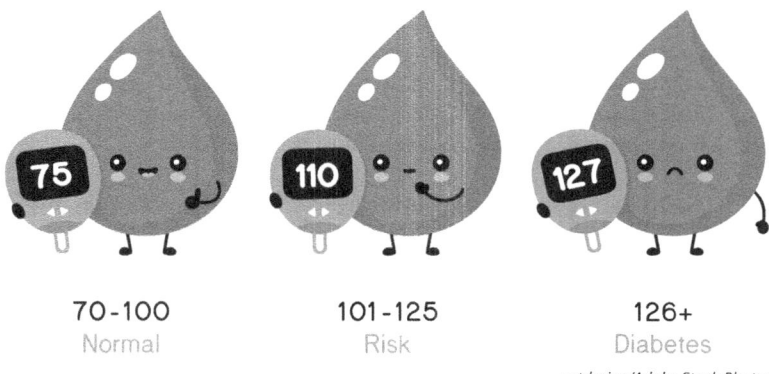

FIGURE 12-2: Fasting blood glucose is an important annual test to determine whether your levels are normal or put you at risk or in the zone for diabetes.

70-100 Normal   101-125 Risk   126+ Diabetes

svtdesign/Adobe Stock Photos

Your annual blood work can also indicate if you have other medical problems like fatty liver or kidney issues.

The preceding list includes traditional blood tests that your doctor orders to measure your metabolic function. Other tests are available to take more detailed measurements of things that may affect your health, including a nutritional panel and DNA testing. Your yearly blood test from your doctor is most likely covered by insurance, whereas the other tests may not be. Currently there are many at-home finger-prick tests that can help assess your nutritional status and genetic predisposition to nutrition-related issues.

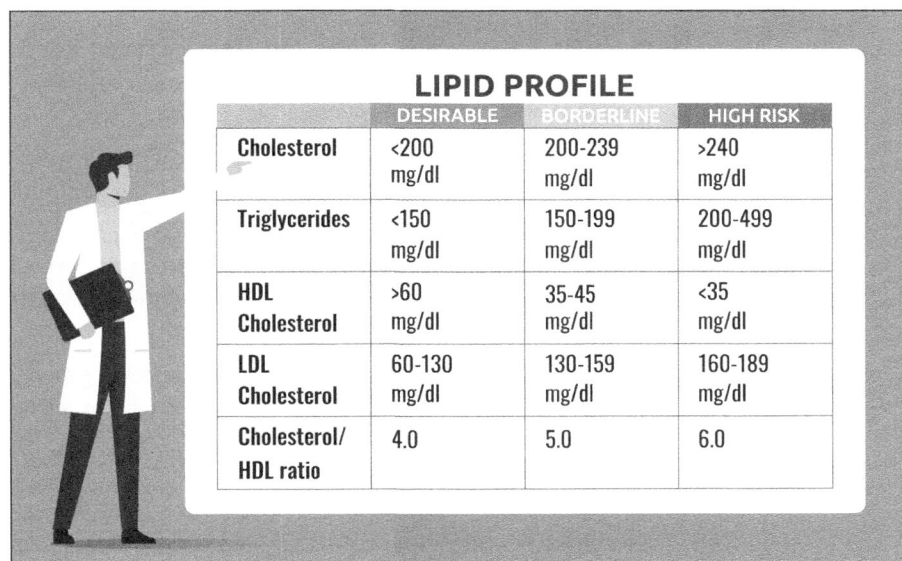

LIPID PROFILE	DESIRABLE	BORDERLINE	HIGH RISK
Cholesterol	<200 mg/dl	200-239 mg/dl	>240 mg/dl
Triglycerides	<150 mg/dl	150-199 mg/dl	200-499 mg/dl
HDL Cholesterol	>60 mg/dl	35-45 mg/dl	<35 mg/dl
LDL Cholesterol	60-130 mg/dl	130-159 mg/dl	160-189 mg/dl
Cholesterol/ HDL ratio	4.0	5.0	6.0

FIGURE 12-3: This chart shows the ranges for lipid profiles in your annual blood work.

Diki/Adobe Stock Photos

Analyzing your annual blood test

Most blood tests reports that you will see in your patient portal or that your doctor will send you have some explanation that you can read it before meeting with your doctor. Most results indicate the normal range of values, your result, and whether your value is out of the normal range. It's important to discuss the results with your doctor because sometimes being out of normal range may not mean anything significant.

Nutrient panel

Because it can be difficult to get an idea of your nutritional status from traditional methods, such as your annual blood test, you can have additional tests to measure many of the micronutrients and other blood factors to get more information. These tests may go beyond what's in your blood to measure intracellular components critical for health.

Here I list some of the companies that do these tests. You should check with your insurance plan to see if they will pay these companies directly or reimburse you for out-of-pocket costs:

>> **Everlywell:** This online company provides about 19 at-home tests and some telehealth options.

>> **Fullscript:** This company (available only in some states) sells supplements from very reliable companies. It also recently began collaborating with labs to offer a variety of testing options.

>> **KBMO Diagnostics:** KBMO offers tests for biochemical markers as well as food sensitivity tests and gut barrier panels.

>> **Labcorp (and Labcorp OnDemand):** This company provides about 75 home blood tests for micronutrients, hormones, blood sugar, weight loss, hormones, and more. You can order these tests without a prescription from your doctor and pay for them directly.

>> **Quest Diagnostics:** This medical laboratory offers more than 144 tests that you can order similarly to using Labcorp, but the choices are more extensive.

>> **SpectraCell:** This company offers micronutrient and other testing. You need your healthcare provider's assistance to have access to the tests. The SpectraCell test measures 31 micronutrients present inside white blood cells, which is where they do their job. The test considers your personal biochemistry and gives insight into where you may have deficits. They also have numerous other available tests, such as lipid profile and some genetic testing.

In some cases, you will need to have blood drawn at a lab. In other cases, you may be able to do a finger prick at home to send directly to them.

One advantage to home testing includes the convenience of not needing a prescription or doctor appointment. It's a good way to learn more about your specific nutritional needs based on valid personal data. At-home tests also make it possible to monitor your nutrient levels over time, and in some circumstances, that may be quite helpful.

It's nice that these companies have these tests that you can order, which enables you to take your health into your own hands. However, choosing which tests will give you the information you need can be difficult. Before wasting too much money on testing without understanding what to do with the results, consult with your trusted healthcare provider.

TECHNICAL STUFF

Precision nutrition is an emerging field of research and practice in which a provider considers your unique characteristics — such as health history, medications, lifestyle, sex, genetics, and race — to help devise a plan of action for you to improve your health, prevent disease, and sometimes to treat disease, especially chronic diseases. You also may have heard of personalized medicine, which is a similar practice for improving disease risk or symptoms using a person's unique characteristics with a wider scope of treating diseases.

Genetic testing

DNA testing can provide insight into how your body digests, absorbs, metabolizes, and excretes food and nutrients. It's known that genetic variation can affect food tolerances and requirements. Understanding your unique nutrition-related genetic makeup may be helpful for developing a personalized nutrition plan to improve your health.

The science of nutritional genomics (or nutrigenomics) is concerned with the impact of dietary components on the genome (all your genes), the proteome (all your proteins), and the metabolome (all metabolites). Nutrigenomics analyzes gene-nutrient interactions, which includes how genes regulate intake and metabolism of nutrients and how nutrients influence expression of genes (nutrigenetics). Figure 12-4 shows a visual representation of this idea.

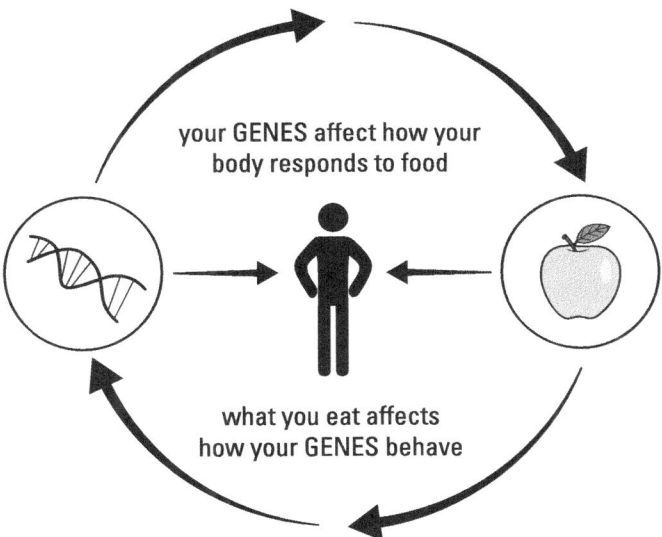

your GENES affect how your body responds to food

what you eat affects how your GENES behave

FIGURE 12-4: Nutritional genomics is how your food effects your DNA.

Epigenetics is the study of gene modifications that are not related to actual change in your DNA. DNA can be modified by food and environmental factors, and these modifications may be reversible but also can be passed down to offspring and further generations. Changes in epigenetic modifications may be part of the mechanism of the onset of chronic diseases and their progression. For example, diets high in sugar and fat may cause methylation or other modifications to genes that contribute to diabetes, obesity, cancer, and non-alcoholic fatty liver disease.

The field of epigenetics is emerging, and tools are being developed to analyze these effects of the gene–nutrient interactions. DNA is made of four nucleotides — adenine, thymine, cytosine, and guanine — that are linked together to make the strand of DNA. Single nucleotide polymorphisms (SNPs) are when just a single nucleotide is replaced by another in a strand of DNA. These are common, and you may have many of these — even millions — in your genome (all of your DNA). SNPs can be measured to help identify genes that may be associated with diseases, affect metabolism, respond to certain nutrients, and be involved in health and disease. Many tests measure multiple polymorphisms that may affect things like eating behavior and metabolism.

Common SNPs that can be used as biomarkers for nutrition-related health include the following. Some of these can influence what you eat or should eat (nutrigenomics), and some are influenced by the foods that you eat (nutrigenetics).

>> **MTHFR (methylenetetrahydrofolate reductase):** Variations in this gene alter folate metabolism. As a result, a person may require supplements. MTHFR may be linked to increased breast cancer risk.

>> **VDRs (vitamin D receptor genes):** This affects availability of vitamin D and may increase the risk for osteoporosis in postmenopausal women who don't take calcium.

>> **FTO (fat mass and obesity-associated gene):** This gene is associated with body mass index and obesity risk. High-fat diets might make the effect worse.

>> **APOE (apolipoprotein E):** This is linked to cholesterol levels, increased risk for heart attack, and increased Alzheimer's disease. People with this polymorphism (and perhaps others) should decrease the intake of saturated fats from the diet.

>> **CYP1A:** This gene is linked to liver metabolism of certain drugs and food substances. It may influence caffeine metabolism.

>> **CYP1A2:** This gene is associated with caffeine-related hypertensive response.

>> **Leptin receptor gene:** This one is linked with increased risk of type 2 diabetes.

>> **ACE (angiotensin converting enzyme genes):** This gene may require that a person needs more sodium intake compared to recommended amounts.

Metabolomics is also a branch of genomics that helps identify metabolites (or biomarkers) in bodily fluids and uses them to understand alterations in metabolism. This is a good tool for investigating the effects of food on health. How food and nutrients interact and change metabolism is another component of developing a personalized precision nutrition plan. You may run across tests that measure these metabolites and offer interpretation.

The field of nutrigenomics is complex and still emerging, as data supports some of its uses, and the number of companies that do analysis and give advice about what you should or shouldn't eat or supplements you should use grows. At the time of writing, there are more than 40 of these companies globally, with about 20 in North America. It is an extremely exciting area of nutrition, but it still has a long way to go.

TIP

Most of the companies in this field give information on different nutrients (macronutrients, vitamins, and minerals). They will let you know if you're likely to have gluten and lactose sensitivities. Your genes can tell you if your metabolism will speed up on alcohol and caffeine. They may recommend a list of genetics superfoods that best match your DNA information and may offer insight into predisposition to stress eating, cravings, or food preferences or how to manage stress with food and lifestyle choices. Some offer in-person counseling and diet plans.

Nutrigenomics is a recent innovative and potentially powerful area of understanding nutrition and health. It is a particularly huge area of research. On an individual level, the ability to create personalized nutrition plans offers lots of potential.

WARNING

As with anything you might be doing on your own, always consult with your healthcare provider before loading up on alternative supplements based on results of genetic testing. It is always best to meet with a healthcare provider to determine the best fit for your nutritional and supplement needs. The reason this is so important is because it's possible to take too much — or too little — of a vitamin or other supplement; either situation can result in side effects. In addition, supplements can interact with your medications negatively, so you need the help of a professional to watch for possible interactions.

Finding Sources for Ordering Supplements

When researching information online, it is important to weed out the sponsored ads from good websites for information. In Chapter 17, I recommend some good informational website. In this section, I provide a few websites for ordering supplements.

When shopping for and deciding where to buy supplements, take the following things into account:

>> Read the container label and look for the USP, NSF, or ConsumerLab seal that means the product has been third-party certified for safety, purity, and dose.

>> Read the supplements fact label (see Chapter 13) and verify that what is in the product matches the label on the front.

>> Choose trusted brands that follow GMP (Good Manufacturing Practices) and that are reputable.

>> Read the entire label, including what other ingredients are in the product. You may want a vegan product or something with no fillers, for example.

>> Look at the recommended dose. Sometimes you may need only one pill and sometimes two or three are required.

>> Check the cost if that's important to you so you can compare and choose the most cost-effective one for you. Food-based or whole food supplements will be more expensive, but they offer better absorption and usually are easier on the stomach than synthetic supplements or those made in a lab.

If you go to an online vitamin store, read very carefully! If they make claims, check to see if there are studies to support the supplements' use. Distinguish between scientific studies and marketing studies.

Here are some websites that I suggest for ordering supplements:

>> **Fullscript:** This is the number one website for ordering vitamins and supplements that are "clean" and reputable. You need a healthcare provider to set you up with an account, but then you can reorder anytime. Your provider can also order many tests from Fullscript.

>> **Reliable and third-party certified brands with proprietary websites:** Some of these are also found in stores:

- Amazon Elements
- Centrum
- Costco brands, such as Kirkland
- CVS or Walgreens
- Gaia
- Garden of Life
- Life Extension

- Megafoods
- Metagenics
- Nature Made
- New Chapter
- Nordic Naturals
- Now
- Olly
- Pure Encapsulation
- Thorne

IN THIS CHAPTER

» **Checking out the Supplement Facts panel**

» **Discovering the wealth of information on the rest of the label**

» **Understanding the FDA regulations for the label and health claims**

» **Making smart purchase decisions**

Chapter **13**

Reading Labels and Understanding Dosages

To be sure that you get the right supplements and the correct doses, you need to put on your reading glasses and look at the fine print on the bottles. The labels on your bottle of calcium, for example, have loads of good information about the supplement, including the form of calcium, the amount of calcium in each pill, the serving size (how many to take), the health benefits (that the manufacturer claims), and the Supplement Facts panel. In addition, you find warnings, directions, disclaimers, information about the packaging, and possibly third-party certification.

In this chapter, I describe the items that you find on your supplements panel in more detail. I present examples of the Supplement Facts panel and go into detail about what information is included and why. I talk about how to interpret the information on this panel — and the other information on the bottle — so that you can make an informed decision about whether to buy and use a particular supplement. You have many factors to consider while making your decision, including whether the supplement contains the chemical form in the amount that you need. You must also consider whether the health claims for the product fit your needs, what other ingredients are in the pill, and even whether you feel confident that the supplement is responsibly manufactured.

Gleaning the Key Information from the Supplement Facts Panel

Supplements have a *Supplement Facts* panel that appears on the bottle and contains information similar to the Nutrition Facts labels you see on foods. Both types of panels follow Food and Drug Administration (FDA) guidelines. The guidelines describe the requirements for companies, which are determined by The Nutrition Labeling and Education Act of 1990 and amendments that have been made over the years.

The Supplement Facts panel is clearly highlighted on the bottle and looks something like Figure 13-1. You will find these five details that the FDA requires on the bottle (not necessarily on the supplement panel, though):

>> A statement of identity — in this case, the dietary supplement's name

>> Quantity of contents statement, which includes the amount of the dietary supplement and the full Supplement Facts panel

>> Nutrition labeling, including anything found on a Nutrition Facts label — for example, 5 grams of sugar that might be found in a gummy vitamin

>> An ingredient list that tells you every other ingredient used in the supplement

>> Name and place of business of the manufacturer, packer, or distributor

Because it's best to get as many nutrients as possible from dietary sources, you should also pay attention to Nutrition Facts labels on foods. They include a lot of good information. For example, you can find out what amount is considered a serving size, how many calories the food has per serving, and how much sodium, cholesterol, fat, protein, and carbohydrates (including fiber and added sugar) that the food contains. The FDA also requires food companies to add information about Vitamin D, calcium, iron, and potassium; you find this at the bottom of the label, as shown in Figure 13-2.

Evaluating the essential ingredients of your supplement

Knowing what you're ingesting when you take a supplement is important, so make sure to study the ingredients in the Supplement Facts panel. The ingredients must have two identifiers, including

>> The recognizable common name, such as Vitamin D

>> The chemical name and form in parentheses after the common name

Supplement Facts

Serving Size 1 Gelcap
Servings Per Container 100

	Amount Per Serving	% Daily Value
Vitamin A (as retinyl acetate and 50% as beta-carotene)	900 mcg	100%
Vitamin C (as ascorbic acid)	90 mg	100%
Vitamin D (as cholecalciferol)	20 mcg (800 IU)	100%
Vitamin E (as dl-alpha tocopheryl acetate)	15 mg	100%
Thiamin (as thiamin mononitrate)	1.2 mg	100%
Riboflavin	1.3 mg	100%
Niacin (as niacinamide)	16 mg	100%
Vitamin B_6 (as pyridoxine hydrochloride)	1.7 mg	100%
Folate	400 mcg DFE (240 mcg folic acid)	100%
Vitamin B_{12} (as cyanocobalamin)	2.4 mcg	100%
Biotin	3 mcg	10%
Pantothenic Acid (as calcium pantothenate)	5 mg	100%

Other ingredients: Gelatin, lactose, magnesium stearate, microcrystalline cellulose, FD&C Yellow No. 6, propylene glycol, preservatives (propylparaben and sodium benzoate).

FIGURE 13-1: A Supplement Facts panel for a multivitamin.

Sign System/Adobe Stock Photos

Nutrition Facts (standard panel)

6 servings per container
Serving size 1 cup (230g)

Amount per serving
Calories 245

	% Daily Value*
Total Fat 12g	14%
Saturated Fat 2g	10%
Trans Fat 0g	
Cholesterol 8mg	3%
Sodium 210mg	9%
Total Carbohydrate 34g	12%
Dietary Fiber 7g	25%
Total Sugars 5g	
Includes 4g Added Sugars	8%
Protein 11g	
Vitamin D 4mcg	20%
Calcium 210mg	16%
Iron 3mg	15%
Potassium 380mg	8%

*The % Daily Value (DV) tells you how much a nutrient in a serving of food contributes to a daily diet. 2,000 calories a day is used for general nutrition advice.

Nutrition Facts (dual column)

2 servings per container
Serving size 1 cup (230g)

Calories	Per serving 245	Per container 490
	% DV*	% DV*
Total Fat	12g 14%	24g 29%
Saturated Fat	2g 10%	4g 20%
Trans Fat	0g	0g
Cholesterol	8mg 3%	16mg 5%
Sodium	210mg 9%	420mg 18%
Total Carb.	34g 12%	68g 24%
Dietary Fiber	7g 25%	14g 50%
Total Sugars	5g	10g
Incl. Added Sugars	4g 8%	8g 16%
Protein	11g	22g
Vitamin D	4mcg 20%	8mcg 40%
Calcium	210mg 16%	420mg 32%
Iron	3mg 15%	6mg 30%
Potassium	380mg 8%	760mg 16%

*The % Daily Value (DV) tells you how much a nutrient in a serving of food contributes to a daily diet. 2,000 calories a day is used for general nutrition advice.

Nutrition Facts (simplified)

6 servings per container
Serving size 1 cup (230g)

Amount per serving
Calories 245

	% Daily Value*
Total Fat 12g	14%
Saturated Fat 2g	10%
Trans Fat 0g	
Cholesterol 8mg	3%
Sodium 210mg	9%
Total Carbohydrate 34g	12%
Dietary Fiber 7g	25%
Total Sugars 5g	
Includes 4g Added Sugars	8%
Protein 11g	

| Vit. D 4mcg 20% | Calcium 210mg 16% |
| Iron 3mg 15% | Potassium 380mg 8% |

*The % Daily Value (DV) tells you how much a nutrient in a serving of food contributes to a daily diet. 2,000 calories a day is used for general nutrition advice.

Nutrition Facts (linear)

6 servings per container
Serving size 1 cup (230g)

Calories per serving **245**

Amount/serving	% Daily Value*	Amount/serving	% Daily Value*
Total Fat 12g	14%	**Total Carbohydrate** 34g	12%
Saturated Fat 2g	10%	Dietary Fiber 7g	25%
Trans Fat 0g		Total Sugars 5g	
Cholesterol 8mg	3%	Includes 4g Added Sugars	8%
Sodium 210mg	9%	**Protein** 11g	

Vitamin D 4mcg 20 · Calcium 210mg 16% · Iron 3mg 15% · Potassium 380mg 8%
Thiamin 13% · Riboflavin 9% · Niacin 12%

*The % Daily Value (DV) tells you how much a nutrient in a serving of food contributes to a daily diet. 2,000 calories a day is used for general nutrition advice.

FIGURE 13-2: A typical Nutrition Facts panel.

maradaisy/Adobe Stock Photos

For example, a bottle of calcium and vitamin D would say "Vitamin D (as Chole-calciferol)" and "Calcium (as Calcium Carbonate)." Sometimes when you're looking for the best form of a vitamin or mineral, these specific names can make a difference to you. In the case of calcium, calcium citrate is more absorbable than calcium carbonate, and this may be important if you are older, taking medications for gastroesophageal reflux disease (GERD), or need to be able to take the supplement with or without food.

The next item to look for is the amount of the nutrient (or nutrients) your supplement contains. This quantity is listed as the amount per serving size and is usually expressed as micrograms (mcg), milligrams (mg), grams (g), or international units (IU).

TIP

The panel lists serving size separately and tells you how many pills, capsules, gels, gummies, scoops, or milliliters of a liquid to take for one serving. In some cases, this serving size can range from one up to as many as six pills or capsules in a day, so reading this information carefully is important.

Getting enough: The % Daily Value

The Supplement Facts panel also converts the amounts in the supplement to *the percent of daily value — % Daily Value* (or *%DV*). This information is in the far-right column. Daily value is the recommended amount of the nutrient based on a daily intake of 2,000 calories per day. The %DV is how much a single serving of the supplement is as a percent of the total amount needed per day.

REMEMBER

The daily value and percentage are a fine estimate for most people, and you need no further calculations if you eat fewer or more calories each day or on some days. For example, on the supplement label for the calcium I use, the vitamin D is 20 mcg, which is 100 under the % Daily Value column. However, each pill (one serving size) has 600 mg of calcium, with the % Daily Value of 46. So, if you intend to get 100 percent of your calcium each day, you need to get the rest (the remaining 54 percent) through food sources.

Recognizing the other ingredients in your supplement

The FDA requires that manufacturers list all food ingredients that would appear on a Nutrition Facts label for foods if the amount is greater than zero. The manufacturers must let consumers know whether the supplement contains any calories, fats, carbohydrates, protein, sodium, vitamin D, calcium, iron, or phosphate.

Figure 13-3 shows a sample Supplements Facts panel for an imaginary omega-3 supplement. You can see that the label includes calories, fat, vitamin A, and vitamin D.

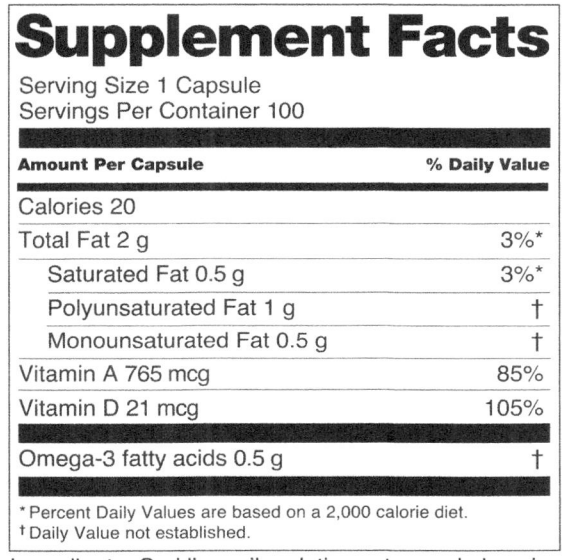

FIGURE 13-3:
A Supplement Facts panel for an imaginary omega-3 supplement.

REMEMBER

If you like taking gummy vitamins that are made with sugar, the number of calories (or the sugar itself) might make a difference in your overall diet. One of my clients takes two multivitamin gummies; two hair, nail, and teeth gummies; and two calcium/vitamin D gummies every day. The calories involved add up to more than 100, and the gummies include 25 grams of sugar.

Minding serving sizes

Paying attention to the serving size listed on the label is important because it tells you how many of the supplement pills, capsules, gels, gummies, scoops, or milliliters of a liquid to ingest. When a serving size is two tablets, that means that all the quantities and % DV listed are for those two pills. If you take only one pill — which may be indicated sometimes — then the quantities and %DV are simply divided by two (half of the totals). Be sure to always check for serving size, because it may be greater for food-based supplements than for synthetic ones.

Differentiating Supplement Names, Forms, and Amounts

Vitamins are sometimes listed by other names, which might be a chemical form of it or a precursor. (A *precursor* is a form that's converted to the active vitamin by your body.) For example, vitamin A includes retinol, retinal, retinyl esters, and retinoic acid. These as well as beta-carotene are "preformed" vitamin A and are converted to vitamin A in your cells. Table 13-1 shows a list of common vitamins and their chemical names.

TABLE 13-1 ## Common Vitamins and Their Aliases

Common Name	Chemical Names
Vitamin A	Retinol, retinal, retinoic acid
Vitamin B1	Thiamine
Vitamin B2	Riboflavin
Vitamin B3	Niacin (or nicotinic acid)
Vitamin B5	Pantothenic acid
Vitamin B6	Pyridoxine (includes pyridoxal and pyridoxamine)
Vitamin B7	Biotin (also known as Vitamin H)
Vitamin B9	Folic acid (or folate)
Vitamin B12	Cobalamin (includes several forms — for example, methylcobalamin)
Vitamin C	Ascorbic acid
Vitamin D	Cholecalciferol (vitamin D3) and ergocalciferol (vitamin D2)
Vitamin E	Tocopherol (and its derivatives, such as tocotrienols)
Vitamin K	Phylloquinone (vitamin K1) and menaquinone (vitamin K2)

The most frequently used units of measurements of vitamins and minerals that are used on supplement labels are milligrams, micrograms, grams, and international units (IUs). Some vitamins that have historically listed IUs are currently being changed to mg or mcg. Be sure that you read labels carefully because there is a big difference between mg and mcg! A mg is 1,000 times that of a mcg! Table 13-2 offers a look at common abbreviations and measures.

TABLE 13-2

Common Abbreviations and Measures

Abbreviations of Units	What They Mean
g or gm	grams
mg	milligrams
mcg	micrograms
mg NE	milligrams of niacin equivalents
mcg DFE	micrograms of dietary folate equivalents
mcg RAE	micrograms of retinol activity equivalents
IU	international units

Examining the Info Outside the Supplement Facts Panel

If you look at all the other information on the supplement packaging, you will see that there is so much information — some of which is very important to consider when making your decisions. Some examples are understanding what other ingredients might be in the supplement or the health claims of the supplement. Or you might wonder if the product is vegan or vegetarian. In this section, I try to fill you in on every detail found on these products so that you can make a good decision about what supplements are for you.

Deciphering other ingredients

Directly under the Supplement Facts panel is the *other ingredient* list. This may contain a lot of words that you don't understand. In general, I believe that fewer other ingredients indicates that the product is cleaner because it contains less of what doesn't actually make up the supplement.

The government has guidelines for what is considered an ingredient. The Dietary Supplement Health and Education Act (DSHEA) uses the term *ingredient* to refer to the compounds used in the manufacture of a dietary supplement. For example, when calcium carbonate is used to provide calcium, calcium carbonate is an *ingredient* and calcium is a *dietary ingredient*.

If something is listed in the Supplement Facts panel, it doesn't have to then be listed in the other ingredients list also. The term *ingredient* also includes substances such as binders (chemicals that help keep the pill's shape), colors, excipients (the vehicle or medium, such as microcrystalline cellulose or polyethylene glycol), fillers added to increase the pill's size (such as starch, lactose, or dical-cium phosphate), flavors, dyes, and sweeteners. The other ingredients are listed in order of quantity by weight. This section may also include a list of possible allergens — for example, it could say "Contains: Soy."

Distinguishing legitimate claims

A vitamin or supplement bottle may also contain health claims. According to the Council on Responsible Nutrition, a supplement label can contain three types of legal claims:

>> **Nutrient content claims:** Tell you how valuable the dosage of vitamin or mineral is as a supplement. For example, a vitamin B12 label may say "a good source of vitamin B12." A vitamin E label might say "high in antioxidants."

>> **Structure/function claims:** Describe the basic benefits of the product on a particular structure or function in the body. As an example, my women's multivitamin says, "Supports energy metabolism, immune and bone health." A calcium/vitamin D3 supplement could say, "Vitamin D3 helps calcium absorption" or "Calcium builds strong bones."

The FDA mandates that these claims must also include a statement on the label that says "These statements have not been evaluated by the Food and Drug Administration. This product is not intended to diagnose, treat, cure or prevent any disease." This statement simply means that the manufacturer is following the law.

Here are examples of structure/function claims you may encounter:

- Supports urinary tract health

- Helps maintain cardiovascular function

- Helps to maintain cholesterol levels that are already within the normal range

- Promotes joint health

- Helps maintain a healthy blood sugar level as part of a healthy diet

- Supports a healthy weight loss plan

- Supports immune health

- Mood support

>> **FDA-authorized health claims or qualified health claims, which must be approved by the FDA:** An FDA committee reviews the scientific evidence for the claim and decides whether a relationship exists between the substance

and reduced risk of a disease. Since 1990, only 12 of these types of claims have been approved.

Notice the distinction between the phrase *reduces the risk* and the phrase *prevents disease*. (The latter cannot legally be used as a health claim.) An example of a valid health claim is "Adequate calcium throughout life, as part of a well-balanced diet, may reduce the risk of osteoporosis."

Looking for third-party certification

Supplement companies are required to follow FDA established Good Manufacturing Practices (GMPs) to help ensure the quality of their dietary supplements. FDA may periodically inspect facilities that manufacture supplements; however little standardization of dietary supplements seems to exist across the brands.

Determining the quality and safety of individual products can be difficult for consumers to do. Luckily, three certification programs exist in the United States that independently evaluate the overall quality of supplements for these criteria: identity, purity, strength, and composition.

There are other certifications that you may see as well, including USDA Certified Organic, Non-GMO Project Verified, Gluten-Free, Kosher, and Halal. In addition, NSF Certified for Sport and Informed Sport are certifications used to assure that supplements have been tested for prohibited substances in sports (for example, low levels of steroids and stimulants), which are prohibited by WADA (World Anti-Doping Agency).

Table 13-3 shows you the three organizations that conduct third-party certifications with their identifying mark, which is added to the supplement container for the products they certify. I highly recommend looking for products that have these marks on their label.

Discovering directions for use

Be sure to carefully follow the instructions you find in the directions for use section of the supplement's packaging. The information in this section may include items such as

» Adult and children's doses

» Number of pills to take

» When to take them

» Whether to take them with food

TABLE 13-3

Third-Party Certifiers

Certifier	Certifier's Mark
ConsumerLab.com	
NSF International (NSF)	
US Pharmacopeial Convention (USP)	

You may also find encouragement to discuss your medications and supplement intake with your healthcare provider or admonishments not to exceed the recommended dose.

Watching the warnings

If you take too many different vitamins and supplements — or too much of any one supplement — you may be at risk for side effects. In addition, you should talk to your healthcare provider to make sure that any supplements you're taking do not interfere with your medications.

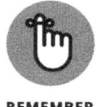

REMEMBER

Taking too many supplements or having them interfere with your medications can be bad. Here are a few examples, taken from the FDA website:

>> Vitamin K can interfere with the ability of the blood thinner warfarin to prevent blood from clotting.

>> St. John's wort may increase the breakdown of some medicines and reduce their effectiveness. For example, you should not take this supplement if you are on certain antidepressants.

>> Vitamins C and E and other antioxidants could interfere with some types of cancer chemotherapy.

Paying attention to expiration dates

Interestingly, the FDA does not require expiration dates on vitamin or other supplements. However, many companies choose to add them. How long a supplement lasts can depend on its form, its contents, and how you store it. A pill or capsule may last longer than a gummy or oil.

The potency and stability of a supplement also depends upon the particular vitamin or mineral. For example, some vitamins are more vulnerable to light or air and will lose potency. Losing potency is not dangerous or toxic. It just means that you're getting less of the supplement than you think you're getting. For example, if you have a deficiency of vitamin B12, and you aren't getting enough from a supplement, then this may not bring your body's B12 content up to normal levels, which could have health consequences such as the physical, neurological, or psychological problems associated with B12 deficiency.

REMEMBER

You should find recommendations for ideal storage conditions on the supplement container, and you should follow the recommendations for each supplement that you take. If you do find an expiration date on the packaging, experts generally believe that, if stored properly, the supplement can last up to two years beyond this date. However, if you notice mold or a bad smell, you should not take the supplement. Dispose of it properly by dropping it at your local pharmacy or other appropriate place in your neighborhood.

Getting the Best Bang for Your Buck

Whether you are walking down the supplement aisle of your local pharmacy or health food store or you go online to websites that sell vitamins and supplements, the incredible number of choices can be overwhelming. You have many things to consider when choosing a supplement. Some of the online or health food store brands are often considered better than the drugstore brands, but they may not be.

TIP

Here are some ideas to keep in mind when shopping around for the right supplements for you:

>> Always consult with your healthcare provider to decide which supplements you need.

>> Discuss potential interactions between medicines and other supplements with your healthcare provider.

>> Read labels carefully to choose the correct vitamin (or combinations) and amounts.

>> Choose a reputable brand, preferably with a third-party certification mark.

>> Look for cleaner, or purer, supplements that may appeal to you. For example, you can look for those with fewer fillers or that are gluten free or vegetarian.

>> Consider the cost. If all other things are equal among your choices — cost may be the deciding factor.

Chapter **14**

Integrating Supplements into Your Daily Life

All through this book, I've frequently mentioned that it's good to eat nutritious foods to get most of your important nutrients. Even if you eat a well-balanced diet, you may find yourself in the position of needing supplements to improve your metabolism and health. In this chapter, I talk about how to focus on improving your food intake and ways to incorporate supplements into your daily routine.

Getting the Most Nutrients from Your Foods

The way to get the most nutrients from your foods is by eating according to the science-based recommended guidelines in the Dietary Guidelines for Americans (DGA). The new edition for the next five years will be published at the end of 2025. At the time of writing, the guidelines are from the DGA 2020–2025, so that's what some of the information in this chapter is based on.

The United States Department of Agriculture (USDA) and Department of Health and Human Services (HHS) are responsible for the DGA focused on a balanced dietary pattern to promote overall health. The idea is to get most of your nutrient needs from food to be healthy and to prevent chronic diseases including obesity, heart disease, diabetes, neurodegenerative diseases, and cancer.

The DGA suggests the three dietary patterns designed to help you get your nutrients:

>> **The Healthy U.S.-Style dietary pattern (HUSS):** This pattern allows for a wide variety of foods and is easy for Americans to follow. It has the following characteristics:

- It's based on healthier forms of typical American foods.

- It focuses on fruits and vegetables — generally five servings a day.

- Lean protein (poultry, fish, eggs, beans) is recommended.

- Skim or low-fat dairy is included.

- Whole grains (brown rice, whole grain bread, whole grain pasta) rather than processed grains (white rice, white bread, sugary cereals, regular pasta) are recommended.

- It includes some healthy fats from vegetable oils, nuts, and seeds.

- It's recommended that you limit added sugar, salt, and saturated or too many fats.

>> **Healthy Mediterranean–style dietary pattern:** This diet is inspired by the way people eat in Mediterranean countries because it lowers rates of chronic illnesses. Compared to the HUSS, this way of eating is

- Higher in fruits, vegetables, healthy fats, and seafood

- Lower in dairy and red and processed meats.

The Mediterranean Diet consists of about 50 percent carbohydrates (from fruits, vegetables, dairy, and grains), 15 percent protein, and 35 percent fat. The DGA describes intake ranges more broadly as 45 percent to 65 percent from total daily calorie intake, 10 percent to 35 percent from protein, and 20 percent to 35 percent from fats.

>> **Healthy Vegetarian Dietary Pattern:** This dietary pattern differs from the other two because it doesn't include any meat, poultry, or seafood. Here are some characteristics of this diet:

- More plant-based protein, including legumes (beans and lentils), meat substitutes from soy and other products, nuts, and seeds

- Dairy and eggs for more protein (if not vegan)

- Whole grains, fruits, and vegetables

Building a Healthy Plate for Well-Balanced Meals

One easy way to know if you are eating well is by using the plating method. There are several versions of this plate. Two that I like are available on the MyPlate website (www.myplate.gov) or the Harvard Health website (https://nutrition source.hsph.harvard.edu/healthy-eating-plate/). The latter is the one I use in my practice because of the details and focus on limited dairy.

Here are the key recommendations on the foods you should be eating and the portion sizes of each from these plates and other similar versions:

>> Fill half your plate with nonstarchy vegetables and/or fruit.

>> A quarter of your plate (about one cup) should be filled with mostly whole grains beans, lentils, bread, cereals, pasta, rice, and other grains and starchy vegetables including potatoes, peas, and corn. Avoid processed grains and foods made from white flour as much as possible.

>> The other quarter of your plate (or 4 ounces) should be good lean protein, including fish, chicken, eggs, turkey, beans, legumes, tofu, and other soy-based products. Avoid fried meats, deli meats, bacon, and too much beef.

>> You need some, but not too much, healthy oils, including vegetables oils (canola, avocado) and olive oil. Limit butter and lard. Studies show that extra-virgin olive oil is the best option because it's high in omega-3 fatty acids. Some vegetable oils may contain more omega-6 fatty acids. Another guideline is that oils that are solid at room temperature (butter, lard, coconut oil) should be limited. The quantity of oils the DGA recommends is about 5 to 6 teaspoons per day for women and 6 to 7 teaspoons per day for men. The Harvard Healthy Plate differs in that it doesn't state any limitation on healthy fats. In my practice, I include things like hummus, guacamole, peanut butter and salad dressings in this category and tell my clients to use about two tablespoons as a portion size. For example, 2 tablespoons of peanut butter or 1 ounce of nuts is about 3 teaspoons of oil.

>> Drinks shouldn't have added sugar. Stick to water, seltzer, tea, coffee, diet drinks, and only small amounts of 100 percent juice (if any).

>> Limit dairy to 2 servings a day and use mostly low-fat or skim dairy. If you're a vegetarian and use dairy, then using skim or low-fat dairy can be an excellent source of protein, and you may want to up the amount you consume. This is an important consideration for children who need protein, calcium, and vitamin D for growth and development.

This way of eating is good throughout all life stages, and it's an easy way to plan meals when you think about what and how much should be on your plate. You can make variations and adjustments based on your budget, cultural traditions, lifestyle, and personal preferences regarding food. It is easier than counting calories or weighing and measuring your food when planning and preparing your healthy meals.

Here are some additional guidelines:

>> Limit alcohol. Recent studies argue that there are no health benefits to alcohol, so it's best not to consume it at all. However, if you do, the DGA recommends not more than one drink per day for women and two for men.

>> Limit added sugars to less than 10 percent of percent daily value (%DV).

>> Limit saturated fat to less than 10 percent of DV.

>> Limit sodium to less than 2,300 milligrams per day.

Planning Your Restaurant and Take-Out Meals

Eating in restaurants has always been a challenge, but these days, many restaurants are more willing to cater to individual food preferences or allergies. You can eat healthily in a restaurant, and I encourage you to tell the server exactly what you need. If you have allergies, it may be helpful to create a card listing allergens that affect you so you can hand it to the waitstaff or chef so that your needs are absolutely clear. My father had heart disease, and 20 or 30 years ago, he would drive the waitstaff crazy telling them exactly how he liked the food. He would bring his own condiments and low-fat cheese to his neighborhood restaurants so that he didn't have to rely on the limited available options.

TIP

Here are some of the things you can say to your server in a restaurant to make your meal healthier:

>> Please do not add any butter.

>> What kind of oil do you use?

>> Is there X (for example, garlic, sugar) in this dish?

>> Is the food fried?

>> Can I get this without the sauce?

>> Please put the salad dressing on the side.

>> Can you leave the cheese off the dish?

Here are some suggestions for choices you can make when you're eating in a restaurant or ordering takeout:

>> Choose grilled, steamed, or baked foods instead of fried.

>> Choose lean proteins such as chicken, turkey, fish, tofu, tempeh, or beans. All of these are good sources of protein and lower in fat and calories than other options including beef, deli meats, and fried foods.

>> If something comes with dressing or gravy, ask for these things on the side. Salad dressings, butter, sour cream, gravy, and sauces can be high in sugar, salt, and fats.

>> Choose whole grains instead of processed grains. Examples include brown rice, quinoa, or farro instead of white rice and whole wheat toast over white bread. Eating whole grains increases your fiber and nutrient intake.

>> Share dishes with your friends or dates. This helps to reduce the amount you eat and add variety to your experience.

>> Order smaller portions, such as appetizers or sides instead of a large main dish. This helps prevent overeating.

>> Look for the vegetable-heavy options on the menu. These will increase your intake of vitamins, minerals, and plant polyphenols.

>> Skip the complementary bread or chips. Both those things can add unwanted calories to your meal without offering much in the way of nutrition. If you want an appetizer and are with other people, share one to reduce your portion.

>> Skip or share desserts. A couple spoonfuls of chocolate mouse or one half of a cookie may satisfy your need for something sweet and spare you the calories from sugar and fats.

Here are some tips for eating healthily from a variety of cuisines:

>> American

- Pick the grilled options; turkey burgers; a baked potato instead of french fries; salads with grilled shrimp, chicken, or tofu; or house-roasted turkey sandwiches.

- Avoid fried foods, deli meat sandwiches, bacon, and cheesy creamy things such as macaroni and cheese.

>> Mediterranean

- Choose salads, grilled fish, hummus (not too much), whole wheat pita bread, quinoa, and roasted vegetables.

- Avoid fried foods, like falafel.

>> Italian

- Avoid fried dishes and cheesy and creamy dishes like chicken or eggplant parmigiana.

- When ordering vegetables, ask for them to be steamed rather than sautéed in olive oil.

- If you're having pizza, have one slice and a big salad. Too many slices will add up to too much cheese and too many calories.

>> Mexican

- Mexican food generally contains a lot of good ingredients, including beans and loads of vegetables.

- Avoid the cheesy dishes, such as enchiladas.

- Avoid sour cream and too many chips and guacamole.

- Good choices include grilled meats, fajitas, tacos, and burritos without added cheese.

>> Indian

- Indian food is often filled with vegetables and lentils, which are very heathy.

- Roti and other breads tend to be made from whole wheat and are pan fried, but you may want to limit the quantity you eat.

- Choose tandoori, which is grilled meats and dal (lentils) or chickpea-based curries.

- » French
    - Avoid rich sauces and buttery, creamy dishes.
    - Choose lean proteins and vegetable options.
    - French cuisine is known for omelets, which are a good option, as long as they're light on cheese.
- » Asian
    - Dishes are often filled with vegetables and can be healthy.
    - When you're eating at a Japanese restaurant, choose vegetable and sushi rolls, sashimi, salads, soups, or stir fries.
    - When you're eating at a Thai restaurant, focus on grilled meats or seafood and opt for curries with vegetables. Avoid dishes with coconut milk if possible.
    - When you're eating at a Chinese restaurant, avoid fried dishes and heavy sauces. Ask for steamed versions of the options.

REMEMBER

Eating out at restaurants doesn't mean that you have to stray from your healthy eating habits. Imagine the visual of the healthy plate and order similar foods and portion sizes. Always ask questions of the server and order the healthier choices on the menu. Moderation is key. If you have few choices, pick the best option or split a dish with your dinner partner.

Understanding Timing and Consistency of Supplements

Some supplements need to be taken daily, and others may not. Water-soluble vitamins need to be taken every day because what you do not absorb gets excreted in the urine. B vitamins and vitamin C fall into this category.

Fat-soluble vitamins can accumulate in your body fat, so you may not need supplements every day. For example, if you're deficient in vitamin D, you can take it every day — perhaps as much as 1,000 international units (IU). Or you can take a larger dose once a week. If you are vitamin D deficient, your doctor might prescribe as much as 50,000 IU per week.

You probably don't need a mineral supplement every day because you don't need large amounts of these to begin with. If you have a deficiency in a mineral, then you may need to take it every day. A common deficiency is iron in menstruating women, so that may be one situation where you need the supplement every day. Another example may be magnesium. You may use magnesium to help you sleep every night or for muscle cramping.

Protein, amino acid, or creatine supplements may need to be taken every day depending on why you are taking them. If you're an athlete or work out a lot, you may need to take them for muscle strength and building. If you're a vegan or vegetarian, you may need extra protein from a supplement.

If you have a medical condition such as Crohn's disease or celiac where you have a decreased absorption of nutrients or dietary limitations, you may need a supplement every day.

REMEMBER

No matter what vitamins and supplements you use, you should discuss with your healthcare provider.

Reviewing Intake Safety and Interaction Information

There are important guidelines for taking any supplements, so be sure to read the labels and do your research. The Supplement Facts panel on the packaging has information about the supplement active ingredients as well as other ingredients. Know what you are taking and the amounts. Always look for independent third-party certifications on the packaging to assure good quality, purity, and safety of your supplement.

In the remainder of this chapter, I talk about how to take supplements if you are also taking medications. Some supplements may interfere with the absorption or function of the medication. I also talk about how some medications may change your needs for supplements, the best timing for taking supplements, and how to be sure that you're getting enough.

Taking supplements with your medications

There are too many scenarios of supplements interfering with medications to address all of the possible interactions. If you're on a medication, always make sure to speak to your pharmacist or healthcare professional to find out if there are any interactions with a particular supplement or botanical.

The way in which each drug and various supplements interact may not always be well understood. Often the interaction affects the absorption or perhaps the metabolism of the medication, and that can result in reduced efficacy or side effects.

In this section, I offer some examples of medication and supplement interactions. In some of these cases, it may be helpful to take a supplement and in some cases it may not be. What I share isn't an exhaustive list, so make sure to check with your doctor.

>> **Statins:** Statins interfere with cholesterol synthesis in your cells, which is that same pathway that will lower CoQ10 synthesis. Deficiency in CoQ10 can affect energy level and cause muscle pain. Taking a CoQ10 supplement may be helpful.

>> **Metformin:** Can reduce the absorption of vitamins B9 and B12, leading to changes in metabolism. In addition, taking supplements of B9 and B12 can improve the response to metformin in type 2 diabetes.

>> **Proton pump inhibitors:** Proton pump inhibitors (or PPIs, such as Prilosec or omeprazole) are remedies for GERD and stomach ulcers. These can decrease absorption of vitamin B12 absorption and alter calcium and magnesium metabolism. The effect on calcium could be correlated with an increase in osteoporotic fractures. Taking supplements may help.

>> **Birth control pills:** According to the World Health Organization (WHO), several nutrients may be affected by birth control pills, including folate, B6, B12, C, magnesium, and zinc. It could be a good idea to take these vitamins or a multivitamin while taking birth control pills.

>> **Diuretics:** Diuretics such as Lasix and Bumex can cause a loss of magnesium. However, other types, such as spironolactone (for example, Carospir and Aldactone), increase potassium or magnesium. This may create an electrolyte imbalance that includes potassium, magnesium, and calcium.

If you're elderly or taking diuretics while having other health issues, consult your doctor about recommended supplements.

It is not recommended to take supplements on your own!

>> **Thyroid medications:** Medications like Synthroid or Armour Thyroid may not be absorbed as well or be as effective if you take a magnesium supplement.

>> **Antibiotics:** These can interfere with your gut bacteria and lower vitamin K. Magnesium and antibiotics can interact and bind together in the stomach, decreasing the effectiveness of both.

>> **Methotrexate:** Some people take this for rheumatoid arthritis, psoriasis, or as part of cancer treatment. A folate supplement may be recommended — 5 mg once a week on the day after you take your methotrexate. Taking it at

WARNING

the same time can stop the medication from working properly. You may need more folate during the week if you are still experiencing side effects.

- ❯❯ **Sulfonylureas:** The absorption of diabetes medications like Amaryl, Diabeta, and Glucotrol can increase if you also take magnesium, leading to blood sugar going too low. Also, these medications can cause a decrease in your body's natural magnesium, which over time could be a problem in a diabetic.

- ❯❯ **Calcium blockers:** Blood pressure medications like Norvasc, Calan, and Verelan may not be good to take with magnesium because it may also lower blood pressure. The combination may lower blood pressure too much.

- ❯❯ **Gabapentin:** This medication, which is for nerve pain and seizures, isn't absorbed as well when it's taken too close to a dose of magnesium. Consequently, effectiveness may be reduced. Taking them two hours apart will help.

Be aware that the following supplements can have undesirable interactions with some medications:

- ❯❯ **Zinc:** Zinc can bind to certain antibiotics, reducing their absorption and effectiveness.

- ❯❯ **Magnesium:** Magnesium can interfere with levodopa/carbidopa (medications used to treat Parkinson's disease), antibiotics, bisphosphates, high blood pressure medications, muscle relaxers, diuretics, anticoagulants, digoxin, diabetes medications, antacids, gabapentin, and ketamine.

- ❯❯ **Vitamin B6:** Vitamin B6 can increase breakdown of levodopa and decrease its effectiveness.

- ❯❯ **Vitamin D:** Chronic use of steroids can reduce calcium absorption and increase urinary excretion, leading to bone breakdown. If you're on steroids, your doctor will most likely recommend a calcium and vitamin D supplement (enhances calcium absorption and metabolism). Some studies show that vitamin K2 also helps protect bone loss with steroid use.

- ❯❯ **Selenium:** High selenium intake may reduce effectiveness of some cancer drugs, so speak with a doctor if you're in chemotherapy treatment and have been using selenium.

- ❯❯ **Vitamin A:** High doses of vitamin A can lead to toxicity when you take a supplement and are using retinoid medications.

- ❯❯ **Garlic:** Garlic has antiplatelet effects so it could increase risk of bleeding if you're also using an antiplatelet medication.

- ❯❯ **Vitamin C:** Vitamin C has the ability to neutralize free radicals, so high doses could interfere with certain chemotherapeutic agents. On the other hand, there are studies showing positive effects of intravenous vitamin C as a treatment or in combination with other medications on some cancers.

>> **Turmeric (curcumin):** Turmeric can increase risk of bleeding if you're taking antiplatelet or anticoagulant medications.

>> **Probiotics:** Probiotics may alter the effects of some immunosuppressants such as cyclosporine.

>> **Caffeine:** Caffeine is generally safe, but it may affect metabolism of antipsychotic medications such as clozapine.

>> **Coenzyme Q10:** CoQ10 may lower blood pressure, which can possibly increase effects of blood pressure medication, including beta blockers.

>> **Melatonin:** If you're taking melatonin to aid with sleep, do not take additional sleep drugs because there could be risk of excessive sedation.

>> **Calcium:** The absorption of thyroid medications can be decreased by calcium.

>> **St John's wort:** This supplement can interfere with selective serotonin reuptake inhibitor (SSRI) and monoamine oxidase inhibitor (MAOI) antidepressants. St. John's wort works by increasing serotonin levels, which can decrease the effectiveness of these drugs and lead to the accumulation of too much serotonin, a condition called serotonin syndrome. In fact, St. John's wort can also interfere with migraine medications, statins, digoxin, birth control pills, seizure medications, and many others.

>> **Vitamin E:** This vitamin can increase the risk of bleeding, so you should not take it with anticoagulants like Warfarin.

>> **Furanocoumarins:** These chemicals in grapefruit juice inhibit an enzyme (CYP3A4) in the liver and small intestines that metabolizes many drugs — as many as 80 — including certain statins, immunosuppressives, blood thinners, cancer drugs, opioids, and bone meds (Prolia).

Planning timing in relation to meals

Some supplements are better taken with food. Always check the supplement label for directions for use if you're unsure. Also talk to your healthcare professional about any special instructions, especially if they prescribed the supplement.

The supplements that should be taken with food are the fat-soluble vitamins (A, D, E, K) and any multivitamins, including prenatal vitamins. It's best if the food includes some fat because it will help with the absorption of these fat-soluble vitamins from the gut. CoQ10, fish oil, curcumin, and some other herbs (for example, Boswellia serrata extracts and CBD) are also fat soluble and best taken with foods. Magnesium, vitamin C, iron, or SAMe taken with food can reduce the risk of getting an upset stomach.

Water-soluble vitamins, including the B vitamins, do not need to be taken with foods. Vitamin C is an exception because sometimes it causes stomach upset, and taking with food can help avoid the issue. Vitamin B12 is a water-soluble vitamin, but it's better absorbed if taken in conjunction with a meal. It's also better absorbed if taken sublingually (under the tongue).

Getting the correct amount

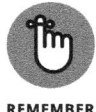

REMEMBER

Always read labels and understand the Recommended Dietary Allowance (RDA) before taking a supplement. Remember that the RDA is what you should be getting daily from *all your sources* of this nutrient. If, for example, you need 1,200 mg of calcium each day, then you can add up what you get from food. If it's an incomplete amount, add a calcium supplement to get to 1,200 mg.

If you take the Swiss cheese off your turkey sandwich, your calcium amount goes down by 221 mg. If you eat only one yogurt, then you lose about 111 mg. A supplement of about 300 mg of calcium would then give you 1,200 mg for the day.

DETERMINING NEED FOR A CALCIUM SUPPLEMENT

Here's an example of how to figure out whether you need a calcium supplement. Imagine you're having the following meals on a particular day:

- **Breakfast:** Two eggs, ¼ cup of cottage cheese, whole wheat toast, ½ cup of blueberries

- **Lunch:** Sandwich with three slices of turkey, one slice of Swiss cheese, lettuce, and tomato and an Apple

- **Dinner:** Baked salmon (7 ounces), brown rice, roasted broccoli, and carrots

- **Snacks:** Two cups low-fat plain yogurt and strawberries.

Using a calcium calculator (https://www.osteoporosis.foundation/educational-hub/topic/calcium-calculator) or an app such as MyFitnessPal, you can log your food and calculate total calcium. The preceding example is equal to 1,200 mg of calcium. Therefore, you would not need a supplement.

You can figure out your amount for any other nutrient in a similar way.

If you're a vegetarian, vegan, or have other dietary restrictions or preferences, you may have deficits of some nutrients. To determine if you are getting the nutrients you need from the foods that you eat, you can keep a food diary and do an assessment of your intake using an app. You can also look at the results of your annual blood test that measures some important vitamins and minerals and ask your doctor if anything is out of normal range. If you are not assessing your intake but feel like you may not be getting everything that you need, a multivitamin may help ensure that you are getting enough of essential vitamins and minerals.

Food tracker apps can help you plan your meals as well as determine your macro- and micronutrient intake. They all work similarly in that you must enter your foods so the app can calculate the nutrient information of the food you've consumed. The apps are basically calorie counters but with much more information available. Tracking may take some getting used to, but it gets easier with time. However, if calorie counting triggers you, it's best to not use it!

Some of the apps are free or have an option to upgrade to a paid premium version with more features. Others have a subscription fee to use them at all.

Some apps include the option to connect a device that measures activity, such as an Apple Watch or Fitbit. If you're trying to lose weight, this sometimes backfires because the calorie allowance will increase. It's very hard to exercise off any excess calories.

REMEMBER

You usually have to estimate your food intake, and most people tend to underestimate their food. When your exercise tracking device is attached or if you're estimating calories burned in some other way, those numbers tend to be overestimated. Combined, the underestimation of calories and overestimation of activity may lead to a miscalculation of how much food you should eat each day. Remember that these apps are a guide and need to be tweaked a bit when using.

Here are some of the free apps for food tracking. Check your devices app store for each of these options:

>> **MyFitnessPal:** Many of my clients use this one. It tracks macros and many micronutrients. You can set goals, create recipes to determine their nutrition facts, and create meal plans. It has more than 14 million verified foods in its database. You can share your diary with friends and attach your exercise device. If you pay for an account, there are many other benefits.

>> **Cronometer:** This app is packed with information to track your diet, exercise, and health data. It can track up to 84 nutrients or compounds. You can use it to set goals, create recipes, and more.

>> **Lose It!** This app includes a large database of foods — 50 million! It has a barcode scanner and photo capabilities, and it's simple to use. It's a great option if your goal is to lose weight.

>> **MyNetDiary:** This calorie counter lets you select a type of diet, such as keto, vegan, or low carb. You can set goals, it has a barcode scanner, and it gives you access to recipes.

>> **LifeSum:** This app offers expert advice on what and how much to eat based on your goals and lifestyle. The app asks in-depth questions to determine your protein, carb, and fat intake and offers advice on personalized eating habits. It also has a barcode scanner and nutritional information on millions of food items.

>> **MyPlate:** This weight-loss tracker is an excellent calorie counter with many of the features you need to track, analyze, and plan your diet. The MyPlate website (www.myplate.gov/myplate-plan) helps you create a plan to follow for weight control or weight loss. This website will help you figure out your daily caloric needs based on your height, weight, sex, and activity level. It also gives information about how much to eat to keep your weight stable or to lose if you need to.

Noom is another great app for tracking diet and lifestyle habits, especially if you're trying to reach weight-loss goals. It has many great features and also attempts to personalize the experience with daily messages and educational and motivational information. There is no free version, so you must pay for this app.

Two other subscription-based apps are Weight Watchers, which is very good and has a history of helping people lose weight based on a point system, and Ate Food Diary, which uses a photo-based food diary to help you easily track your intake.

Avoiding overdoses

Vitamins and minerals supplements are best for addressing deficiencies in nutrients. There is often no real advantage to taking more vitamins or minerals that are recommended. Most studies looking at advantages of supplements show that they work best when the subjects are deficient in that nutrient.

If you're taking a supplement, be sure to stick to one that is a dose equal to the RDA or daily value (the amount of a vitamin or nutrient that a person should get for optimum health) so that you don't suffer from side effects. Even some of the water-soluble vitamins can have side effects in large doses. Let your health professional know how much you're taking so that they can help keep you in a safe range.

Normal intake of fortified foods and a multivitamin is considered safe because most multivitamins consider that you will be getting some nutrients from your foods. There is a wide margin of safety when it comes to multivitamin products and fortified foods.

Americans often get too much of certain nutrients, including sugar, salt (sodium), and fats. These are nutrients to be aware of as you plan your meals because too much sugar and fat can lead to obesity and other chronic diseases.

TIP

Some vitamins and minerals have upper limits of what you should take, so pay attention to these values. In some cases, your doctor may recommend a high dose because you have a specific medical condition; otherwise, do not exceed the RDA.

Here are some of the side effects of taking too much of certain supplements:

>> **Vitamin D:** Adults who exceed 4,000 IU of vitamin D for a period of time may experience side effects. You cannot get too much D from sunlight and food, so it is only through additional supplements that you need to be careful not to get too much. Too much vitamin D can cause hypercalcemia, a buildup of calcium in your blood. This buildup can cause kidney issues. Early symptoms of hypercalcemia include loss of appetite, nausea, vomiting, diarrhea, and constipation. Over days or weeks, other symptoms might include excessive thirst, fatigue, pain, headaches, confusion, and irregular heartbeat.

>> **Vitamin A:** It's easy to get a lot of vitamin A from foods and supplements. Too much can cause drowsiness, irritability, nausea, and vomiting. In smokers, it may also cause an increased risk of lung cancer.

>> **Folic acid:** This nutrient is found in many enriched grain products and has helped reduce birth defects. However, having more than 1,000 micrograms (mcg) per day on a regular basis from supplements plus fortified foods might hide a vitamin B12 deficiency in older people. It can also cause bloating, loss of appetite, nausea, and vomiting.

>> **Calcium:** Too much calcium can result in hypercalcemia that can cause nausea, vomiting, confusion, itching, irregular heartbeat, or kidney issues.

>> **Iron:** After menopause, a woman's needs for iron are reduced to 8 mg per day. Too much iron can cause constipation, nausea, vomiting, stomach pain, and diarrhea. Overdoses can cause low blood pressure, liver failure, lung injury, and coma.

>> **Vitamin B3 or niacin:** This vitamin is sometimes taken in large doses to lower cholesterol. Too much can cause red, itchy skin, high blood pressure, stomach pain, and liver damage.

>> **Vitamin B6:** In high doses, vitamin B6 can cause irreversible nerve damage. Other side effects include ataxia, heartburn, nausea, and vomiting and sensitivity to light.

>> **Vitamin C:** In high doses for an extended period of time, vitamin C can contribute to kidney stones. Other side effects might include heartburn, diarrhea, headaches, nausea, or vomiting.

>> **Vitamin E:** You aren't likely to get too much vitamin E from food, but if you take a supplement and get too much, it can get be in your liver and tissues. This can affect blood clotting and cause hemorrhages.

>> **Zinc:** You need enough zinc to support cell processes, but if you get too much, you may experience nausea, vomiting, diarrhea, or stomach cramps.

WARNING

Always seek medical advice if you're taking supplements and experience side effects or unanticipated changes in how you feel. Other possible side effects could include changes in mood, appetite, or frequency in urination.

TIP

If you or someone in your home takes too much of a supplement and you need to talk to someone, you can reach the 24/7 poison control hotline at 1-800-222-1222.

Chapter **15**

Special Considerations for Various Life Stages

Supplements are important throughout life, and your needs depend on your age, sex, and lifestyle as well as according to your health situation, including whether you're pregnant or lactating. Getting what you need throughout the life changes from food plus supplements will help you stay healthy, prevent chronic diseases, and age well. A healthy lifestyle of good nutrition, exercise, work–life balance, and controlling stress supports metabolic health and determines any supplements you may need. It's difficult to discuss what supplements you may need without talking about food and nutrition.

In this chapter, I first cover general dietary guidelines and then talk about specific recommendations based on stages of life.

General Government Guidelines

The U.S. government offers several very good resources for information about dietary recommendations and vitamin and supplement intake. These guidelines include information on safety and efficacy of specific nutrients throughout a person's lifespan.

The best and most up-to-date resource for dietary recommendations throughout the lifespan is the Dietary Guidelines for Americans (DGA). This document is updated every five years with the latest scientific information on all the important nutrients you require, how to get them primarily from foods, and when it might be important to supplement for health and to prevent chronic diseases. It is jointly created by the U.S. Department of Agriculture (USDA) and the Department of Health and Human Services (HSS) with the guidance of a team of nutrition scientists. Outside peers in the fields of nutrition and medicine review the guidelines. The DGA is also used to create federal nutrition and food programs and to develop educational materials for the public. You can find the guidelines at www.dietaryguidelines.gov.

In addition, the National Institutes for Health (NIH) Office of Dietary Supplements (ODS) provides information about every nutrient and supplement you can imagine. It is an evidence-based source for most of what you need to know, including safety and efficacy throughout the lifespan. The fact sheets for the different dietary supplements are located at https://ods.od.nih.gov/factsheets/list-all.

The U.S. Food and Drug Administration (FDA) is one of the organizations within HHS. The FDA is responsible for regulating dietary supplement products and dietary ingredients. The set of regulations fall under the umbrella of the Dietary Supplement Health and Education Act of 1994 (DSHEA). Manufacturers and distributors of supplements are responsible for assuring the quality and safety and proper labeling of their products according to government standards and regulations. The FDA has the authority to act against any misbranded or adulterated dietary supplement after it is already on the market.

The FDA maintains a Dietary Supplement Ingredient Directory, where you can look up ingredients used in supplement products to see what the FDA reports about it. This website is also the place to look to find out whether any actions have been taken regarding the ingredient. You can find this directory at www.fda.gov/food/dietary-supplements/information-select-dietary-supplement-ingredients-and-other-substances.

Here are some other useful government sites that provide information about nutrition, vitamins, and supplements:

>> **The Centers for Disease Control and Protection (CDC):** Provides information on micronutrients (www.cdc.gov/nutrition/features/micronutrient-facts.html?CDC_AAref_Val=https://www.cdc.gov/nutrition/micronutrient-malnutrition/micronutrients/index.html), nutrition, and much more health information

>> **The National Center for Complementary and Integrative Health (NCCIH):** is one of the 27 institutes of the NIH that has a searchable list of herbs and supplements (www.nccih.nih.gov/health/herbsataglance) where you can look up herbs, their uses, and potential side effects

>> The **U.S. Preventive Services Task Force (USPSTF):** Has a searchable database of published recommendations from a volunteer panel of national experts

>> **NIH Dietary Reference Intakes (DRI):** An authoritative source on the relationship between the food you eat and nutrition and health that's issued by the Food and Nutrition Board of the National Academies

WHAT ARE THE DIETARY REFERENCE INTAKES

DRI is the overall term for the reference nutrient values used to plan and assess nutrient intakes of healthy people. The DRI vary by age and sex. The four subcategories of the DRI are the following:

- **RDA:** The RDA are what you may think of when you try to get your daily nutrients. This is the average daily amount that is sufficient to meet the nutrient requirement of most (97 percent to 98 percent) healthy individuals.

- **Adequate Intake (AI):** This is the amount of a nutrient you need to be sure to meet a level that will provide you with enough of that nutrient. It's used for those nutrients when there isn't enough evidence to develop an RDA.

- **Estimated Average Requirement (EAR):** This is the average daily intake that is estimated to meet the requirements of half of healthy individuals. This can be used to assess the nutrient intake of individuals or groups and to plan diets.

- **Tolerable Upper Intake Level (UL):** This is the maximum daily intake that you should take of a nutrient to avoid negative health effects.

Dietary Guidelines for Specific Groups

The DGA is published by the USDA and the HHS and are updated every five years. The information provided at the time of this writing is up to date. Most of the recommendations will remain the same from one version to another, with some updates based on new scientific information. These guidelines are interesting to read as a consumer, but they're mostly meant as guidelines for federal nutrition policies, educational programs, and government programs like the school lunch programs. The DGA is a large document that provides science-based information on diet and nutrition that promotes health and can reduce the risk of chronic diseases.

REMEMBER

Some of the basic guidelines for healthy eating were created to be sure that you get your important macro and micronutrients from food. Here are some key takeaways from the DGA:

>> Follow a healthy diet at each stage of life.

>> Choose nutrient-dense food and drinks according to your preferences, traditions, and budget.

>> Choose foods from all the food groups — fruits, vegetables, grains, dairy, and protein.

>> Stay within reasonable calorie limits depending on your weight, height, age, and activity level.

>> Limit foods and drinks high in added sugars to no more than 10 percent of your daily calories.

>> For people aged two and older, limit saturated fats to less than 10 percent of daily calories.

>> Adults should limit sodium to less than 2,300 milligrams per day.

>> Limit alcohol to maximum of one drink per day for women and two drinks for men. Recent studies suggest that there are no health benefits to alcohol intake and that it is better to avoid altogether.

>> Always encourage healthy eating in infants and toddlers and avoid added sugar for those under two years old.

>> Incorporate a variety of proteins including seafood, lean meat, poultry, eggs, legumes, nuts, seeds, and soy.

- » Make your grains whole grains when possible. The DGA suggests making half of your grains whole grains to increase fiber and nutrients. Often grains are fortified, which is helpful for getting essential vitamins and iron.

- » Drink and eat low-fat or fat-free dairy products including milk, yogurt, and cheese or fortified soy milk.

- » Opt for good fats like oils rich in unsaturated fats such as olive or canola oils instead of solid fats (at room temperature) like butter or lard.

- » Limit red meat and processed meats because they contain saturated fats and are correlated with risk of some chronic diseases.

- » Select foods with healthy fats, such as avocados, nuts, and fish. Limit trans fats.

- » Watch your portion sizes to prevent overeating and manage caloric intake.

- » Stay away from sugary drinks. Choose water, seltzer, unsweetened tea, and coffee.

Recommendations for infants and toddlers

It is recommended that for about the first six months of life, infants be exclusively fed breast milk, if possible. The idea behind this is that breast milk has all the necessary nutrients (except possibly vitamin D and iron), bioactive substances, and immunity that supports health, growth, and development. This also protects the gut and helps support the microbiota and gut lining.

If breastfeeding isn't possible, an FDA-approved iron-fortified formula is a good substitute.

The American Academy of Pediatrics (AAP) recommends that all infants get 400 IU of vitamin D daily. Breastfed infants may need a supplement. Nonbreastfed infants and children who don't get enough sunlight or vitamin D–fortified foods may also need a supplement. Over a year of age, children need 600 IU of vitamin D daily.

At about six months of age, infants are introduced to nutrient-dense foods. This is when they are also introduced to potentially allergenic foods to determine whether they have a reaction. Infants and toddlers should be encouraged to eat a variety of foods and textures from all food groups. It is particularly important to be sure that they get foods rich in iron and zinc, especially if they are getting breast milk.

TIP

Here are some additional recommendations:

>> Avoid foods and drinks with any added sugar and do not offer honey before a child is one year old.

>> Limit sodium intake.

>> When weaning from breast milk or formula, follow a healthy diet, including

- Vegetables and fruits with potassium, vitamin A, and vitamin C

- Meat, poultry, eggs, seafood, nuts, and seeds for protein, iron, zinc, good, and fats

- Beans and lentils for protein and fiber

- Yogurt and cheese for protein, calcium and D

- Grains and iron-fortified infant cereal

- Small amounts of fluoridated water

WARNING

Cow's milk or nut milks including soy should not be introduced until after 12 months of age. At that time, whole cow's milk helps meet calcium, potassium, vitamin D, and protein requirements. Juice is not necessary.

TIP

The American Academy of Pediatrics (AAP) recommends that children who eat a balanced diet do not need additional supplements unless they are premature, breastfed, or have a health condition.

Your pediatrician may suggest an iron supplement for breastfed infants between the ages of four and six months.

Table 15-1 gives the current RDA and AI for carbohydrates, fats, proteins, vitamins, and minerals for infants and toddlers.

Recommendations for children and adolescents

Recommendations for children and adolescents between the ages of 2 and 18 have the primary goals of promoting healthy growth and development and creating healthy long-term habits. Another goal is to prevent obesity and chronic diseases, which are on the rise in children. A good dietary pattern and lifestyle is similar for this group as it is for every age group. This includes a variety of nutrient–dense foods along with regular physical activity and limiting screen time.

TABLE 15-1 **RDA and AI for Infants and Toddlers**

Nutrient	0 – 6 months	7 – 12 months	1 – 3 years
Macronutrients			
Carbohydrates (g/day)	60 (AI)	95 (AI)	130 (RDA)
Protein (g/day)	9.1 (AI)	11 (RDA)	13 (RDA)
Total fat (% of daily kcal)	31 (AI)	30 (AI)	30% – 40% (AMDR*)
Fiber (g/day)	No AI/RDA	No AI/RDA	19 (AI)
Micronutrients			
Calcium (mg/day)	200 (AI)	260 (AI)	700 (RDA)
Iron (mg/day)	0.27 (AI)	11 (RDA)	7 (RDA)
Zinc (mg/day)	2 (AI)	3 (RDA)	3 (RDA)
Vitamin A (mcg/day)	400 (AI)	500 (RDA)	300 (RDA)
Vitamin C (mg/day)	40 (AI)	50 (RDA)	15 (RDA)
Vitamin D (mcg/day)	10 (AI)	10 (AI)	15 (RDA)
Vitamin E (mg/day)	4 (AI)	5 (RDA)	6 (RDA)

* Acceptable Macronutrient Distribution Range

TIP

Healthy foods should include the following:

>> Fruits and vegetables

>> Whole grains

>> Lean proteins (chicken, fish, beans, and eggs)

>> Low-fat dairy

>> Limited added sugar — less than 10 percent of daily calorie intake

The RDA for macronutrients and micronutrients varies according to age and sex. Most children and adolescents can theoretically get all of their nutrients from food. However, many children and teens do not eat well or sufficient amounts. Sometimes they may eat too much, but not enough nutritious food, which may mean they're overfed but undernourished. If a child is not getting the RDA for essential nutrients, then a supplement is needed to meet these goals.

Table 15-2 includes the RDA for macronutrients and essential vitamins and minerals for children and adolescents.

TABLE 15-2 Macronutrient and Micronutrient RDA for Children and Adolescents

Nutrient	1 – 3 years	4 – 8 years	9 – 13 years	14 – 18 years
Macronutrients				
Carbohydrates (g/day)	130	130	130	130
Protein (g/day)	13	19	34	52 (M)/46 (F)
Total fat (% of daily kcal)	30% – 40%	25% – 35%	25% – 35%	25% – 35%
Fiber (g/day)	19	25	26 (F)/31 (M)	26 (F)/38 (M)
Micronutrients				
Calcium (mg/day)	700	1,000	1,300	1,300
Iron (mg/day)	7	10	8	11 (M)/15 (F)
Zinc (mg/day)	3	5	8	11 (M)/9 (F)
Vitamin A (mcg/day)	300	400	600	900 (M)/700 (F)
Vitamin C (mg/day)	15	25	45	75 (M)/65 (F)
Vitamin D (mcg/day)	15	15	15	15
Vitamin E (mg/day)	6	7	11	15
Folate (mcg/day)	150	200	300	400
Magnesium (mg/day)	80	130	240	410 (M)/360 (F)
Phosphorus (mg/day)	460	500	1,250	1,250
Potassium (mg/day)	3,000	3,800	4,500	4,700
Sodium (mg/day)	1,200	1,500	1,800	2,300

Recommendations for adults

The focus for adults aged 19 to 59 is to maintain good health and do your best to prevent chronic diseases that are prevalent in the United States, including obesity, hypertension, heart disease, diabetes, cancer, neurodegenerative diseases, and stroke. Specific recommendations are to follow one of the three recommended dietary patterns: Healthy U.S.-Style (HUSS), Mediterranean, or vegetarian. Each of these dietary patterns will help you to prioritize fruits, vegetables, whole grains, and lean proteins. To these, you want to add some — but not too much — healthy fats such as olive oil, avocados, and nuts. Be sure to limit added sugar to less than 10 percent of your calories each day. Also keep sodium to less than 2,300 mg/day. Lastly, saturated fats should be kept low at less than 10 percent of your daily calories.

TIP

The word *diet* can have two different meanings depending on how it is used. Most people may think of a diet as a temporary, restrictive eating plan used to lose weight or address another situation. *Dietary pattern* refers to a broader and long-term way of eating to support health and wellness.

If you eat the right amount of food and choose variety from all the food groups, you may not need supplements. If, however, you eat too little, too much, too much fast food, or otherwise do not get the RDA for vitamins and minerals, you may need supplement help! Table 15-3 gives the recommended macronutrients and micronutrients for adults between the ages of 19 and 59.

It is generally recommended that adults older than 50 may need a multivitamin. I always recommend this in my practice for a few reasons. First, if you're older than 50, you may eat less and may not be getting everything you need from your food. Second, your absorption of some micronutrients may decrease. Third, if you're taking medications, you may need more of a nutrient — for example, using a statin may increase your need for CoQ10. Lastly, if you have specific dietary restraints or preferences and have to exclude certain foods from your diet, you may need supplements.

TABLE 15-3   **Macronutrient RDA for Adults (19–59 years)**

	Males	Females
Macronutrient		
Energy (kcal/day)	2,400 – 3,000	1,800 – 2,400
Protein (g/day)	56	46
Carbohydrates (g/day)	130	130
Total fat (% of total kcal)	20% – 35%	20% – 35%
Fiber (g/day)	38	25
Micronutrient		
Vitamin A (mcg/day)	900	700
Vitamin C (mg/day)	90	75
Vitamin D (mcg/day)	15	15
Vitamin E (mg/day)	15	15
Vitamin K (mcg/day)	120	90
Calcium (mg/day)	1,000	1,000 (1,200 for ages 51 – 59)

(continued)

TABLE 15-3 *(continued)*

	Males	Females
Iron (mg/day)	8	18 (8 for ages 51 – 59)
Zinc (mg/day)	11	8
Magnesium (mg/day)	400 – 420	310 – 320
Folate (mcg/day)	400	400
Potassium (mg/day)	3,400	2,600
Sodium (mg/day)	2,300 UL	2,300 UL

There are some vitamins in particular to pay attention to in this age group, especially if you have special dietary patterns or health issues. The following list includes vitamins and mineral supplements that may be helpful for adults:

>> **Multivitamins:** A multivitamin can help to fill in any gaps in nutrition from your food. This is recommended especially for people older than 50 or if your dietary intake isn't balanced.

>> **Vitamin D:** Many Americans are deficient in vitamin D, which supports bone health, immunity, calcium, and mood regulation. If you don't get enough sun exposure or live in a northern climate (particularly in the winter), you may need a supplement. Your doctor can test you for vitamin D and let you know if you need a supplement.

>> **Omega-3 fatty acids:** EPA and DHA, which usually come from fish oil or algal oil supplements, support heart health, reduce inflammation, and can aid neurological and brain function. If you eat fatty fish two to three times a week, then you may not need supplements of omega-3.

>> **Vitamin B12:** If you're a vegetarian, vegan, or older person, have had weight-loss surgery, or have other absorption issues, you may need vitamin B12 supplements.

>> **Magnesium:** This electrolyte is essential for over 300 biochemical reactions and important for muscle and nerve function, energy, and bone health. If you have muscle pain or fatigue or sleep issues, a magnesium supplement could help.

>> **Probiotics:** Healthy gut bacteria are correlated with positive health outcomes, including mental health, digestion, skin health, and immunity. Eating fermented foods (yogurt and kimchi), fruits, vegetables, and whole grains provides prebiotics for a healthy gut. Adding a probiotic can help with general gut health and if you have gastrointestinal (GI) issues such as irritable bowel syndrome (IBS).

- >> **Vitamin C:** This antioxidant can help with immunity, skin, and wound repair. If you eat fruit and vegetables, you may get enough. If you have a cold or other virus, extra vitamin C may reduce the severity of your illness.

- >> **Zinc:** Zinc is important for immunity and wound healing. Vegans and vegetarians or people with GI disorders may need more zinc.

- >> **Iron:** Iron is essential for producing hemoglobin, and a deficiency can cause immune issues. Menstruating women, vegetarians (and other people who don't eat red meat), and athletes or others who are very active may need extra iron.

- >> **Calcium:** Calcium is important to build strong bones throughout life. If you don't eat dairy, you may need extra calcium.

- >> **Coenzyme Q10:** Levels of CoQ10 decrease with age, and it's important for energy production and as an antioxidant. Also, if you take statins, you may need this supplement.

- >> **Fiber supplements:** Fiber is important for GI health and helps to control blood cholesterol and sugar levels. If you don't get enough fiber from fruits, vegetables, and whole grains, you may experience constipation. You can get more from supplements of psyllium fiber, a plant-based fiber.

Recommendations while pregnant and nursing

While a woman is pregnant and nursing, eating well and using supplements is key for the health of both the parent and baby. Nutrient needs increase when a person is pregnant. If you're pregnant or trying to get pregnant, you should take a prenatal vitamin to be sure that you have all the vitamins and minerals needed, especially folic acid.

REMEMBER

Folic acid is important at the very beginning of pregnancy to prevent neural tube defect and spina bifida. The CDC and other organizations recommend that "women capable of becoming pregnant get 400 mcg of folic acid daily" (www.cdc.gov/folic-acid). It is often recommended that you be sure to get enough folic acid at least one month before getting pregnant. These vitamins are sometimes prescribed by a doctor, but they're also available over the counter.

TECHNICAL STUFF

The macronutrient needs — calories from carbohydrates, fats, and protein — change during pregnancy and are best fulfilled by eating more food. Caloric needs stay the same as prepregnancy levels during the first trimester. But in the second and third trimesters, energy needs increase as the fetus grows. How many calories a person needs while pregnant depends on where they start. The increase is 340 kcal/day more than the usual intake during the second trimester and an extra 450 kcal/day during the third trimester.

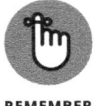

REMEMBER

If you are overweight or obese, you want to avoid gaining excess weight during your pregnancy. Therefore, you may need only a modest increase in calories during the second or third trimester. Too much weight gain can increase risks of gestational diabetes, high blood pressure, and preeclampsia.

Protein needs increase from about 50 grams/day to 71 grams/day. Fat intake doesn't need to increase, but you should focus on increasing the amount of omega-3 fatty acids for fetal eye and brain development.

While breastfeeding your baby during the first six months, your caloric needs go up by about 330 kcal/day. After six months, it takes more energy to produce more milk synthesis for your growing infant, so add about 400 kcal/day to your intake.

The keys to supporting maternal health and development of the fetus or infant are summarized in Table 15-4. Specific nutrient needs that increase are folate, calcium, iron, iodine, choline, and omega-3s. Taking a prenatal vitamin and focusing on nutrient-dense foods are essential. Other tips include

>> Eat fish and seafood two to three times a week to get enough DHA but avoid high-mercury fish (like tuna) and raw fish.

>> Limit caffeine.

>> Do not drink alcohol.

>> Stay hydrated and consume extra calories as needed.

>> Work closely with your healthcare provider to develop a nutrition and supplement plan.

TABLE 15-4   **Macronutrient RDA while Pregnant and Nursing**

	Pregnancy	Lactation
Macronutrient		
Calories (kcal/day)	+340 kcal (second trimester) +452 kcal (third trimester)	+330 kcal (first six months) +400 kcal (after six months)
Protein (g/day)	71	71
Carbohydrates (g/day)	175	210
Fiber (g/day)	28	29
Total fat (% of total kcal)	20% – 35%	20% – 35%

	Pregnancy	Lactation
Linoleic acid (g/day)	13	13
Alpha-linolenic acid (g/day)	1.4	1.3
Micronutrient		
Vitamin A (mcg/day)	770	1,300
Vitamin C (mg/day)	85	120
Vitamin D (mcg/day)	15 (600 IU)	15 (600 IU)
Vitamin E (mg/day)	15	19
Vitamin K (mcg/day)	90	90
Thiamin (B1) (mg/day)	1.4	1.4
Riboflavin (B2) (mg/day)	1.4	1.6
Niacin (B3) (mg/day)	18	17
Vitamin B6 (mg/day)	1.9	2.0
Folate (mcg/day)	600	500
Vitamin B12 (mcg/day)	2.6	2.8
Pantothenic Acid (mg/day)	6	7
Biotin (mcg/day)	30	35
Choline (mg/day)	450	550
Calcium (mg/day)	1,000 (1,300 if <18 years)	1,000 (1,300 if <18 years)
Iron (mg/day)	27	9
Magnesium (mg/day)	350	310
Phosphorus (mg/day)	700	700
Potassium (mg/day)	2,900	2,800
Sodium (mg/day)	1,500	1,500
Zinc (mg/day)	11	12
Iodine (mcg/day)	220	290
Selenium (mcg/day)	60	70

If you're on any medications and become pregnant, it's important to discuss your pregnancy with your doctor as soon as possible. If you have had weight-loss surgery, you may have additional requirements because you may be absorbing fewer nutrients or eating less food and getting less from your diet than needed. If you are on weight-loss medications or are pregnant or trying to get pregnant, discuss what additional supplements might be important for you to take.

Specific nutrients and their functions to be aware of include

>> **Folic acid:** This nutrient is essential for development of the neural tube, which becomes the baby's spinal cord and brain. Getting enough folic acid prevents neural tube defects such as spina bifida. You can get folic acid from fortified cereals, leafy greens, citrus, and beans.

>> **Iron:** Iron is critical to produce hemoglobin. Pregnancy increases your blood volume, and you need more hemoglobin, which binds oxygen in the blood. Most iron will probably come from foods that contain iron, including meat, fish, poultry, lentils, beans, and iron-fortified cereals or grains.

>> **Calcium:** Calcium is important for bone health in both the parent and the baby. Calcium is found in dairy, fortified plant milks, leafy greens, and fortified foods.

>> **Vitamin D:** This vitamin helps with calcium absorption and immune function. You get vitamin D from sunlight, fatty fish, and fortified foods. It isn't always easy to get enough from foods, though, so supplements are important. In addition, people who are overweight or obese may need higher doses of vitamin D.

>> **Omega-3 fatty acids:** DHA and EPA are important for the mother's health and for the baby's brain and eye development. The best sources are salmon, mackerel, sardines, seaweed, algae (spirulina), chia seeds, flaxseeds, hemp seeds, walnuts, canola oil, and supplements.

>> **Iodine:** Iodine is necessary for synthesizing thyroid hormones, which are essential for metabolism and brain development. Iodized salt is a good source, but iodine also comes from seaweed, dairy, seafood, and eggs.

>> **Vitamin B12:** This vitamin is essential for red blood cell production and the baby's nervous system. Good sources are meat, dairy, and eggs. Vegetarians need to supplement vitamin B12.

>> **Vitamin A:** Vitamin A is important for fetal growth, eyes, skin, and immunity. Great sources are liver, sweet potatoes, carrots, and dark leafy greens.

>> **Magnesium:** This electrolyte is important for muscles and bones and regulating blood sugar. The best sources are from nuts, seeds, whole grains, and leafy greens.

>> **Zinc:** This mineral supports immunity and cellular growth. The best sources are meat, shellfish, legumes, seeds, and nuts.

Recommendations for older adults

As you get older than 60, some things happen that change your needs and intake. For example, you may eat less and therefore not get enough of some nutrients. Your blood B12 levels may decline with age because less may be absorbed from your diet. Women's iron needs change once they stop menstruating. You also may lose muscle mass, so it's important to eat enough protein and exercise to maintain muscle.

The goal as you age is to stay healthy and prevent chronic disease, stay strong, and ultimately maintain your independence. DGA recommendations for meeting this goal include these:

>> Increase your fiber intake to support digestion and heart health.

>> Get adequate calcium and vitamin D because of increased needs due to higher osteoporosis risk.

>> Many older adults should aim for less than 2,300 mg/day of sodium.

>> Prioritize protein-rich foods (animal and plant-based) to maintain muscle mass and prevent frailty.

>> Stay hydrated and maintain a healthy sodium intake to manage blood pressure.

>> Maintain a healthy weight.

>> Stay physically active and work on balance to reduce fall risk.

Table 15-5 shows the recommended amounts of macronutrients and micronutrients for older adults.

TABLE 15-5 RDA for Adults (60+ years)

	Males (60+)	Females (60+)
Macronutrient		
Energy (kcal/day)	2,000 – 2,600	1,600 – 2,000
Protein (g/day)	56 – 75*	46 – 75*
Carbohydrates (g/day)	130	130
Total fat (% of total kcal)	20% – 35%	20% – 35%
Fiber (g/day)	30	21
Micronutrient		
Vitamin A (mcg)	900	700
Vitamin C (mg)	90	75
Vitamin D (mcg)	20 (increases from 15 for better bone health)	20 (same increase)
Vitamin E (mg)	15	15
Vitamin K (mcg)	120	90
Calcium (mg)	1,200 (increases for bone health)	1,200
Iron (mg)	8	8
Zinc (mg)	11	8
Magnesium (mg)	420	320
Folate (mcg)	400	400
Potassium (mg)	3,400	2,600
Sodium (mg)	2,300 UL (ideally lower for heart health)	2,300 UL
Vitamin B12 (mcg)	2.4 (emphasis on fortified foods or supplements due to reduced absorption with age)	2.4

* Some studies suggest higher protein intake (1.0 – 1.2 g/kg body weight) for muscle maintenance and prevention of sarcopenia in older adults.

TIP

If you're older than 60, consider these supplements:

>> **Vitamin D:** You need this to help absorb calcium and support immune function and muscle strength.

>> **Calcium:** Take calcium to keep bones strong and prevent osteoporosis.

>> **Vitamin B12:** This vitamin is necessary for energy, red blood cell formation, and neurological health.

>> **Omega–3 fatty acids:** A fish oil supplement supports heart health, joints, cognitive function, and reducing inflammation.

>> **Magnesium:** This electrolyte supports overall metabolism including muscles, nerves, bones, and energy.

>> **Probiotics:** Probiotics support gut health.

>> **Vitamin C:** This vitamin is known for its antioxidant ability, collagen production, and immune support.

>> **Vitamin K2:** K2 regulates calcium distribution and supports bone and cardiovascular health.

>> **Zinc:** Absorption of zinc may decrease with age, which can increase risk of infection and slow wound healing.

>> **Coenzyme Q10:** Cellular CoQ10 decreases with age, which can lead to fatigue, muscle weakness, and increase risk of heart disease. Also, if you take statins, you may need a CoQ10 supplement.

REMEMBER

It is always important to eat a balanced diet and try to get nutrients from foods when possible. If you choose to take supplements, check with your healthcare provider to be sure that you are taking the right product, the best dose, and that there are no interactions with your medications. And remember that supplements are not meant to treat disease.

5

The Part of Tens

Chapter **16**

Ten Myths about Vitamins and Supplements

The ten top myths about supplements in this chapter are the most common. However, this list is limited to myths about vitamin and mineral supplements. I only touch on all the myths about herbal, amino acid, protein, and other supplements available everywhere. The marketing material involved in the $177 billion global supplement industry is large and daunting. Companies often quote their own studies as evidence that something works. Some companies don't even attempt to show evidence that a product is good for you. It can be overwhelming, but at least the ten myths about vitamin and mineral supplements give you a place to start!

B12 and Other Vitamins Will Give You Energy

B12, also known as cobalamin, is an essential vitamin for red blood cell formation, cell metabolism, nerve function, and the production of DNA. Specifically, B12 and other B vitamins catalyze enzymatic reactions that convert food to glucose, which provides your body with energy. For this reason, a deficiency in B12 can result in fatigue, low blood pressure, muscle weakness, stiffness, spasticity, shakiness, and, most seriously, megaloblastic anemia. This type of anemia reduces the number of red blood cells and the amount of oxygen in circulation around the body.

A simple blood test can tell you if your B12 level is normal. If it is normal, taking a B12 supplement will not have any effect on your energy level. As you age, the absorption of B12 from the stomach decreases, and many people need to take a supplement to alleviate a deficiency. Other reasons for deficiencies where you may need a supplement are celiac, bowel diseases, following a vegan diet, taking certain medications (including some antacids or chemotherapy), and having HIV. In these cases, supplements and sometimes injections of B12 can improve energy levels.

Other vitamins and minerals are also important at the molecular and cellular levels related to energy, fatigue, and cognition. Those include the other B vitamins, vitamin C, iron, magnesium, and zinc. These have a critical role in cellular energy production, oxygen transport in the blood, brain cell structure and function, and nervous system function.

WARNING

When levels of any of these vitamins and minerals are below what your body needs, there is an increased chance you may experience physical and mental fatigue. Be sure to get enough of these through food and supplements along with enough calories (which also provide energy). If you get enough, taking more will not make a noticeable difference!

TIP

If your B12 or other B vitamin levels are normal, additional supplements will not give you extra energy. The excess over normal levels will be excreted in the urine.

Everyone Needs Supplements

More than half of Americans take one or more dietary supplements daily or on occasion, and the reasons vary. Whether you need a supplement depends on your food choices and intake, your health status, your stage of life, and perhaps your lifestyle or where you live. Therefore, no one answer applies to everyone!

TIP

If you eat a well-balanced diet with a variety of foods and are healthy, then you may get everything you need from your daily intake, in which case, you don't need any extra vitamins or minerals. It is always best to get your nutrients from foods because foods contain other healthy things like fiber and water.

There are times when dietary restrictions or health conditions make supplements important. For example, being pregnant means you need more folic acid and iron than what you get from your diet. In this case, you'll be prescribed prenatal vitamins to avoid deficiencies. Aging adults, who may eat less or absorb nutrients less efficiently, may need a multivitamin (usually recommended over 50 years old). If you don't see the sun much and your vitamin D is low, you need a vitamin D supplement. Breastfed babies also need vitamin D.

There are times when a multivitamin is a good "insurance policy" for getting vitamins and minerals that you need to keep your metabolism happy and at its peak performance. Most adults get a blood test during their yearly physical. Some important nutrition-related measures include a lipid panel, blood glucose and HbA1C, and checks on levels of iron, calcium, magnesium, phosphorous, 25-hydroxyvitamin D, B6, and B12. If the levels are low, the recommendation is often to eat more foods high in these nutrients or to take a supplement.

TIP

People who are pregnant or nursing will be prescribed a prenatal vitamin. People older than 50 need to be sure to get recommended amounts of B12 because absorption goes down with age. And if you're 50 or older, taking a multivitamin may help improve cognitive function, memory, and related mental skills. Other medical conditions may be reason to take a multivitamin. Be sure to consult with your healthcare provider.

WARNING

Supplements include vitamins, minerals, and botanicals, some of which may have side effects in high doses or in someone with certain medical conditions or treatments. Before taking supplements, you should check with your healthcare provider to be sure there are no interactions with your current medications.

More Is Better

According to the FDA, more than half of Americans take dietary supplements. Most vitamins and minerals have tolerable upper limits (UL), which should be taken very seriously. Going over the UL can cause side effects or toxicity. The fat-soluble vitamins A, D, E, and K are stored in your body fat and can accumulate. For example, too much vitamin D can trigger extra calcium absorption and lead to kidney stones, muscle or abdominal pain, or mood disorders. Excess calcium may enhance the risk of heart disease and stroke.

t's true that B vitamins are water soluble, and there are no upper tolerable limits (ULs) for *most* of them. Because excess of these vitamins is excreted in the urine, they don't accumulate in the body. However, niacin and B6 have ULs, and there are side effects of taking too much. Choline, which is neither a vitamin nor a mineral but is often lumped in with the B-complex supplements, can also cause side effects in large amounts. Side effects from excess niacin, B6, and choline can cause some people diarrhea, gas, and nausea. Other more serious effects include blurry vision, vomiting, numbness, high blood sugar, liver issues, and skin issues.

Vitamin C and Zinc Prevent Sickness

Numerous studies have shown that vitamin C and zinc are important for innate immunity because they're part of the cellular mechanisms involved in fighting infection. Deficiencies in vitamin C and zinc can reduce immunity and make you more vulnerable to viral infection. In addition, exposure to some viruses such as flu and COVID can increase demand for these nutrients. Getting enough vitamin C and zinc from foods will support your immune system to fight off some illness such as viral infections.

But what about taking excess vitamin C and zinc? Recent randomized controlled studies of people with COVID showed no difference in the length or severity of symptoms with intake of vitamin C and zinc. Other studies show no prevention of illness with supplementation of C and zinc; however, there is some evidence that C may reduce the severity of some viral diseases like colds and flu.

Dietary Supplements Are Not FDA Regulated

The Food and Drug Administration (FDA) regulates supplements under the Dietary Supplement Health and Education Act of 1994 (DSHEA). This is a different set of laws than for conventional foods and drugs. There are requirements set by the Federal Food, Drug, and Cosmetic Act as amended by DSHEA that manufacturers are responsible for the quality and quantity of the ingredients in their products and the safety and labeling to meet the government guidelines. Once these products reach the public, the FDA can act against any adulterated or misbranded dietary supplement.

There are third-party certifiers that test supplement products. These are NSF International (NSF), USP (United States Pharmacopeia), and ConsumerLab. They analyze products for their contents to verify that they match their labels — that the supplement is indeed what it says on the label and that the amounts are correct. See Chapter 4 for more information on this.

Supplements Aren't Necessary If You Eat a Healthy Diet

If you eat a variety of fruits, vegetables, whole grains, lean protein, some dairy, and healthy oils, chances are good that you're getting the nutrients you need from your food intake. However, there are situations and conditions when you may need to supplement your dietary intake with more nutrients. The best way to get nutrients from foods is to use fresh or frozen foods, store them correctly, cook them in ways that preserve the nutrients, and pair foods for maximum absorption.

Vegans and vegetarians can't get everything from their food sources and need supplements of essential nutrients, such as B12 and DHA (docosahexaenoic acid), which is an essential omega-3 fatty acid. There are other nutrients that may not be essential (because they can be made in cells), but they've been found to be low when measured in vegans and vegetarians. These nutrients include creatinine, carnosine, iron, and taurine. Supplements for these nutrients may be recommended.

There are other situations where you may not get everything that you need from your food because of dietary limitations or illness. A currently relevant example is in people who take the weight-loss drugs, semaglutides or GLP-1s (such as

Ozempic, Rybelsus, and Wegovy) or have had surgery for weight loss. The weight-loss medications work to increase insulin secretion and slow digestion as well as reduce appetite and lower glucagon levels. These people may eat less and not get all the nutrients they need. In this case, they may require supplements. It's important to seek advice from your healthcare provider to determine your needs.

Vitamin D Prevents Cancer

Researchers are very interested in the connection between vitamin D and cancer because there are some epidemiological studies that show lower rates of some cancers in southern states where there is more sun exposure. Also, vitamin D has been shown in laboratory research studies to have biological properties that may be involved in preventing cancer. Many clinical studies that have been done have mixed results.

A recent five-year study in 25,000 people, called VITAL, showed no effect of taking vitamin D supplements in preventing cancer. Another large study, the Nurses' Health Initiative, showed no correlation between vitamin D supplements and cancer prevention.

Clinical studies to determine whether vitamin D supplementation decreases mortality from cancer are mixed. However, one meta-analysis of 10 randomly controlled trials found a slight decrease (13 percent) in deaths over a three- to seven-year follow-up. The jury is still out on this, but vitamin D has other health benefits, so be sure that you get enough!

Vitamins and Supplements Are Harmless

All of the fat-soluble vitamins, some of the water-soluble vitamins (A, B6, folate, niacin), and some of the minerals (calcium, iron, selenium) have specific tolerable ULs defined by the National Academy of Medicine (NAM, formerly the Institute of Medicine or IOM). If you take these vitamins in doses at or above the ULs, you could experience side effects. Vitamins and supplements can also interfere with each other or medications to reduce the action of the supplement OR the drug. Check out Chapter 13 for more information and examples.

You Get Enough Iodine
by Eating Salty Foods

Iodine is necessary to make thyroid hormone, and a deficiency of iodine can cause hypothyroidism or underactive thyroid. The symptoms include fatigue, slowing of metabolism, and increased sensitivity to cold. Despite iodine fortification of salt, Americans and Europeans experience mild to moderate iodine deficiencies. Worldwide, iodine deficiency leading to goiter affects about 2.2 billion people.

Fortifying salt with iodine has been an effective intervention to reduce the incidence of goiter in the world. But not all countries have fortification programs. In those countries that fortify salt with iodine, most people get enough iodine to avoid deficiencies. Be aware that not all salt is iodized here in the United States, however. Table salt is usually fortified with iodine, but people also use some non-iodized products for cooking, such as kosher salt, sea salt, and Himalayan pink salt. Regular table salt is the best source of iodine; 1 teaspoon offers 310 micrograms of iodine.

Salty foods are pervasive in supermarkets and restaurants. Prepared foods, processed foods, canned foods, and restaurant foods contain a lot of salt. The salt from these sources is generally not fortified with iodine and therefore not a good source for the nutrient. Milk, yogurt, and cheese are good sources of iodine. If you are not using table salt at home, it would be good to be sure that you are getting enough from dairy or your multivitamin.

"Natural" or "Organic" Means
the Product Is Safe

Organic usually refers to foods or products that are made with ingredients that are grown under specific conditions. Organic farmers have restrictions about what kind of additives, fertilizers, genetic engineering, and radiation they can use. They need to feed farm animals food that does not include hormones or antibiotics. For dietary supplements, *natural* means that the ingredients are derived from natural sources, including plants, animals, or algae, with minimal processing.

There are supplements made from natural sources and organic foods. Chemically synthesized vitamins and other supplements are mostly chemically identical to their natural counterpart. However, they're processed very differently, and the finished product may contain other chemicals to stabilize the ingredient or make it into its final form (pill, gel, liquid). Food-based supplements may be absorbed into the body more efficiently than synthetic ones. In addition, food-based supplements may contain other components of the food that make it more available or more effective.

TIP

Getting natural and organic nutrients from whole foods or supplements made from whole foods is almost always a better option than using synthetic supplements.

WARNING

However, just because a supplement is natural and organic, doesn't mean it can't be harmful. Some supplements could be contaminated with heavy metals like lead, mercury, arsenic, or cadmium or with bacteria. You can still take too much of a supplement — even if it is herbal — that can be harmful at high doses. Some may also interact with some medications (see Chapter 13).

Chapter 17

Ten Websites about Vitamins, Supplements, and Botanicals

Aside from the websites for The National Institutes of Health Office of Dietary Supplements (ODS) and the Dietary Guidelines for Americans, which are mentioned frequently throughout the other chapters, there's a wealth of information about vitamins, supplements, and botanicals to be found on the internet. In this chapter, I share a handful of resources you may find helpful for your health and wellness journey.

Harvard T.H. Chan School of Public Health and Harvard Medical School

Harvard Health and Harvard T.H. Chan School of Public Health are good sites for evidence-based information on health, including uses for vitamins and supplements. It is not as extensive as the ODS site, but you can search topics and know that you're getting good information that is well researched.

The first page of this site contains The Healthy Eating Plate, which is a good guideline for a balanced diet of all the nutrients you need. (It includes a version for children as well.) The sidebar has tabs that include all the food groups, as well as vitamins and minerals. Clicking on these tabs takes you to concise articles to help you make decisions about your food and supplement intake.

You can find the Vitamins and Minerals page of the site at https://nutrition source.hsph.harvard.edu/vitamins.

Cleveland Clinic

The Cleveland Clinic is an academic medical center. Its website provides articles of evidence-based information from a team of professional writers, journalists, and academics. The site provides medical and nutritional information, shares links to resources, and debunks health-related myths. The Cleveland Clinic prides itself on providing expert research information and up-to-date information so that you can make the best decisions for yourself.

The site includes more than 300 articles about vitamins. You can depend on the information from the Cleveland Clinic, which you can find at https://health.clevelandclinic.org.

Linus Pauling Institute at Oregon State University

The Linus Pauling Institute was cofounded by Linus Pauling more than 50 years ago to advance research on vitamins and other essential micronutrients. It is now located on the campus of Oregon State University. Part of the institute's mission is to promote the principles of healthy living and healthy aging, and providing information on vitamins and other nutrients to the public is integral to that mission.

The Micronutrient Information Center tab on the website is a source for scientifically accurate information about the roles of vitamins and other dietary components in health. The information on the site is reviewed by multiple scientists and experts who distill published research literature into articles.

The Resource tab provides access to reliable information and sources, including a nutrient index, info on drug-nutrient interactions, books, and other relevant links.

The Health and Disease tab is a searchable link to the latest research on a variety of health and disease issues, possibly including a list of recommendations about supplements. You can find the site at `https://lpi.oregonstate.edu`.

WebMD

WebMD is an easily searchable and reliable website for medical information. You can search most medical conditions that you can think of, and the site provides a lot of information including relevant information about prevention and treatment that may include vitamins or other supplements.

The Drugs and Supplements tab has links to drugs, supplements, a pill identifier, and interactions. The supplement section alphabetically lists vitamins, minerals, herbs, amino acids, teas, and much more, and each item's page offers an overview, uses, side effects, precautions, dosing, and reviews. The reviews are from people who have used the supplements rather than being scientific evaluations, so be careful interpreting this information. Personal stories may not apply to you.

A section on well-being provides information on aging, children's health, weight management, exercise, and many other topics related to lifestyle and supplements.

You can find the main Vitamins & Supplements page on the WebMD site at `www.webmd.com/vitamins/index`.

Healthline

The Healthline site covers information on all kinds of medical-related topics. You can search for vitamins and supplements to get many interesting and well-researched articles. You can also subscribe to newsletters specific to your interests.

The Health Conditions tab provides information on specific problems, including links to supplement information if there are data supporting use as a preventative or as part of the treatment plan.

The main Vitamins & Supplements page on the Healthline website is at `www.healthline.com/nutrition/vitamins-and-supplements`.

Examine.com

Examine.com summarizes the latest evidence for its articles about nutrition and supplement information. The researchers evaluate diets and supplements for efficacy in a variety of health conditions. They provide good guidance for use of supplements to address health and wellness issues. The organization behind the site has no ties to industry or advertisements, so the information should not be biased.

The downside of this website compared to the others in this chapter is that it's a fee-based site. You can get a monthly, yearly, or lifetime subscription.

Visit `www.examine.com` to find out more.

ConsumerLabs

ConsumerLabs is an independent, advertisement-free website for information on supplements. The website is divided into the following categories:

>> **Product Reviews:** This section has a searchable list of supplements with articles addressing information such as when the supplement may be appropriate, how much you should take, how much is too much, specifics about the supplement, and best products.

>> **Health Conditions:** This section has an alphabetical list of conditions that links to articles that may answer questions about which supplements may be helpful.

>> **Brands:** Brands are listed alphabetically and linked to product reviews and information to help you find a brand that suits your needs.

>> **Warnings:** This tab provides up-to-date information about recalls or warnings for specific products.

>> **Answers:** Information on this page addresses common questions consumers have about supplement products.

>> **News:** Any recent news, news releases, and testimonials about ConsumerLab are included here.

Mayo Clinic

The Mayo Clinic website offers evidence-based information and expert advice on vitamins and supplements. The Health Library tab on the site has a section for drugs and supplements that is easily searchable. The entries list what the current research says and what the Mayo Clinic's take is on the vitamin or supplement. It also offers information about the potential interactions between vitamins and drugs. There is more to explore on the site, which you can find at www.mayoclinic.org.

Memorial Sloan Kettering Cancer Center

Memorial Sloan Kettering Cancer Center's website has a lot of information on it. The About Herbs section includes vitamins and supplements with special attention to information for patients and caregivers as well as healthcare professionals. It provides evidence-based information on vitamins, supplements, herbs, and botanicals with a focus on support for managing symptoms and side effects of cancer treatment. If you're dealing with a cancer diagnosis, you may find this site very helpful. You can find it at https://www.mskcc.org.

American Botanical Council

The American Botanical Council is a good source for information on botanicals and herbal medicines. It provides science-based information to educate and promote the responsible use of herbs and botanicals. Some areas of the site offer open access, but you need to become a member to see all the information. The site is at https://herbalgram.org.

Glossary

For more terms and definitions, refer to information from the National Institutes of Health Office of Dietary Supplements.

A1C (or HbA1C): A blood test that measures average blood sugar over three months and is used to diagnose prediabetes and diabetes.

Absorption: When protein, fats, carbohydrates, and other nutrients are digested in the gastrointestinal (GI) tract and move into the bloodstream.

Adequate Intake (AI): This is a value used when there isn't enough scientific information to establish an Recommended Daily Allowance (RDA) or Estimated Average Requirement (EAR). It's based on existing evidence or observations as an intake to maintain adequate nutrition for most people in a particular life stage and gender group.

Alpha-tocopherol: The most active form of vitamin E, an antioxidant.

Amino acids: Molecules that are the building blocks of proteins.

Antioxidant: Substances that protect cells from free radical damage and reduce inflammatory processes in the cells.

Ayurvedic: An ancient type of medicine using herbs and botanicals, diet, and lifestyle to address health issues.

B vitamins: Essential vitamins — biotin, folate, niacin, riboflavin, thiamin, pyridoxamine, cobalamin, and pantothenic acid — needed for cell function.

Beri-beri: A disease caused by a deficiency in thiamin or vitamin B1.

Bioavailability: How well the body can use a nutrient after ingested.

Biotin: Essential B vitamin found in egg yolk, liver, and yeast.

Black cohosh: Plant-derived compound used to reduce hot flashes and other symptoms of menopause.

Blood sugar: Glucose is the sugar broken down to create cellular energy. It comes from food and the storage form (glycogen) in the liver.

Blood-brain barrier (BBB): A cellular barrier that prevents substances from crossing from the blood vessels to the brain tissue.

Calcium: An essential mineral needed for bones, teeth, nerve, and enzyme function. Found in dairy, fortified foods, and some vegetables.

Carotenoids: Over 600 types of compounds, including alpha-carotene, beta-carotene, beta-cryptoxanthin, lycopene, lutein, and zeaxanthin, found in green, red, yellow, and orange foods that form Vitamin A and may act as antioxidants.

Cholesterol: Biochemical synthesized by your cells or absorbed from foods that is a structural part of cells and a precursor of some hormones and vitamin D. Too much in your blood is a risk factor for heart disease.

Clinical trial: A research study to test the safety and efficacy of a drug or supplement in people.

Cobalamin or B12: A B vitamin responsible for nerve cell and production of red blood cells, metabolism of carbohydrate, fat, and protein.

Collagen: A protein in skin, bone, tendons, and cartilage.

Control group: The group in a clinical trial that does not receive the treatment and is used for comparison to test group.

Copper: An essential trace mineral, present in several foods, that is often a cofactor in several enzymatic functions and supports brain function and immune functions.

Daily Value (DV and %DV): DVs are the recommended amounts of nutrients to consume each day. The %DV is the percent of a nutrient in one serving of the food or supplement. It's based on a 2,000 calorie per day intake.

Dietary fiber: Nondigestible carbohydrates, cellulose, hemicellulose, pectin, and lignin found in grains, fruits, vegetables, nuts, seeds, and legumes that help keep you satiated and may lower risk of some diseases. It can be soluble (in water) or insoluble fiber.

Dietary Guidelines for Americans (DGA): a document updated every five years by the U.S. Department of Health and Human Services and the U.S. Department of Agriculture as a guideline for improving health.

Dietary Reference Intake (DRI): A set of recommendations used to plan and evaluate the nutrient intake of healthy people. They include the Estimated Average Requirement, Recommended Dietary Allowance, Adequate Intake, and the Tolerable Upper Intake Level.

Double blind study: Where the subject and researcher of a study do not know who is getting treatment (the test drug or supplement) or the placebo.

Echinacea: A plant used for colds, flu, and some infections.

Efficacy: Ability of an intervention such as a dietary supplement to be beneficial under the best conditions, such as in a clinical trial.

Electrolyte: Minerals such as calcium, sodium, potassium, and chloride that help maintain fluid balance in and around the cells and involved in cell metabolism.

Enzyme: A protein that catalyzes a biochemical reaction.

Epidemiologic study: Research studies of causes, patterns, and control of a disease at a population level.

Estimated Average Requirement or EAR: See DRI.

Fat soluble: Something that dissolves in fat, such as the fat-soluble vitamins A, D, E, and K.

Folate or folic acid (B9): A B vitamin found in leafy greens, fruits, beans, and supplements and fortified foods (folic acid form).

Food and Drug Administration (FDA): Regulates dietary supplements by acting against any unsafe product after it reaches market.

Free radical: A molecule that has one unpaired electron that is reactive and can protect or harm us.

Gamma-aminobutyric acid or GABA: A chemical that works by decreasing nerve cell impulses in the brain and causing inhibition of nerve function.

Ginger: A plant root used in cooking and for some medical conditions.

Glucosamine: Found naturally in fluid around joints and as a supplement.

Glutamine: A nonessential amino acid important in immunity and nerve function.

HDL cholesterol: High-density lipoprotein — the "good cholesterol" — that moves cholesterol away from tissues and arteries and to the liver.

Herb: A plant used for cooking or medicinal purposes.

Homocysteine: An amino acid that, when high, can increase risk of disease.

Inorganic: A substance that is not from a plant or animal — for example, minerals.

Institute of Medicine (IOM), now known as the National Academy of Medicine, NAMA nonprofit, nongovernmental organization that provides independent advice on biomedical science, health, and medicine to the public and decision-makers.

Iodine: A mineral needed to make thyroid hormones that control metabolism and other functions.

Iodized salt: Fortified salt to help prevent deficiency of iodine.

Iron: A mineral needed to make red blood cells, proteins, and enzymes and also needed for cell growth and development.

LDL cholesterol: Low-density lipoprotein — the "bad" cholesterol — found in blood.

Lutein: A carotenoid good for the eyes.

Lycopene: A carotenoid found in tomatoes, watermelon, and other colorful fruits.

Macronutrients: Proteins, fats, and carbohydrates.

Magnesium: A mineral needed for normal function of muscles, nerves, bones, and the immune system; maintaining normal blood sugar and blood pressure; energy; and protein metabolism.

Malabsorption: Reduction in nutrient absorbance that can lead to malnutrition.

Megaloblastic anemia: Caused by folate or B12 deficiency.

Meta-analysis: A review of the results from many research studies that statistically determines the combined effect of the studies and outcomes.

Metabolism: Chemical reactions in your cells that produce energy and basic materials needed for important life processes.

Micronutrients: Vitamins and minerals needed in small amounts.

National Institutes of Health (NIH): Federal government organization comprised of 27 institutes or centers that conduct biomedical research.

Niacin (nicotinamide or B3): A B vitamin important for cell function.

Nurses' Health Study: A long-term study started in 1976, of more than 280,000 participants, for determining the risk factors of major chronic disease.

Nutrient content claim: A label on a dietary supplement stating "fortified," "high," "rich in," "excellent source of," "good source of," or "high potency."

Nutrition: Eating, digesting, and absorbing nutrients from food to maintain the body, grow new cells, repair tissues, and supply energy. Also, the science of food, diet, and health.

Observational study: A type of research study where there is no treatment given and people are assessed for a specific amount of time and certain outcomes are measured.

Office of Dietary Supplements (ODS): A department in the NIH that evaluates scientific information, supports research, and is a good online resource for evidence-based information about dietary supplements.

Omega-3 fatty acid: A monounsaturated fat essential for energy and tissues, present in olive (and other) oils and fish.

Oxidative damage: Normal chemical changes in the body's cells. Too much can lead to risk of chronic diseases such as heart disease, diabetes, age-related issues, and cancer.

Pantothenic acid (B5): Essential for metabolism of food, red blood cells, hormones, and fats and support of nerves.

Peer-reviewed journal: A scientific publication where articles are reviewed by experts in the field before publishing.

Pernicious anemia: When the body cannot make intrinsic factor, which is in the stomach and is necessary to absorb B12 into the body. It is an autoimmune disease and causes low

B12, which leads to red cell dysfunction and less oxygen delivered to cells and tissues (called megaloblastic anemia).

Physicians' Health Study: A long-term study conducted to see whether various nutritional supplements can prevent heart disease, cancer, and age-related eye diseases in men in the United States.

Phytochemicals or phytonutrients: A general term for chemicals naturally produced by plants (*phyto*).

Placebo-controlled study: In a clinical study, the dietary supplement or drug is compared to an inactive ingredient called the placebo.

Polyphenols: Over 8,000 plant biochemicals that have healthy benefits.

Potassium: A mineral important for nerves, muscles, and the heart.

Protein: Made from amino acids and necessary for cell and tissue structure, enzymes, and antibodies

Provitamin or precursor: A substance found in food that converts to a vitamin in the body.

Pyridoxine (B6): Plays a critical role in protein metabolism, brain development, and the production of neurotransmitters.

Randomized clinical trial (RCT): The best type of clinical trial that can be done to prove effect of a treatment. The researchers and subjects do not know which study group is getting the treatment or the placebo (called blinded).

Recommended Dietary Allowance (RDA): The average amount of a nutrient a healthy person needs each day. Varies by age, sex, pregnancy, and breastfeeding.

Retinal/retinaldehyde: The form of vitamin A needed for vision.

Retinoid: A type of vitamin A including retinol, retinal, and retinoic acid. Synthetic retinoids are manufactured for use in treating acne, psoriasis, and other skin disorders.

Retinol: A form of vitamin A found in animal products (meat, dairy, fish).

Riboflavin (B2): A vitamin that is needed for growth, cell function, and to make energy from food. Also acts as an antioxidant.

Saponin: A substance found in some plants. Saponins may help lower cholesterol and may have anticancer effects.

Scientific literature: Published peer-reviewed original research.

Selenium: A trace mineral needed for enzyme production, thyroid function, fertility, and immune support.

Statistically significant: A mathematical measure of the difference between treatment groups in a study that is greater than what might have happened by chance.

Structure/function claim: A claim on a dietary supplement or food label that tells how it may affect your body. It cannot mention a specific disease and does not require FDA approval.

Thiamin (B1): Needed for many metabolic processes including energy production, cell, muscle, and nervous system function.

Triglyceride: A type of fat in your blood. High levels increase your risk for heart disease and stroke.

United States Pharmacopeia (USP): A nonprofit organization that sets standards for the quality of medicines, food ingredients, and dietary supplements.

Upper Limit (UL): The highest amount of a nutrient consumed per day considered safe for most people. Taking more than this can cause risk.

U.S. Department of Agriculture (USDA): A government agency responsible for food safety and improving nutrition, health, and agriculture by providing education, management, financial programs, and more.

Valerian: A plant root that can be used as a mild sedative or sleep aide.

Vitamin: An essential nutrient needed for healthy body function that your body cannot make, including A, D, E, K, C, and the B vitamins.

Water-soluble vitamins: B vitamins and vitamin C that dissolve in water and are excreted in urine.

Whole grain: Unprocessed grains that contain vitamins, minerals, and fiber and may lower heart disease, obesity, and type 2 diabetes.

World Health Organization (WHO): Part of the UN concerned with worldwide health issues.

Zinc: A mineral essential for supporting immunity, wound healing, DNA synthesis, and biochemistry for growth and development.

Index

A

A1C, 309

AAP (American Academy of Pediatrics), 278

Abbott, 19

abdominal obesity, 33

absorption, 309

The Academy of Nutrition and Dietetics, 58

acai berry, 125

acetylcholine, 80, 101, 161

acupuncturists, 4

acute inflammation, 149

adaptive immune system, 155

adaptogens, 118

adenosine triphosphate (ATP), 23, 25, 30, 34, 78, 79, 133

Adequate Intake (AI), 43, 277, 281, 309

adolescents, RDA for, 280–282

adults, RDA for, 17, 282–285, 289–291

age, impact on metabolism, 28–29

aged garlic extract (AGE), 185

age-related macular degeneration (AMD), 152, 166, 215

alanine, 137

alcoholism, 201–202

allicin, 185

all-trans-retinol, 165

aloe vera, 122

alpha tocopherol. *See* vitamin E (tocopherol or alpha-tocopherol)

alpha-hydroxy acids (AHA), 212

alpha-linolenic acid (ALA), 158, 176, 195, 206, 287

Amazon Elements, 244

AMD (age-related macular degeneration), 152, 166, 215

American Academy of Pediatrics (AAP), 278

American Academy of Sleep Medicine, 124

American Botanical Council, 307

American Dental Association, 164–165

American Dietetic Association, 232

American Institute for Cancer Research, 96

American Nutrition Association, 4, 58

American Society for Nutrition (ASN), 58

American Thyroid Association (ATA), 106

The American Journal of Clinical Nutrition, 57

amia, 123

amino acids
  branched-chain amino acids (BCAA), 139, 142
  defined, 309
  essential amino acids, 137–141
  for long COVID, 220
  non-essential amino acids, 137
  RDA, 137
  role of, 32, 132, 137–143
  supplements, 141–143

Amway, 19

amylase, 30, 31, 140

anabolic reactions, 22, 23

analytical epidemiology, 56

anemia, 16, 17, 40, 97, 312–313

animal studies, 52–53, 148

anthocyanidins, 154

anti-aging products, 77, 125, 168–169

anti-inflammation, 149–150

anti-inflammatory foods and supplements, 151

antioxidants. *See also specific antioxidants*
  as anti-inflammatories, 17
  for boosting immunity, 157
  defined, 309
  described, 149–150
  endogenous antioxidants, 150, 151
  examples of, 195
  exogenous antioxidants, 150, 151–152
  for reducing oxidation, 24, 151–152
  sources of, 125, 150

antioxidants *(continued)*
  vitamin A as, 17, 152
  vitamin C as, 17, 25, 84, 152, 157
  vitamin D as, 157
  vitamin E as, 17, 24, 87, 152, 153
  zinc as, 153
anxiety, supplements for help with, 113
apolipoproteins, 32
appetite control, 134–135, 190
apple cider vinegar, 180
Apple Watch, 271
apps, 27, 114, 271, 272
AREDS (National Eye Institute Age-Related Eye Disease Studies), 215
arginine, 137, 138, 139, 140, 176
artichoke leaf extract, 124
ascorbic acid (vitamin C). *See* vitamin C (ascorbic acid)
ashwagandha, 18, 115, 118, 206, 210, 219
Asian ginseng, 115
ASN (American Society for Nutrition), 58
asparagine, 137
aspartate, 80
aspartic acid, 137
assessment (of needs for vitamins and supplements), 229–230
astragalus, 115, 117
ATA (American Thyroid Association), 106
Ate Food Diary, 272
atherosclerosis, 188–189
athletes, supplements for, 17, 170–171
ATP. *See* adenosine triphosphate (ATP)
autoimmune diseases, 209–210
ayurvedic, 309

B

B cells, 98, 140
B vitamins. *See also specific B vitamins*
  as added to breakfast cereals, 12
  for cognitive and mental health, 18
  defined, 309
  for diabetes/prediabetes, 206

  for long COVID, 221
  for mental health and cognitive disorders, 210
  RDA and food sources for, 78
Bacopa monnieri, 186
bariatric surgery, supplementing after, 190, 202–203
basal metabolic rate (BMR), 27
basil, 185
BBB (blood-brain barrier), 138, 139, 309
BCAA (branched-chain amino acids), 139, 142, 170
beetroot/beetroot juice, 185, 221
behavioral studies, 53
benzoyl peroxide, 212
berberine, 179, 187, 206
beri-beri, 40, 309
beta alanine, 170
beta-carotene, 18, 47, 150, 154
bilberry/bilberry extract, 18, 115
Bill and Melinda Gates Foundation, 166
bioavailability, 18, 48, 60, 150–151, 309
biochemical reactions, 22, 23–24
biochemistry, 22–34
bioidentical, 59
biotin (B7). *See* vitamin B7 (biotin)
birth defects, prevention of, 81–82
bitter orange, 115
black cohosh, 115, 121, 206, 309
blinded studies, 54
blindness
  prevention of, 166
  vitamin A deficiency and, 75–76
blood clotting, vitamin K role in, 24, 26, 89
blood pressure
  high blood pressure, 33
  lowering of, 184–186
blood sugar (glucose)
  in biochemical reactions, 25
  breakdown of, 23
  defined, 309
  production of, 30
  regulation of, 178
blood tests, 37, 186, 238–239

cells
  healthy turnover of, 156
  of immune system, 157
  protection of, 150–151
cellular communication, zinc role in, 103
cellular respiration, 78, 79
Centers for Disease Control (CDC), 42, 45, 151,
    173, 180, 276
Centrum, 19, 244
certification
  for manufacturing of supplements, 224–225
  of nutritionists, 4
  of supplements, 13, 18, 58, 60–61, 224, 255–256
Certified Gluten-Free, 69, 225
Certified Nutrition Specialist (CNS), 4
Certified Vegan, 13, 69, 225
ceruloplasmin, 108
chamomile, 115, 119, 122, 124, 214
chaste tree berry (vitax), 115, 206
Cheat Sheet, 3
children, RDA for, 17, 280–282
chiropractors, role of, 4
chloride, 11, 26, 92, 108
cholecystokinin (CCK), 30
cholesterol
  defined, 310
  in fat metabolism, 32
  HDL cholesterol, 33, 311
  LDL cholesterol, 33, 311
  lowering of, 186–187
  manufacture of, 23
choline, 25, 77, 287
chondroitin sulfate, 17
chromium, 179
chromium picolinate, 206
chronic diseases, 173
chronic inflammation, 149
chylomicrons, 32, 33
chymotrypsin, 32
cinnamon, 115, 118, 179, 185, 206
circulatory health, herbal supplements for, 121
citrulline, 176
CL (ConsumerLab). See ConsumerLab (CL)

Cleveland Clinic, 138, 304
clinical studies/clinical trials, 148, 310
ClinicalTrials.gov, 58
clove oil, 165
CNS (Certified Nutrition Specialist), 4
cobalamin (B12). See vitamin B12 (cobalamin)
Cochrane Library, 57
Cocoa Supplement and Multivitamin Outcomes
    Study (COSMOS), 193
coenzyme Q10 (CoQ10)
  for adults, 285, 291
  for cognitive and mental health, 162
  for diabetes/prediabetes, 206
  drug–supplement interactions, 269
  as endogenous antioxidant, 150
  for heart health, 17, 188, 207
  for lowering blood pressure, 185
  for mitochondrial health, 176
cofactors (coenzymes), 24–25
cognitive health, supplements for, 18, 65,
    113, 120, 210
cohort studies, 54, 56
colds, supplements for prevention and reduction
    of symptoms of, 83, 221–222
collagen, 25, 135, 143, 169–170, 208, 310
collagen supplements, 135–136, 170
colon cancer, protection from, 96
conjugated linoleic acid, 190
Consortium for Advancing Research on Botanical
    and Other Natural Products (CARBoN), 20
ConsumerLab (CL), 13, 57, 58, 60, 113, 224,
    256, 299, 306
control group, 310
cooked foods, benefits of, 48, 50
copper
  in biochemical reactions, 25
  as cofactor, 24
  deficiencies in, 108
  defined, 310
  as essential mineral, 11
  function of, 92, 108
  for immune response, 26
  RDA, 108
  sources of, 108

diseases *(continued)*
  heart disease. *See* heart disease
  inflammatory diseases, 149–150
  metabolic disorder, 33
  neurodegenerative diseases, 192–195
  targeting preventable chronic ones, 173–196
  Tay-Sachs disease, 28
  Wilson's disease, 28
DNA
  repair of, 102
  synthesis of, 25
docosahexaenoic acid (DHA), 158
dong quai, 121
dopamine, 80, 101, 138, 159
dosages, 247–258, 270–272
dose-response studies, 52, 54
double blind study, 310
DRI (Dietary Reference Intake), 42, 277, 310
drug–supplement interactions, 226, 266–269
DSHEA (Dietary Supplement Health and Education Act) of 1994. *See* Dietary Supplement Health and Education Act (DSHEA) of 1994
DV and %DV (Daily Value), 310

E

EAR (Estimated Average Requirement), 43, 277, 311
echinacea, 16, 18, 115, 117, 222, 310
efficacy, 114, 310
EGCG (epigallocatechin-3 galate), 119, 190
eicosapentaenoic acid (EPA), 158
elastin, 143
elderberry/elderberry extract, 18, 115, 117, 222
electrolytes, 159, 160, 187–188, 310
endogenous antioxidants, 150, 151
endorphins, 101
energy, amino acids role in provision of, 141, 142
energy metabolism, role of food in, 174–177
enzymatic reactions, 22, 24–25, 100
enzymes, 140, 310
eosinophils, 98
ephedra, 115

epidemiological studies, 55–56, 148, 311
epigallocatechin-3 galate (EGCG), 119, 190
epigenetics, 193, 241–242
epinephrine, 80, 101, 138
erythropoietin, 26
essential minerals, 11–12, 91–109. *See also specific essential minerals*
essential vitamins, 73–90
Estimated Average Requirement (EAR), 43, 277, 311
estrogen, 29
European mistletoe, 115
The European Food Safety Authority, 57
evening primrose/evening primrose oil, 115, 119, 122, 217
Everlywell, 239
evidence-based information, seeking it out, 57–58
Examine.com, 58, 306
exercise, impacts of and recommendations for, 29, 46
exogenous antioxidants, 150, 151–152
eye health
  eye dryness, 40
  protection against eye damage, 166
  supplements for issues with, 215

F

FAD (flavin adenine dinucleotide) coenzyme, 25
familiar hypercholesterolemia, 28
fat soluble, 311
fatigue, supplements for help with, 113, 178–179
fats, RDA, 19, 281, 282, 283, 286, 290
fat-soluble vitamins, 10, 18, 32, 33, 73, 74, 84, 88, 150, 202, 265, 269, 300, 311
fatty liver, 34
FDA (U.S. Food and Drug Administration), 12, 13, 18, 41, 61–62, 114, 116, 148, 155, 181–182, 224, 248, 255, 276, 299, 311
FDA Modernization Act of 1997 (FDAMA) Health and Nutrient Content Claims page, 61
Federal Food, Drug, and Cosmetic Act, 299
fenugreek, 115, 121, 123, 190, 219
fermented foods, benefits of, 50

feverfew, 115

fiber. *See also* dietary fiber

  RDA, 281, 282, 285, 286, 290

  for treatment of diabetes, 180, 206

  for treatment of GI distress, 211

  types of, 182–183

fibrin, 26

fibrinogen, 26

fish oil, 17, 151, 181–182, 187, 220

Fitbit, 271

fitness supplements

  examples of, 112

  as percent of supplement sales, 65

5-hydroxy-tryptophan (5-HTP), 141

flavin adenine dinucleotide (FAD) coenzyme, 25

flavonoids, 128

flaxseed and flaxseed oil, 115, 187

flu, supplements for prevention and reduction of symptoms of, 221–222

folate or folic acid (B9). *See* vitamin B9 (folate or folic acid)

folinic acid, 176

food

  benefits of cooked foods, 48, 50

  benefits of fermented foods, 50

  benefits of raw foods, 48

  getting the most nutrients from, 259–265

  getting what you need from, 47–50

  metabolization of, 174–177

  supplements as better taken with, 269–270

food allergy testing, 20

Food and Nutrition Board, 18, 35, 40, 42

food diary/food record, 40, 133

food fortification, 37

food tracker apps, 271

Framingham Heart Study, 47, 186

free radicals, 82, 84, 87, 88, 104, 106, 122, 123, 127, 144, 149, 150, 151, 167, 215, 268, 311

FTC (Federal Trade Commission), 13, 18, 42, 62

Fullscript, 240, 244

functional medicine practitioners, role of, 4

furanocoumarins, 269

G

Gaia, 19, 244

gallstones, 34

gamma-aminobutyric acid (GABA), 80, 101, 138, 141, 159, 311

garcinia cambogia, 115, 124, 190

Garden of Life, 19, 69, 244

garlic, 115, 118, 121, 151, 165, 185, 207, 222, 268

gastric lipase, 32

gastrointestinal issues, probiotics for people with, 17

Gaucher disease, 28

gene regulation, supplements for, 193–194

general health, support of, 147–171

generally recognized as safe (GRAS), 155

genetic testing, 20, 241

ghrelin, 29, 134

ginger, 115, 118, 119, 120, 151, 180, 185, 211, 311

ginkgo/gingko biloba, 115, 120, 210

ginseng, 115, 216, 219

glossary, 309–314

GLP-1 (glucagon-like peptide-1), 20, 30, 134, 190–191, 202–203

glucagon, 30

glucomannan, 190

glucosamine, 16, 17, 208–209, 311

glucose. *See* blood sugar (glucose)

glutamate, 80, 101, 138

glutamic acid, 137, 151

glutamine, 137, 139, 140, 171, 211, 311

glutathione, 151, 153

Gluten-Free certification, 255

gluten-free products, 20

glycerol, 32

glycine, 101, 137, 138, 151, 214

glycogen, 25, 30

glycolic acid, 169, 212

glycolysis, 30, 78

GNC, 19

goals, identification of health goals, 67

goiter, 14, 40

J

Johns Hopkins University, 190
joint health, supplements for, 16, 17, 64, 208–209

K

kava, 115
KBMO Diagnostics, 240
keratin, 143
keto diet, 236–237
kidney stones, avoidance of, 95
Klean Athlete, 69
Korean ginseng, 121
Kosher certification, 20, 255
Krebs cycle, 23, 25, 78, 79–80, 141

L

Labcorp (and Labcorp OnDemand), 240
labels
  FDA specification for, 181–182
  reading, 247–258
  types of claims that may be seen on, 61–62
lactase, 31, 140
lactating, supplement recommendations for
    women while, 15, 17, 37, 74, 93, 102, 106, 108,
    163, 187, 224. *See also* nursing
lactic acid, 169
lactoferrin, 221
L-arginine, 185, 207, 216, 219
lavender/lavender oil, 115, 123, 124, 215
L-carnitine, 221
L-citrulline, 219
L-cysteine, 143
LDL (low-density lipoprotein) cholesterol, 33, 311
lemon balm, 120, 214
leptin, 29
leucine, 137, 139, 140, 142
licorice root, 115, 165
licorice root extract, 211
Life Extension, 19, 244
life stages, needs for supplements per,
    17, 278–291

lifestyles, needs for supplements per, 17
LifeSum (app), 272
lingual lipase, 32
linoleic acid, 287
The Linus Pauling Institute, 57, 83,
    221–222, 304–305
lipase, 31, 32, 140
lipid panel, 186, 239
lipids, 32
lipoproteins, 32, 33
liver health, herbal supplements for, 123–124
longevity, life choices that contribute to, 46
longitudinal studies, 52–53, 54
Lose It! (app), 27, 272
lovastatin (monacolin K), 116
L-theanine, 214
L-tryptophan, 141, 214
lutein, 154, 311
lutein zeaxanthin, 18
luteolin, 128
lycopene, 48, 154, 311
lysine, 137

M

maca root, 121, 219
macronutrients, 40, 311
macrophages, 98
magnesium
  for adults, 284, 291
  benefits of, 160
  for body fluid balance, 26
  for bone/joint health, 164, 208
  for cognitive and mental health, 18
  deficiencies in, 99, 160
  defined, 312
  for diabetes/prediabetes, 206
  drug–supplement interactions, 268
  as essential mineral, 11
  function of, 92, 99–102
  good forms of, 225
  for heart health, 183, 187–188, 207

monosaccharides, 30

mood regulation, supplements for, 85, 102, 113, 120, 142

MTHFR genetic mutation, 80

mTOR pathway, 140

mugwort, 115

multivitamins, 17, 284

muscle function, supplements for, 86, 100–101, 133–134

mushrooms, 179

MyFitnessPal (app), 27, 271

MyNetDiary (app), 272

MyPlate (app), 12, 16, 41, 223, 232, 261, 272

N

N-acetyl cysteine (NAC), 195, 219, 221, 222

NAD (nicotinamide adenine dinucleotide), 25, 157

NADP (nicotinamide adenine dinucleotide phosphate), 25, 157

nail health, supplements for, 81, 143

National Academies of Science Engineering, and Medicine, 18, 42

National Academy of Medicine (NAM) (formerly Institute of Medicine or IOM), 35, 84

National Center for Complementary and Integrative Health (NCCIH), 114, 126, 277

National Eye Institute Age-Related Eye Disease Studies (AREDS), 215

National Health and Nutrition Examination Survey (NHANES), 47, 230

National Institutes of Health (NIH), 12, 42, 43, 57, 85, 114, 115, 155, 276, 303, 312

National Research Council, 40

"natural," myth about, 301–302

natural ingredients, 59

natural kill (NK) cells, 98

Nature Made, 19, 69, 245

Nature's Bounty, 69

naturopathic doctors, role of, 5

neem sticks, 165

nerve function/system, supplements for, 95, 101, 159–162, 194

Nestle, 19

nettle, 119, 123

neural tube defects (NTD), 81

neurodegenerative diseases
 examples of, 193
 supplements for, 193–195

neuropeptide (NYP), 30

neurotransmitters. *See also specific neurotransmitters*
 classes of, 80
 defined, 80
 described, 101
 examples of, 159
 functions of, 138
 magnesium role in regulation of, 101
 number of, 138
 synthesis of, 81

neutrophils, 98

New Chapter, 19, 69, 245

NHANES (National Health and Nutrition Examination Survey), 47, 230

NHS (Nurses' Health Study), 47, 152, 153, 312

niacin (nicotinamide or B3). *See* vitamin B3 (niacin or nicotinamide)

nicotinamide adenine dinucleotide (NAD), 25, 157

nicotinamide adenine dinucleotide phosphate (NADP), 25, 157

NIH. *See* National Institutes of Health (NIH)

nitric oxide, 138, 140

NK (natural kill) cells, 98

Non-GMO Project Verified, 13, 69, 225, 255

non-heme iron, 97

noni, 115

Noom (app), 27, 272

Nordic Naturals, 69, 245

norepinephrine, 80, 101, 138

NOW, 19, 69, 245

NSF Certified for Sport, 255

NSF International (NSF), 13, 58, 60, 113, 224, 256, 299

NTD (neural tube defects), 81

Nurses' Health Study (NHS), 47, 152, 153, 312

nursing, supplement recommendations for women while, 285–286, 297. *See also* lactating

nutrient content claim, 62, 312
nutrient deficiencies
  addressing, 37
  commons ones, 198–200
  development of, 197–198
nutrients, as distinguished from foods and supplements, 19
nutrition
  defined, 312
  and genetic testing, 20
  growing areas of, 20
  personalized nutrition, 20
  precision nutrition, 240
  study of, 52
Nutrition Facts labels, 248, 249
nutritional biochemistry, 21
nutritional genomics (nutrigenomics), 241, 242, 243
nutritional recommendations
  government responsibilities for, 41–42
  history of, 40–41
nutritional science, 51–56
nutritionist, 3, 4
The Nutrition Labeling and Education Act of 1990, 248
NYP (neuropeptide), 30

O

obesity, 33, 189
observational studies, 148, 312
Office of Dietary Supplements (ODS), 12, 20, 43, 57, 115, 276, 303, 312
older adults, RDA for, 289–291
Olly, 245
omega-3 fatty acids
  for addressing heart disease, 181
  for adults, 284, 291
  for bone/joint health, 208, 209
  for brain health, 17
  defined, 312
  for diabetes/prediabetes, 206
  for heart health, 17, 207

  for immune function, 158
  for menopausal symptoms, 217
  for mental health and cognitive disorders, 210
  as percent of supplement sales, 64
  for skin conditions, 213
  for supporting athletic activities, 171
  for vegetarian lifestyles, 17
  for vision health, 18
  while pregnant and nursing, 288
ORAC (oxygen radical absorbance capacity), 155
oral health, supplements for, 164–165
oregano, 118
Oregon State University, The Linus Pauling Institute, 83, 304–305
organ function, vitamin E role in, 87
organic products
  myth about, 301–302
  use of, 20
osteocalcin, 89
osteopenia
  prevention of, 163
  supplements for, 207–208
osteoporosis
  prevention of, 16, 17, 163
  supplements for, 207–208
other ingredient list, 253–254
oxidation reactions, 24
oxidative damage, 312
oxidative phosphorylation, 23, 78, 100
oxidative stress
  consequences of, 149
  reduction of, 149–155
oxygen radical absorbance capacity (ORAC), 155

P

panax ginseng, 219
pancreatic amylase, 30
pancreatic lipases, 32
pantothenic acid (B5). *See* pantothenic acid (B5)
parathyroid hormone (PTH), 94
parsley, 185

as percent of supplement sales, 64

for skin conditions, 212, 213

use of, 17, 158–159, 185

progesterone, 30

proline, 137

proteases, 32, 140

protein

for bone formation, 27

defined, 313

good forms of, 225

importance of, 132

intake of, 132–136

RDA, 19, 134, 281, 282, 283, 286, 290

sources of, 133

for supporting athletic activities, 170

synthesis of, 25

protein supplements

as percent of supplement sales, 64

shopping for, 136–137

prothrombin enzyme, 24

proton pump inhibitor, 160

provitamin or precursor, 313

PTH (parathyroid hormone), 94

PubMed, 57

PUFAs (polyunsaturated fatty acids), 158

Pure Encapsulation, 19, 69, 245

purified cytoplasm of pollen (PCP), 217

pyridoxal phosphate coenzyme, 25

pyridoxine (B6). *See* vitamin B6 (pyridoxine)

PYY (peptide YY), 134

Q

QAI (Quality Assurance International), 225

quality (of supplements), assessment of, 60–63

quality control, as limitation of supplement, 18

quercetin, 222

Quest Diagnostics, 240

R

RAE (retinol activity equivalent), 75

randomized clinical trial (RCT), 53, 56, 148, 313

randomized crossover trials, 53–54

raw foods, benefits of, 48

RBCs (red blood cells), formation of/production of, 25, 26

RD (Registered Dietitian), 4

RDN (Registered Dietitian Nutritionist), 4

reactive nitrogen species (RNS), 149

reactive oxygen species (ROS), 126, 149, 150, 151–152

Recommended Dietary Allowance (RDA)

for adolescents, 280–282

for adults, 283–285, 290

of B vitamins, 78

of calcium, 93, 161, 163, 281, 282, 283, 285, 287, 290

for children, 282

of chloride, 108

of copper, 108

defined, 42, 313

as DRI, 277

of essential amino acids, 137

evaluating your current diet for reaching, 223

for females, 43

importance of following, 18, 270

for infants, 281

of iodine, 106, 287

of iron, 96, 281, 282, 284, 287, 290

of magnesium, 98, 99, 161, 282, 284, 287, 290

for males, 44

of manganese, 109

origin of, 40–41

of phosphorous, 105, 282, 287

of potassium, 105, 161, 282, 284, 287, 290

of protein, 19, 134, 281, 282, 283, 286, 290

of selenium, 106, 287

of sodium, 107, 282, 284, 287, 290

of sulfur, 109

for toddlers, 281

updating of, 35

use of essential vitamin and mineral supplements to meet, 9

of vitamin A, 74, 281, 282, 283, 287, 290

of vitamin B1, 287

U

ubiquinol, 151

ubiquinone, 151

UL (Tolerable Upper Intake Level), 43, 277

UNICEF, 166

United States Pharmacopeia (USP), 58, 60, 113, 224, 256, 299, 314

United States, top ten causes of death in, 45

Upper Limit (UL), 18, 43, 314

U.S. Department of Agriculture (USDA), 13, 41, 225, 260, 276, 278, 314

U.S. Department of Health and Human Services (HHS). *See* HHS (U.S. Department of Health and Human Services)

U.S. Federal Trade Commission. *See* FTC (Federal Trade Commission)

U.S. Food and Drug Administration (FDA). *See* FDA (U.S. Food and Drug Administration)

U.S. Preventive Services Task Force (USPSTF), 277

USDA Certified Organic, 13, 69, 225, 255

V

vaginal dryness, supplements for, 218

valerian/valerian root, 115, 124, 214, 314

valine, 137, 139, 142

vegan lifestyle
  described, 233–235
  supplements with, 17, 47

vegetarian diet. *See also* Healthy Vegetarian dietary pattern
  benefits of, 16, 47
  described, 232–233
  supplements with, 17, 47

vegetarianism, 232–233

vision health
  maintenance of, 165–167
  supplements for, 18, 75–76, 215

vitamin A
  as antioxidant, 17, 152
  in biochemical reactions, 24
  deficiencies in, 75, 166
  drug–supplement interactions, 268
  for immune response, 18, 26, 157

overview, 74–77
preformed vitamin A (retinoids), 74, 75
provitamin A (carotenoids), 74, 75
RDA, 74, 281, 282, 283, 287, 290
side effects of taking too much, 273
for skin conditions, 212, 213
sources of, 166
for vision health, 18, 165–166
while pregnant and nursing, 288

vitamin B. *See* B vitamins; *specific B vitamins*

vitamin B1 (thiamine)
  in biochemical reactions, 24
  defined, 314
  for energy metabolism, 174
  for mitochondrial health, 176
  RDA, 287

vitamin B2 (riboflavin)
  in biochemical reactions, 25
  defined, 313
  for energy metabolism, 174
  for lowering blood pressure, 184
  for mitochondrial health, 176
  RDA, 287

vitamin B3 (niacin or nicotinamide)
  as anti-inflammatory and anti-aging, 157
  in biochemical reactions, 25
  defined, 312
  for energy metabolism, 174
  for helping control cholesterol, 187
  RDA, 287
  side effects of taking too much, 273
  for skin conditions, 212

vitamin B5 (pantothenic acid)
  in biochemical reactions, 25
  defined, 312
  for hair, nail, and skin health, 81
  RDA, 287
  for skin conditions, 212

vitamin B6 (pyridoxine)
  in biochemical reactions, 25
  for breaking down homocysteine, 79
  defined, 313

X

xerophthalmia, 40

Y

Y aminobutyric acid (GABA), 80
yerba matte, 190
yohimbe, 115

Z

zinc
  for adults, 285, 291
  as antioxidant, 153
  in biochemical reactions, 25
  as cofactor, 24
  for colds and flu, 222
  deficiencies in, 103, 104
  defined, 314
  drug–supplement interactions, 268
  as essential mineral, 12
  function of, 92
  good forms of, 225
  for immune response, 18, 26, 219
  for long COVID, 220
  for men's sexual health, 219
  myth about, 298
  overview, 102–104
  RDA, 102, 281, 282, 284, 287, 290
  side effects of taking too much, 274
  for skin conditions, 212, 213
  sources of, 102, 153
  toxicity from, 104
  for vision health, 18
  while pregnant and nursing, 289
  for women's sexual health, 216
zinc citrate or picolinate, 206

About the Author

Shelley B. Weinstock, PhD, CNS, FACN, is a nutritional biochemist and has a consulting company and nutrition practice in New Jersey and New Mexico. She has held faculty and staff appointments at Barnard College at Columbia University, the Institute of Human Nutrition at Columbia University, Vagelos College of Physicians and Surgeons, and Montclair State University. She maintains an active research focus, has a number of published articles in peer-reviewed scientific journals, and has presented at national meetings.

Dr. Weinstock consults for organizations in the nonprofit, industry, and academic sectors. She has served as a chief scientific officer for a nutraceutical start-up company focused on the clinical development of novel nutritional products and has been on the boards of other nutrition-related start-up companies. She also currently consults for the Langer/Jaklenic labs at MIT on an innovative vitamin fortification project to help people in need worldwide.

She spends much of her time on her personalized nutrition practice, where she sees clients with a variety of nutrition-related health issues. In her practice, Dr. Weinstock focuses on identifying clients' areas of concern and establishing appropriate health goals to develop a food-first approach as part of a personalized health plan.

She earned her BA at Bard College, her PhD at the Massachusetts Institute of Technology, and her post-doctoral fellowship at the Harvard School of Public Health. In her spare time, she is a potter.

Author's Acknowledgments

I want to thank the editors at Wiley for making this an extremely efficient process. In particular, Jennifer Yee and Charlotte Kughen were delights to work with and responsive to my needs. Also, special thanks to Silvia Solan, MS, for her expert content editing. I could not have done this book without this team.

Thank you to my parents, Sharon and Jack, for those early years of nourishment, literally and figuratively, that shaped my interests.

Thanks to my children, Kate and Max Bartick, who were forced to grow up eating healthy and organic foods and chew on vitamin C — although we always had cookies in the house! They are my biggest accomplishment, and they feed my heart every day.

The places where I pursued my education — at Bard, MIT, and Harvard School of Public Health — are all amazing institutions in different ways. They provided me with the background to forge ahead and pursue a tough and exciting career path.

My appreciation to my family and friends for their continuous support and for letting me interview them about their habits for using supplements. It truly takes a village to feel successful in work and life. There are too many people to mention, but I want to acknowledge those who are my confidantes, morning calls, walking partners, travel partners, and pottery pals.

Thank you to my longtime friends, Dr. Eileen Hoskin and Dr. Randi Fain for their expert advice in their fields throughout the years and for this book.

I want to give a special mention to my friend and mentor, Professor Robert Langer, who has helped shape my career since I began at MIT. Our scientific collaborations have resulted in exciting and life-changing opportunities for me. My conversations with him and his wife, Dr. Laura Langer, over the years have influenced this book's recommendations on health and wellness.

Lastly, my gratitude and love to Dr. Robert B. Geller, for his patience, support, and his expert opinions and advice on science, medicine, writing, and life in general.

Dedication

To Kate and Max, my mother, Sharon and in memory of my father, Jack.

Publisher's Acknowledgments

Acquisitions Editor: Jennifer Yee
Project Editor: Charlotte Kughen
Technical Editor: Silvia Solaun

Production Editor: Magesh Elangovan
Cover Image: © KucherAV/Getty Images

Printed and bound by CPI Group (UK) Ltd, Croydon, CR0 4YY

10/06/2025

14686747-0001